Encephalitis Lethargica

Encephalitis Lethargica

DURING AND AFTER THE EPIDEMIC

Edited by

JOEL A. VILENSKY, PhD

Department of Anatomy and Cell Biology
Indiana University School of Medicine
Fort Wayne, IN

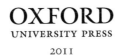

OXFORD
UNIVERSITY PRESS

2011

OXFORD
UNIVERSITY PRESS

Oxford University Press, Inc., publishes works that further
Oxford University's objective of excellence
in research, scholarship, and education.

Oxford   New York
Auckland   Cape Town   Dar es Salaam   Hong Kong   Karachi
Kuala Lumpur   Madrid   Melbourne   Mexico City   Nairobi
New Delhi   Shanghai   Taipei   Toronto

With offices in
Argentina   Austria   Brazil   Chile   Czech Republic   France   Greece
Guatemala   Hungary   Italy   Japan   Poland   Portugal   Singapore
South Korea   Switzerland   Thailand   Turkey   Ukraine   Vietnam

Published by Oxford University Press, Inc.
198 Madison Avenue, New York, New York 10016
www.oup.com

Oxford is a registered trademark of Oxford University Press

Library of Congress Cataloging-in-Publication Data

Encephalitis lethargica: during and after the epidemic/edited by Joel A. Vilensky.
p.; cm.
Includes bibliographical references and index.
ISBN 978-0-19-537830-6
1. Epidemic encephalitis—Epidemiology. 2. Epidemic encephalitis—History. 3. Postencephalitic
Parkinson's disease—Epidemiology. 4. Postencephalitic Parkinson's disease—History.
I. Vilensky, Joel A., 1951–
[DNLM: 1. Parkinson Disease, Postencephalitic—epidemiology. 2. Parkinson Disease,
Postencephalitic—history. 3. History, 20th Century. WL 359 E556 2011]
RA644.E52E53 2011
614.5'9833—dc22
2010015646

1 3 5 7 9 8 6 4 2
Printed in the United States of America
on acid-free paper

Dedicated to the memory of Sophie Cameron,
who died of complications associated with
encephalitis lethargica on May 30, 2006,
at the age of 24 years.

FOREWORD BY OLIVER SACKS

Encephalitis Lethargica: During and After the Epidemic is the story of one of the greatest medical mysteries of the 20th century, a condition that affected millions of people all over the world and became a living death for some of them, until they were "awakened" by the miracle drug L-dopa. Oddly, the epidemic, which was front-page news for more than a decade, has been all but forgotten, and there has not been a comprehensive book on the subject in 75 years. Now, Joel Vilensky and the many eminent contributors to this volume have given us a new perspective on the "sleepy sickness," one that is comprehensive and scholarly but also beautifully organized and vividly written.

While Vilensky was the instigator and driving force behind this enormous project, he has enlisted many knowledgeable colleagues: Lindsay Anderson, Judith Cameron, Jennifer Cook, Paul Foley, Sid Gilman, Sherman McCall, Dana Marlowe, Ravil Mukhamedzyanov, Keith Josephs, Hope Owens, Richard Steele and, not least, Roger Duvoisin, one of the handful of physicians still living who actually saw and treated many hundreds of postencephalitic patients.

The authors have clearly read critically all the monographs written on this epidemic, as well as some 9,000 papers written on encephalitis lethargica in the years that it spread around the world. One can only guess at the thousands of hours spent reading in obscure libraries and forgotten archives—yet the product of all this research is full of life and a fresh perspective which was not possible for me when I wrote *Awakenings* 40 years ago.

Such a perspective may only have become possible now, in the 21st century, for this volume not only revisits the horrible years between 1915 and 1930 when the epidemic raged and the plight of the survivors for decades afterward, but the sporadic return of similar (perhaps identical) diseases since that time, including the recent outbreak in England. While the essential mystery of encephalitis lethargica remains unsolved, some important clues have been added to the story in recent years, which Vilensky evaluates here. He also brings together here a number of (often very poignant) self-reports, never before published or long forgotten. He considers the question of whether "encephalitis lethargica" is in fact a single disease, as has always been assumed, or whether it comprises a range of different disorders with different causes.

The effects of encephalitis lethargica were different in every patient, and often included personality changes or psychiatric disorders, movement disorders, sleep disorders, and almost every other imaginable symptom—many of which occurred only decades later. This often made diagnosis difficult or impossible, and adds further complexity to studying the disease now. Vilensky, therefore, has taken great pains to present this data in an organized form, with many well thought-out tables. This analysis, and the many fine essays on different aspects of the great epidemic, will be invaluable to physicians and researchers, especially if the disease or cluster of disorders we call encephalitis lethargica ever returns in the overwhelming, pandemic form it took in the 1920s. But I think this excellent book will find a much wider readership too, for it is a moving human chronicle with profound implications for anyone concerned with the themes of sickness and health.

Foreword © 2010 by Oliver Sacks

PREFACE

M edical historians are typically historical detectives. We find a medical mystery and try to solve it by either combining information from a number of historical sources or locating the "holy grail" pertaining to the mystery—that is, the one article or book that contains the solution to the mystery that everyone else has overlooked.

Encephalitis lethargica (EL) has been my medical mystery to solve. Although thousands of articles and books were written on the syndrome during the 1920s, definitive knowledge is limited or almost nonexistent. What was it, what caused it, what became of it, and will it return? all remain unanswered questions.

I have known about EL for a very long time but only became interested in it after publishing some descriptions of films taken of EL and postencephalitic parkinsonism (PEP) patients in 2005 (Vilensky et al.). Subsequently, I began to read about the disease and spent a wonderful morning with Dr. Oliver Sacks in his New York office. He, of course, had written about EL and PEP in his 1974 book, *Awakenings*, which later became a motion picture. Dr. Sacks encouraged my work on EL, has continued to provide me with insights into the condition, and wrote the Foreword for this book.

I subsequently began to write articles on various aspects of EL (e.g., its effects on children and its manifestations in the Soviet Union: Vilensky et al., 2007; Vilensky et al., 2008) and was beginning to be recognized as one of the few world experts on the syndrome. Subsequently, in late 2007, during an e-mail exchange with Craig Panner, neurology editor for Oxford University Press (OUP), I asked him simply if OUP might be interested in a book on EL. To my surprise and delight, he said yes; however, because of the enormity of the task, especially in terms of locating, translating, and reading references in many languages, I knew I would need financial support for editorial assistance. I then approached the Sophie Cameron Trust, which had provided some earlier research funds to me, and the Trustees again graciously provided the funds I needed. Subsequently, OUP, the Trust, and I agreed on the terms of the contract and the book process was begun.

I am of course grateful to many people for their assistance with this book, and their names are listed below. I want to first thank all the co-authors who wrote with me the chapters of this book, and who are listed on the Contributors page. Among these Contributors, Dr. Sid Gilman has guided me through the neurology of EL since I first started this project, and his guidance and patience throughout my career is tremendously appreciated.

Special thanks are due Dr. Oliver Sacks, for encouraging my work on EL since he first agreed to spend a morning with me in 2005. And, of course, I thank him for writing the Foreword to this book. His assistant, Ms. Kate Edgar, could not have been more helpful in coordinating my communications with Dr. Sacks.

Messrs. Craig Panner and assistant editor David D'Addona are due much gratitude for their assistance and patience with my impatience to complete this project. Similarly, Ms. Annie Woy's copyediting was superb and project manager Mr. Jais K. Alphonse could not have been more helpful in the final stages of getting this manuscript into book form. I thank both of them most sincerely. Ms. Lowene Stipp continually provided clerical, editorial, and secretarial help else this book would not have been finished on time. Ms. Linda Adams made sure that I spent the funds allocated by the Trust in an approved manner and helped me with all the purchases I made. Mr. Richard Steele, Trustee of the Sophie Cameron Trust, did everything he could to help me with the development and implementation of this book, and I am most grateful to him and to the Trust.

Two librarians at the Ruth Lilly Medical Library, Indiana University School of Medicine, Mr. Michael Wilkinson and Ms. Nancy Eckerman, continuously amazed me with their ability to find and get to me materials from close to 100 years ago from all corners of the world. The project would not have been possible without them.

Ms. Roberta Shadle of the Indiana University Purdue University–Fort Wayne (IPFW) Publishing Department is thanked for drawing the original figures presented in the book. Mr. Gary Travis of the same department taught me enough Photoshop to enable me to work with the figures in the book, and I am very grateful to him for that.

Dr. Kenneth Crews of Columbia University, Ms. Sherri Michaels of Indiana University, Ms. Cheryl Truesdale (IPFW), Dr. John Burnham of Ohio State

University, and Ms. Sherri Feldman of Random House all provided much appreciated assistance pertaining to copyright issues. Also of Columbia, Dr. Stephen Novak is thanked for searching and finding a photograph of Dr. Josephine O'Neal for me.

Mr. Kris Kallmeyer, Ms. Hope Owens, and Dr. Paul Foley all contributed greatly to this book by translating German and French materials for me.

The following individuals/organizations are thanked for allowing me to reproduce the noted images or text. For those images/passages not specifically listed, the material is in the public domain.

Chapter 2: Figure 2.2: permission granted from BMJ Group (License #2247200635708).

Chapter 3: Figure 3.1: Courtesy of and permission granted by Columbia University Medical Center Archives and Special Collections (Dr. Stephen E. Novak). Figure 3.2: Permission granted by Columbia University Press (Mr. Christopher John Williams).

Chapter 5: Figure 5.1 lower images. Permission granted by Springer Publishers. Figure 5.2 Permission granted by the Rhode Island Medical Society (Ms. Sarah Brooke Stevens).

Chapter 6: Figure 6.2: Courtesy and permission via Derby Local Studies Library (Mr. Mark Young).

Chapter 7: Figures 7.1 and 7.2: Permission granted by Hodde Education (Mr. Nick Welton) and Dr. J.V. Kinner Wilson. Figure 7.3: Permission granted by Elsevier (Ms. Kayleigh Harris).

Chapter 8: Figures 8.1 and 8.2. Permission granted by Dr. Oliver Sacks.

Chapter 9. Figure 9.1. Courtesy of Dr. D. Caleton Gajdusek and Dr. Ralph Garruto (DCG-WNG 15-11 of Gadusek Collection).

Chapter 10. Figure 10.5, top. Permission granted by Oxford Journals (Ms. Katherine Randall). Figure 10.5, middle and bottom. Permission granted by BMJ Publishing group (License #2234360723391). Figure 10.6: Permission granted by Oxford Journals (Ms. Katherine Randall).

Chapter 11. Case 11.6: Permission granted by *The Lancet* (via RightsLink).

Joel A. Vilensky

REFERENCES CITED

Vilensky, J. A., Goetz, C. G. & Gilman, S. (2005). Movement disorders associated with encephalitis lethargica: A video compilation. *Movement Disorders, 21*, 1–8.

Vilensky, J.A., Foley, P., & Gilman S. (2007). Children and encephalitis lethargica: A historical review. *Pediatric Neurology, 37*, 79–84.

Vilensky, J. A., Mukhamedzyanov, R., & Gilman, S. (2008). Encephalitis lethargica in the Soviet Union. *European Neurology, 60*, 113–121.

PROLOGUE

The Sophie Cameron Trust is quite a new organization—its story began in 1999. In February of that year, Sophie Cameron, who had just been elected Head Girl of the Royal High Senior School in Bath, returned from a holiday in Venice, Italy. She felt poorly, and several days later she was admitted to the Royal United Hospital in a delirious state. Over the subsequent weeks, her condition worsened dramatically. She developed many of the classical symptoms of encephalitis lethargica (EL), including oculogyric crises, respiratory irregularity, and coma, and was finally discharged home late in 1999, in a minimally aware state. Despite 24-hour care from her family and various professionals, as well as intensive physiotherapy and other treatments, Sophie made little progress, and she died suddenly on May 30, 2006.

During Sophie's illness, her parents, Phillip and Judith, discovered that EL is currently a very rare condition, and it proved frustratingly difficult for them to identify reliable information about it. The many friends of the Cameron family also wanted to learn about EL and to offer practical help. This led them to form the Sophie Cameron Trust. The Trust committee soon realized that not only Sophie, but also others with EL might need assistance, and so the idea of a charitable trust arose. Individuals with the skills that would be needed, in science, medicine, law, accounting, fund-raising, public relations, and management, were already involved, and were willing to donate their time to act as trustees or members of the fund-raising committee. So, in April 2002, the Trust was registered with the Charities Commission in the United Kingdom as charity No. 1092190. The aims of the Trust were set out in the by-laws, and are, briefly, to help people affected by EL and their families, to increase knowledge about EL and its implications among the medical profession and the general public, and to encourage research into the management and causes of EL.

Our first project, which arose directly out of Sophie's illness, was to explore existing treatments, and with the aid of matched funding from two other local charities, the Medlock Trust and the Brownsword Charitable Foundation, we set up a programme to investigate whether intensive physiotherapy could benefit patients in Sophie's position. Next, we needed to make contact with other EL patients—not easy because of medical confidentiality issues. While we considered how best to do this, we focused on raising the profile of EL among the medical profession. In particular, we wanted to see whether we could encourage a broad spectrum of research into EL without preconceptions as to what might be most valuable.

The requirements for developing a useful research programme seemed clear. First, we needed to identify and engage with researchers who were active in the field. Second, we needed to discover whether funding on the relatively small scale that we could provide would prove sufficient to make a difference: we hoped that by providing small grants, we would be able to encourage research into this rare syndrome, stimulating projects that might otherwise never be started and attracting funding from other sources to extend the projects that were successful. Then, at a conference on encephalitis, we met Dr. Russell Dale, who was the lead author of an article describing 20 modern cases of EL, entitled "Encephalitis Lethargica Syndrome: 20 New Cases and Evidence of Basal Ganglia Autoimmunity," published in *Brain*, in 2004.

Through Russell, we also met Dr. Gavin Giovannoni; with others, they were investigating whether EL might be part of a spectrum of autoimmune disorders. We received a great deal of help and encouragement from Gavin, and eventually we asked him if he would act as (unpaid) scientific adviser to the Trust, because we knew that an expert neurologist's input would be needed to evaluate research proposals that we might be asked to fund. Happily, he agreed. His advice proved invaluable, and he has played a key role in helping us to develop the program of research that is described on our website, www.thesophiecamerontrust.org.uk. He also set up the most important single project that the Trust is funding—a national surveillance programme for early identification and study of patients with EL in the UK. This is the only such program currently operating in the world, and its purpose is to gain near-complete, long-term surveillance of EL across the UK. It involves the inclusion of EL on a monthly electronic questionnaire circulated to all neurologists and pediatric neurologists in the UK. We hope that this program will eventually establish the incidence of EL, as well as providing epidemiological information and perhaps insight into the causes of EL. In addition, blood, cerebrospinal fluid, and other samples collected during clinical investigations for diagnostic purposes will be stored for future research, provided that patients or their families give their consent. All patients identified will also receive a letter giving them information about the Sophie Cameron Trust.

From the beginning, the Trust wanted to encourage international cooperation in research on EL, and we established contact with the editor and primary author of this book, Dr. Joel Vilensky, who kindly agreed to act as the Trust's "eyes and ears" for developments relating to EL in the United States and elsewhere in the world. We had the opportunity to meet him in 2008, when he gave a lecture sponsored by the Trust at the Institute of Neurology in London, attended by a number of eminent British neurologists. We were enormously impressed by his encyclopaedic knowledge of EL, and he generously provided an abridged version of his lecture for our website. Thus, when he requested funding for editorial assistance and translation of non–English-language material during the preparation of this book, we were keen to help. We felt that the book would not only provide a comprehensive resource for clinical professionals, but also would be useful to patients, family members, and friends who wanted to understand their experience and place it in a broader context. In addition, we felt that the book would be a memorial for Sophie, and we greatly appreciate the fact that it is dedicated to her.

The Trustees would also like to take this opportunity to thank everyone who has contributed to the Trust; both those who have given their time and skills, and those who have contributed financially or in other ways. Some have preferred to remain anonymous, and others have been acknowledged on our website and in our newsletters, but particular mention here should go to the Royal High School, Bath, and its staff. They gave tremendous help and support to the Cameron family during and after Sophie's illness, as well as generously supporting the Trust by providing facilities for functions and organizing a variety of fundraising activities.

The final part of this Prologue should be dedicated to Judith Cameron, Sophie's mother. During Sophie's illness, Judith wrote a regular column for the *Guardian* newspaper which, focusing on the role of carers, provided an important forum for raising awareness of EL. The following paragraphs are taken from the article that Judith wrote following Sophie's death:

> At 8.55 P.M. on Tuesday, 30th May 2006, I was no longer the mother of four children, but three. My beautiful daughter, Sophie, suddenly died. Seven years earlier, aged only 17, she contracted a rare infection of the brain and a few weeks later, in Intensive Care, suffered a cardiac arrest. The oxygen starvation resulted in irrevocable brain damage and when she finally returned home, she needed 24-hour care. Her condition became stable, and we implemented a rigorous regime of physiotherapy to maintain her body in good physical shape. We prayed that, one day, either through drug or stem cell treatment, something would be discovered that could once again give her a life worth living....

Today I am still working to remove all trace of her awful suffering and yet during those years, I tried hard only to concentrate on the present. It was too painful to dwell on the past and what might have been while I looked after the shadow of who my daughter once was. I was determined to do the best for the daughter I had. But of course Sophie was the little girl I taught to swim, the little girl who held my hand during the births of her younger brother and sister while her Dad took photos. She grew to be the only person in the household, other than me, who noticed when the bin needed emptying or the loo roll replaced. Only now am I slowly allowing myself to recollect the vibrant child I had for seventeen years.

Despite her severe disability, I had always assumed that Sophie would outlive us. I am sure that no mother is ever ready for her child to die. I hate to think that I will never ever see her again—never be able to cuddle or smell her, never be able to show her how much I love her. Any possibility of her getting better has gone. But I can feel that the weight of the seven years of Sophie's illness is starting to lift and I remember again my gorgeous, vivacious, sassy daughter. Although I still weep copiously, I am going to allow myself that privilege of remembering what a fantastic person she was. I will exult in who she was and continue to be proud of being her mother.

Richard Steele
Trustee
The Sophie Cameron Trust
www. thesophiecamerontrust.org.uk

CONTENTS

CONTRIBUTORS

Lindsay L. Anderson, MD
Department of Anatomy and Cell Biology
Indiana University School of Medicine
Indianapolis, IN

Judith Cameron, BS
Journalist
Bath, United Kingdom

Jennifer Cook, MS
Department of Anatomy and Cell Biology
Indiana University School of Medicine
Fort Wayne, IN

Roger C. Duvoisin, MD, FACP
University of Medicine and Dentistry of New Jersey (Emeritus)
New Brunswick, NJ

Paul B. Foley, PhD
Prince of Wales Medical Research Institute
Sydney, Australia

Sid Gilman, MD
Neurologist and former Chairman
Department of Neurology
University of Michigan
Ann Arbor, MI

Keith Josephs, MD
Department of Neurology
Mayo Clinic
Rochester, MN

Dana Marlowe, MD
Department of Anatomy and Cell Biology
Indiana University School of Medicine
Indianapolis, IN

Sherman McCall, MD
Department of Clinical Pathology
US Army Medical Research Institute of Infectious Diseases (USAMRIID)
Fort Detrick, MD

Ravil Z. Mukhamedzyanov, MD
Department Neurology and Rehabilitation
Kazan State Medical University
Kazan, Russia

Hope E. Owens, BA
Department of Anatomy and Cell Biology
Indiana University School of Medicine
Fort Wayne, IN

Oliver Sacks, MD
Neurologist and author of many books, including *Awakenings*
New York, NY

Richard Steele, BSC
Trustee
Sophie Cameron Trust
Bath, United Kingdom

Encephalitis Lethargica

1

INTRODUCTION

Joel A. Vilensky and Sid Gilman

During the 1920s and 1930s, encephalitis lethargica (EL; also known as epidemic encephalitis, von Economo disease, and sleepy sickness) was a major clinical phenomenon, perplexing the medical profession across the world, and spanning thousands of articles and numerous monographs in English, French, German, Italian, and Russian (Fig. 1.1). The most widely cited monograph, *Die Encephalitis lethargica, ihre Nachkrankheiten und ihre Behardlung* (Encephalitis Lethargica: Its Sequelae and Treatment) was published by Constantin von Economo in German in 1929, and in English (translated by K. O. Newman) in 1931 (Fig. 1.2).

The last major monograph on EL prior to the current one was *Encefalite Lethargica Acuta e Cronica*, published in Italian by C. Frugoni in 1935. Most of the monographs on EL from the epidemic period covered essentially the same topics: epidemiology, symptomatology, etiology, transmissibility, sequelae, pathology, and treatment. This volume generally covers these same topics, as well as providing some unique features (e.g., self-reports), and also covers developments in EL since the epidemic period.

Thus, the two major justifications for another monograph on EL, albeit one almost 100 years since the epidemic period, are that there is information to be added to that available during the epidemic period and that there is some importance to understanding this mysterious disease, both because EL may return, and also because understanding EL will contribute to the general understanding of neurologic degenerative diseases.

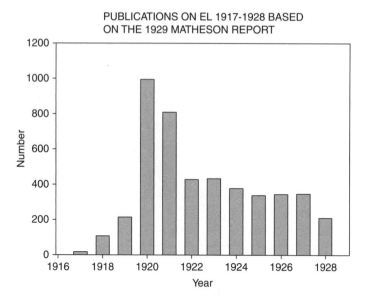

Figure 1.1 Bar chart of all of the references listed in the 1929 Matheson Report on EL for the noted years.

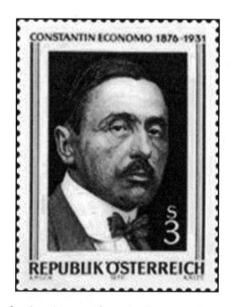

Figure 1.2 Image of an Austrian stamp honoring Baron von Economo.

Encephalitis lethargica may also be important because of its role in 20th-century history. Chapter 12 in *The Throwing Madonna: Essays on the Brain* (1983) by William H. Calvin is titled, "The Woodrow Wilson Story." In it, Calvin described how U.S. President Wilson wanted Germany completely defeated in World War I but, in contrast to his European counterparts, did not want the country to be crushed. Wilson believed that a peace treaty that humiliated Germany would be resented and presumably not last, as it did not. At the 1919 peace conference, he initially argued against the French efforts to try the ex-Kaiser and to force punitive reparations. But, during the peace conference, Wilson became very ill and virtually overnight developed profound changes in personality. It is possible that he suffered a stroke, but Dr. Edwin Weinstein, who wrote, *Woodrow Wilson: A Medical and Psychological Biography* (1981), suggested that Wilson's brain manifestations were either the product of EL or influenza. Following this episode, Wilson proposed that the former Kaiser be tried, and he was contemptuous of all the German delegates. Wilson no longer was willing to listen to advice, groped for ideas, and had lapses of memory. Dr. Weinstein was a Columbia University neurologist who meticulously studied Wilson's medical history, and his opinion must be taken very seriously. And, if so, EL indeed, potentially, had a pronounced effect on the particulars of the Treaty of Versailles and by inference on those conditions that resulted in the rise of Adolf Hitler and World War II. Furthermore, most interestingly, there has been speculation that Adolf Hitler too suffered from EL and subsequently one of its sequelae, postencephalitic parkinsonism (PEP; cf. Chapter 7), and that these disorders affected (caused?) his fanatical behavior (Walters, 1975; Lieberman, 1983).

Three chapters in this book, Chapter 2, "Epidemic-Period Encephalitis Lethargic"; Chapter 3 "Epidemiology"; and Chapter 4 "Pre-1917 History," contain basic information that is not substantially different from that contained in the epidemic-period monographs, although we believe the synthesis and the modern graphics and tables better convey these aspects of EL than do the aforementioned monographs.

The material in Chapter 5, "Post–Epidemic Period," includes tabular summaries of all of the reports of putative EL and PEP cases from around the world published since the epidemic period. In that chapter, we evaluate these reports and suggest criteria by which modern cases should be judged to be similar to EL, as described during the epidemic period.

Chapter 7, "Chronic Encephalitis Lethargica," details the initial reports of the chronic sequelae, especially PEP, and shows the initial confusion pertaining to how PEP related to idiopathic Parkinson disease (PD) and to EL. Many of the articles discussing PEP and PEP patients that have been published since the epidemic period are reviewed. Furthermore, we show that the relationship between EL and PEP may be more complex than currently perceived, and we suggest that neither may be a unitary condition. One of the authors of this chapter (and of Chapters 5, 8, and 10), Dr. Roger Duvoisin, was an active researcher in all aspects of PD during the 1960s and 1970s, including PEP. He was also involved in the initial L-dopa treatment trials in both PD and PEP. Dr. Duvoisin offers a unique contribution to this volume because of his first-hand experience during the period when PEP (and to some extent EL) was a living syndrome and neurologists were actively treating these patients.

Similarly, in Chapter 8, we present a reviewof the use of L-dopa in PEP patients, with an emphasis on the data in Oliver Sacks' 1990 book, *Awakenings*. These data have not been organized in tabular fashion previously. Dr. Sacks not only wrote a Foreword for this book, but also reviewed this chapter and made some contributions to it, although he declined co-authorship.

Chapter 10, "Neuropathology," not only summarizes the older literature on EL and PEP neuropathology, but also provides a review of a computer-based analysis of the locations of the lesions in acute EL conducted by one of the authors (LLA) while a medical student. Furthermore, we evaluate all of the recent descriptions of the central nervous system lesions in PEP patients who died after the epidemic period and also of the recent immunohistochemical analyses of PEP neuropathology. These analyses are given a modern perspective through the co-authorship of Dr. Keith Josephs of the Mayo Clinic, an expert on neurofibrillary tangles in neurodegenerative diseases.

Although some of the monographs from the epidemic period discussed the transmissibility of EL (contagiousness), none selected example reports from all over the world and assembled them as we have done here (see Chapter 6). Although the evidence for person-to person transmission of EL is generally weak, there are surprisingly some very thorough reports that suggest that, in rare situations, the contagiousness of EL was very high.

In Chapter 9, "Etiology," Drs. McCall and Vilensky review both the older presumptive causes of EL (e.g., viruses, botulism) and the newest theories (e.g., autoimmune disease; associated with anti–N-methyl-D-aspartate [NMDA] receptor encephalitis. This chapter also presents a thorough analysis of the relationship between EL and influenza, concluding that, although it is unlikely that influenza caused EL, it is impossible to entirely rule it out. Finally, we suggest here and in other chapters that perhaps some of the confounding findings pertaining to EL have resulted because neither EL nor PEP are unitary conditions.

Undoubtedly, the most unusual chapter in this monograph is Chapter 11, "Self-Reports." We have assembled every self-report we could locate on EL, most by physicians, and presented either the actual self-report as originally written (if it was short) or, in the case of a book, a summary of the account. No previous work has ever compiled these self-reports, and together they offer a unique perspective of the disease, and will contribute to the diagnosis of any putative future cases.

In 1930, Pool wrote:

> It is now about 10 years since von Economo gave an accurate clinical description
> of the disease which has come to be known as epidemic encephalitis. As far as

the historical record of the disease was concerned, this malady was something new, mysterious in its onset, and appalling in its destruction. Its etiology was a matter of conjecture, its pathology merely guessed at, and its sequelae undreamt of. During the intervening years there has been much clinical material for concentrated study of the disease, and yet we must confess that etiology is still obscure, the causative agent still unknown, the pathological riddle still unsolved and of necessity therefore treatment is practically non-existent. (p. 45)

Does the present volume solve the "riddle" of EL, which also has been referred to as the greatest medical mystery of the 20th century? Unfortunately, no: but inroads are certainly made here especially pertaining to diagnosis, pathology, and even treatment. Because sporadic cases of EL continue to be diagnosed (cf. Chapter 5), some synthesis of the old and new material is needed, and this volume fills that need. And, there is the ever-present possibility that EL will reappear on a larger scale, in which case both the old and newer reports on EL will need to be consulted—this volume will serve as a guide to them.

REFERENCES CITED

Calvin, W. H. (1983). *The Throwing Madonna: Essays on the Brain*. New York: McGraw Hill.

von Economo, C. (1929). *Die Encephalitis lethargica, ihre Nachkrankheiten und ihre Behardlung*. Berlin: Urban and Schwarzenberg. (Published in English in 1931: Translated by K. O. Newman; London: Oxford University Press.)

Frugoni, C. (1935). *Encefalite Letargica Acuta e Cronica*. Milan: Societa Editrice Libraria.

Lieberman, A. N. (1983). Adolph Hitler: his diaries and Parkinson's disease. *New England Journal of Medicine, 309*, 375–376.

Matheson Commission. (1929). *Epidemic Encephalitis: Etiology, Epidemiology, Treatment*. New York: Columbia University Press.

Pool, A. (1930). A clinical and pathological study of three cases of epidemic encephalitis. *Journal of Neurology and Psychopathology, 2*, 45–59.

Sacks, O. (1990). *Awakenings*. New York: HarperCollins Publishers.

von Wagner-Jauregg, J., & von Economo's wife. (1937). *Baron Constantin von Economo: His Life and Work*. Burlington: Free Press Interstate Printing Corp. (Translated by R. Spillman.)

Walters, J. H. (1975). Hitler's encephalitis: A footnote to history. *Journal of Operational Psychiatry, 6*, 99–112.

Weinstein, E. A. (1981). *Woodrow Wilson: A Medical and Psychological Biography*. Princeton: Princeton University Press.

2

ENCEPHALITIS LETHARGICA DURING THE EPIDEMIC PERIOD

Joel A. Vilensky and Sid Gilman

Its dramatic advent on a war-torn world, its rapid diffusion to all continents and the islands of the seas, its striking and characteristic pathological picture, its astonishing masquerade in the guise of a myriad of other diseases, its remarkable shifts of group types in succeeding years of its recurrence, and its almost unforetellable course in any individual case has no parallel in the entire field of medicine. And it is doubtful if any plague has ever been visited upon humanity that has claimed so many victims, has so completely covered the earth, and left so many maimed and crippled wrecks in its wake.

(Crafts, 1927, p. 3)

INTRODUCTION

This chapter concentrates primarily on encephalitis lethargica (EL) as described during the epidemic period, especially during the first few years after von Economo's 1917 initial characterization of it.

A PROTEAN DISEASE AND PRIMACY

In 1921, H. F. Smith, working for the U.S. Public Health Service, reported the results of a survey of EL taken in the United States in 1920 (Smith, 1921).

He defined epidemic encephalitis (encephalitis lethargica, nona) as "an epidemic syndrome characterized in most instances by a gradual onset with headache, vertigo, disturbances of vision, ocular palsies, changes in speech, dysphagia, marked asthenia, fever (usually of a low grade), obstinate constipation, incontinence of urine, a peculiar mask-like expression of the face, and a state of lethargy which gradually develops in the majority of the recognized cases into a coma that is more or less profound" (p. 207).

If EL was consistently described as fitting the above description, then many of the diagnostic ambiguities associated with the disease would not have occurred. Among the approximately 9,000 publications on EL from the epidemic period (Peng, 1993), however, many described the symptomatology, but few were in agreement as to the most reliable signs and symptoms associated with the disease. The signs and symptoms that were linked with EL in these many articles include virtually every neurologic sign and symptom described in neurology textbooks. The inconsistency in diagnostic criteria was explained at the time by suggesting that, during different geographic or temporal epidemics, different signs and symptoms predominated and that there were great day-to-day (hour-to-hour) shifts in the symptomatology. Nevertheless, it is difficult for a modern clinician to appreciate why, despite this variability, the clinicians of the period ascribed a unifying designation to the disorder. Our view is that there tended, even with all the variability, to be an emphasis on sleep and ocular muscle disorders, and also that the constellation of symptoms and signs exhibited did not fit any other established neurologic condition. Crafts stated, "And while no other disease, perhaps, presents so many difficulties in diagnosis as does this protean complex, the fact must always be borne in mind, that while it usually offers a very close resemblance to one or another condition, careful and painstaking study and comparison will reveal either some incongruity, some essential symptom lacking or a superabundance of elements, thus offering a definite aid or conclusive basis for differential diagnosis" (p. 60). Thus, indefinite clinical observations were used to make a diagnosis of EL because, at the time there simply were no definitive laboratory tests to confirm a diagnosis. Furthermore, although the unity of the disease was assumed, it also is possible that the variation in symptomatology described reflects either minor or even major variations in etiology and that EL was not a unitary condition (see below and Chapter 12).

To facilitate diagnosis within EL's vast array of symptoms, some clinicians from the period divided the disease into temporal stages and symptom-based types (forms). To illustrate these stages and types, many of the articles and monographs from the period included short case descriptions that exemplified specific stages and/or types. This resulted in the publication of a few thousand (if not more) case reports globally. These reports, although interesting, are less clinically useful than expected because they are very inconsistent, listing specific signs and symptoms for some patients, but not for others, with very variable time frames.

Some of the confusion pertaining to the diagnosis of EL may also relate to the fact that Constantin von Economo's original 1917 article and case descriptions were published in German, at a time when much of the world was at war with Germany and Austria. Strong anti–German sentiment prevailed at the time, and communication between belligerent nations was poor, so that foreign journals were probably not distributed until after the war ended in 1918. Although many non-German language articles about EL were published beginning in 1918 (especially in English), von Economo's original article was not published in English until 1968 (Wilkins & Brody, 1968). However, even then, the actual case histories were not translated, which we suggest has hindered accurate contemporary comparisons with the original syndrome. In contrast to the original article, von Economo's 1929 monograph, *Die Encephalitis lethargica, ihre Nachkrankheiten und ihre Behandlung,* was published in English in 1931 (translated by K. O. Newman). But, by 1931, the EL epidemic period was essentially over.

Here, we present English translations of the seven relatively detailed cases presented on pages 582–583 of *Encephalitis Lethargica,* which was published in *Wiener klinische Wochenschrift,* vol. 30, 1917. In a later paper, published in the same year, *Neue Beitrage zur Encephalitis lethargic* (New Findings on Encephalitis Lethargica), von Economo republished these same cases (with some additional information), along with four new cases.

Case 1: 31-year-old woman

The patient became sick on February 4, 1917, with shivering, headache, and somnolence. On February 26, she was somnolent and slept throughout the day, but it was possible to get her attention by calling her, and she answered in a normal manner; left to herself, she fell asleep again. Total paralysis of the external oculomotor nerve, both eyes being fixed with no movement in the outer angle. There was ptosis, sensitivity to pressure on the eyeballs, and a difference of reflexes on the right side, and her temperature was 36.2°C [97.1°F]. Sleepiness increased to extreme stupor, accompanied by a complete paralysis of the right upper limb. Rigor of both lower limbs with Babinski's present. Temperature 36.8°C [98.2°F]. Pulse 48. On March 24, the stupor continued. Temperature 39.5°C [103.1°F]. Decubitus. No abnormalities of the internal viscera. From then on, there was a slow recovery. On April 4, fever and somnolence had disappeared. The paralysis of the oculomotor nerve began to disappear, as did the paralysis of the upper extremity. Babinski sign was negative. At the beginning of May, the paralysis of the oculomotor nerve had disappeared completely. Only a mild tendency to sleep continued until the end of May, making a total of four months in all, and even after that the patient slept surprising much. The patient showed a mild impairment of her mental functions but this state also improved until the end of June when she died of pneumonia.

At the onset, the spinal puncture showed an increase in pressure but the clear cerebrospinal fluid (CSF) was free of micro-organisms. The protein content was increased: 5.5. The Nonne-Apelt reaction was slightly positive, 43 elements. The Wasserman reaction in the blood and the CSF was negative. The urine findings were normal. Lumbar puncture shortly before death showed normal findings.

Case 2: 17-year-old girl

She became sick on February 3. Her temperature was 39.5°C [103.1°F], and there was headache and stiffness of the neck. Delirious state, from which she could be aroused and answer questions accurately. Paresis of the left abducent nerve. Internal organs without pathological findings. The somnolence increased to deep stupor with rigor of the lower limbs, bilateral clonus of the ankle. The Babinski sign was positive on the right. The temperature reached 42.2°C [108°F]. Findings in the serum and in the CSF were negative, as well as in the urine. A slow improvement appeared beginning of April. The tendency to sleep had lasted 2½ months. After the middle of April, she was alert during daytime but at night became delirious. The positive Babinski sign on the right side persisted. Mid-May she was discharged from the hospital after complete recovery and by this time Babinski sign was negative.

Case 3: 38-year-old male teacher

This patient became severely sick on February 27 with headache and general malaise. On March 1, delirium, confusion, somnolence, and ptosis. Temperature of 37.2°C [99°F]. On being called, he awakened and behaved in an orderly manner. Muscle paresis on looking to the right, nystagmus, facial paresis on both sides, and slightly bulbar speech. He also had slight difficulties in swallowing. During the following days, the somnolence increased and, for hours, the patient was in a deep stupor from which he could not be roused. From the end of March until approximately the end of April, days of deep stupor alternated with other days when the patient could be roused more easily. The persistence of somnolence and ocular paresis disappeared slowly, and the patient was dismissed from the hospital by the end of June without apparent defects. The somnolence lasted 2½ months. Lumbar puncture revealed normal CSF and no increase in pressure.

Case 4: 14-year-old girl

She became ill at the end of March with headache, shivering, diminished consciousness, and singultus. She was admitted to the hospital on March 22. She slept the whole day and showed signs of marked delirium. When spoken to, she answered promptly and was well orientated, but left alone she relapsed into stupor. The cranial nerves were normal. The eyeballs and the neck were sensitive to pressure. Paresis of the right upper limb. Continuous singultus with a contraction of the left abdominal musculature. Temperature: 38.5°C [101.3°F]. The next days showed increasing stupor and rigor of the lower limbs. Babinski sign positive. She died on March 21 with a pre-mortal temperature of 39.8°C [103.6°F]. The Wasserman reaction and CSF were negative. Lumbar puncture did show an increase in pressure, but the CSF was clear and free from organisms, without any pathological findings. The postmortem examination by Prof. von Wiesner showed increased fluid in the subarachnoid space. The leptomeninges were bloody, and the cerebral cortex spotwise hyperemic, particularly on the right hemisphere where there was an edematous swelling. Anterior and posterior horns of the upper cervical column showed some congestion.

Case 5: 26-year-old woman

She was admitted to the hospital on March 22. Confused speech for two days, and she fell asleep whenever she was standing or walking. At the University Hospital, the patient resembled a somnambulist, and it was possible to wake her up and she was able to pay attention for short periods. After that, she immediately relapsed into her somnolent state. Her temperature was 36.4°C [97.5°F]. The physical findings were questionable, with ptosis and paresis of the right rectus internus. Otherwise, there were no pathological findings in the area of the nervous system or in the in the internal organs. In the evening of the day of admission, there appeared a primary edema followed by death. The Wasserman reaction and CSF were negative. Lumbar puncture showed a slight increase in pressure–clear–several spinal fluid samples without microorganism or coagulated fibrin. Several elements – 12. Postmortem examination (Prof. von Wiesner): hyperaemia of the brain and the leptomeninges with spotted hyperemia in the medulla and the grey matter of the dorsal spinal cord. Acute pulmonary edema.

Case 6: 38-year-old woman

She became ill on March 17th with a temperature of 39.5°C [103.1°F] and coryza. After two days, these symptoms disappeared. We noticed ptosis, especially on the right side, and at times she suffered from diplopia. Her mother reported that whenever she stood or sat, she fell asleep immediately and at night she suffered from delirium. This also occurred during the day. She started speaking loudly while arising from sleep. In the hospital, the patient sat in a chair most of the day and a call was enough to wake her up. She then gave correct and clear answers, and she could be carried back to bed. During the night, she spoke a lot. The clinical examination revealed a bilateral ptosis of the eyelids, more so on the left side. The rectus internus was bilaterally slightly paretic. There was a diplopia of the extreme lateral gaze and an upward gaze palsy. The rest of the physical and neurological examination was negative. The body temperature was 36.5°C [97.7°F]. Urine, and Wasserman test in serum and CSF were normal. The somnolence was very variable during the first ten days in the clinic. The gaze palsy had disappeared together with the ptosis, and at the beginning of May, the patient was able to leave the hospital without deficit.

Case 7: 32-year-old-woman

32-year-old-widow; always healthy, becomes ill suddenly after Christmas with headache, nausea, pain in arms and legs. The next day, vertigo and staggering gait. Admission January 9. Strong ataxic nodding movements of the head and the trunk; choreatic unrest; visual paralysis on the left, visual paralysis upwards, abducent nerve paresis to the right, nystagmus; coarse ataxia of both upper and lower extremities. Clonic reflexes, Babinski on both sides positive, abdominal wall reflexes lacking. Mentally, peculiarly dazed, long reaction times, and sees continually a number of persons around herself; forced-laughter. Temperature 36.2 C [97.2°F]. On the 10th of January, amblyopic to the right, only light and dark are distinguished. Patient sleeps usually; peculiar stupor, aroused she is not alert. Only at the beginning of February is there improvement of the mental stupor condition, the amblyopia, and the eye muscle disturbances, except for some nystagmus; and, the appearances of the ataxia of the head and trunk faded. Ataxia of the upper extremities with spastic paresis and ataxia of the lower extremities with Babinski still present. Wassermann-reaction negative. Urine normal. Eye condition: to the right of opticus normal, to the left temporally paled.

Case 8: 56-year-old woman

She became sick with a feverish cold at the beginning of March. In addition, she complained of back pain and coughing. After two weeks of treatment, she recovered completely. On March 18, she had a sensation of foreign body in her eyes. Sometime afterwards, she had diplopia, uncoordinated gait, and her eyelids drooped. At that time, she fell asleep quite frequently when sitting during the daytime for short or longer periods according to a report of a friend and sometimes only for a few minutes. When the patient arrived on April 6 for hospitalization, the symptoms of drowsiness disappeared but she showed a complete bilateral ptosis, paralysis of the rectus internus muscles on both sides, and paresis of the eye muscles when trying to look up. Reaction of the pupils was normal and the remainder of the neurological examination was also normal. The Wasserman reaction in serum and CSF were negative. CSF clear, no increase in pressure. Total protein according to Nissl: 1.0. None-Apelt weakly opalescent. In the urine, the sugar content up to 1 percent but this disappeared after a proper antidiabetic diet. Whether or not diabetes had existed prior to the disease could not be determined. The paresis of the oculomotor nerves improved rapidly, and on May 5, the ptosis was much less. By making an effort of the frontal musculature, the eyes could be opened completely and, when looking sideways, the movement of the eyeballs was normal. At that date, the patient was discharged.

Case 9: 16-year-old girl

She became ill with headache and fever at the end of April but the symptoms lasted only one day. Subsequently, for the next two weeks she was permanently somnolent. The eyelids drooped again and again, and whenever she sat down she fell asleep. From that time, she had strabismus. When admitted to the hospital on June 6, she was no longer somnolent but suffered from bilateral ptosis of moderate degree, both eyes showed a divergent strabismus and eye movements upwards were limited. The left pupil was wider than the right. Reaction to light was prompt. Neurological examination did not reveal other pathological findings, apart from the absence of the pointing reaction of the right arm when testing vestibular function. The Wasserman test in blood and CSF was negative. Lumbar puncture did not show an increase in pressure, and the spinal fluid was clear, without protein and no increase of cells. No bacteria were present. The disturbance of the eye muscles decreased rapidly, so that, after three weeks, except for the slight ptosis of the left eye, nothing abnormal could be noticed.

These three cases, Nos. 6, 8, and 9 are of special interest because the drowsiness, especially in the last two cases, was not connected with diminished consciousness. The somnolence was a symptom independent of the severity of all the other symptoms. It appeared as a physiological drowsiness and was so perceived by the relatives. I would like to lay stress on this independence of the drowsiness, which is independent of diminished consciousness. If it is not always so clear in all cases, in those instances in which consciousness was severely impaired, the symptom of somnolence was not so obvious. In cases in which the meningism was rather dominant and exceptional, when the lumbar puncture revealed pleocytosis, a diagnosis of meningitis was made. Such cases are represented by the two following cases whose postmortem examination confirmed the diagnosis of encephalitis.

Case 10: 14-year-old girl

At the beginning of May, she became ill with fever, headache, earache, lack of appetite, and, at times she was delirious. Three weeks after the onset of the disease, she developed difficulties in swallowing, it being reported that food was regurgitated through the nostrils. On June 1, the patient was admitted to a hospital. She was confused and could not swallow. The rest of the cranial nerves were normal. No stiffness of the neck, no chronic sign, no hyperalgesia or tendon reflexes were present, nor were they normally increased. Babinski sign was negative. In the afternoon, the temperature reached 37.2°C [98.9°F]., she had visual hallucinations, some stiffness of the neck, and hyperkinesias of the lower limbs. Abdominal muscles were intensively contracted, and she had pulmonary edema. In the evening of the same day, she died. Postmortem examination findings: pia mater and arachnoid were in spots severely infected, the brain was swollen and, on cutting, an increased amount of fluid escaped. The vessels were bloody, the medulla was soft, liquefied, and covered with petechiae. The anterior horns of the spinal cord, especially in the subcortical area, were swollen. The gray matter was diffusely hyperemic. Hypostatic pneumonia. Degeneration of the liver parenchyma and moderate hyperplasia of the spleen.

Case 11: 12-year-old boy

He was admitted to the hospital on April 20 in a comatose state with a temperature of 37.6°C [99.7°F], persistent delirium, and restlessness. When the eyes were open—but without verbal communication—he did not react to calling and was lying awake day and night in his bed. The eyes were directed to the right in a slight ocular deviation. He could not look to the left. The other cranial nerves were normal. Babinski sign was positive on both sides. He did not have stiffness of the neck or Kerning's sign. Moderate hyperalgesia of the skin was seen when the skin folds were pinched. During the next days, the meningism increased. The Wasserman test and CSF remained negative. Lumbar puncture showed an increase in pressure. The spinal fluid was slightly yellowish, and the Nonne-Apelt reaction showed a slight opalescence. Total protein according to Nissl: 2.0. Cell count 100. Slight veil of coagulation. No germs. The patient died on April 28. The diagnosis was suspected tuberculous meningitis. During a postmortem examination performed by Prof. von Wiesner, an acute encephalitis was found. The brain was edematous, the leptomeninges were not discoloured but showed a diffuse, severe infection of all blood vessels. Diffuse hyperemia of the brain. The gray matter of the brain, on cutting, showed multiple tiny petechiae. The spinal cord showed an increase in fluid content, and was soft. The anterior horns were reddish-gray.

Below we present the key symptomatology of each of these cases.

1. Flu symptoms, hypersomnolence (with easy awakening), ophthalmoplegia, ptosis, paralysis of upper extremity, lower–limb rigidity and Babinski; moderate recovery after 4 months
2. Flu symptoms, hypersomnolence (with easy awakening), ophthalmoplegia, lower–limb rigidity and Babinski; complete recovery after 3 months
3. Flu symptoms, hypersomnolence (with easy awakening), ophthalmoplegia, facial paralysis, dysphagia; complete recovery after 2.5 months
4. Flu symptoms, delirious, diminished consciousness, singultus, upper extremity paresis, rigidity of lower extremities; died
5. Hypersomnolence (with easy awakening), ophthalmoplegia, ptosis; died
6. Flu symptoms, hypersomnolence (with easy awakening), ophthalmoplegia, ptosis, diplopia, deliria; complete recovery in 2 months
7. Flu symptoms, hypersomnolence, dazed, limb pain, ataxia, ophthalmoplegia, nystagmus, Babinski; gradual improvement
8. Flu symptoms, hypersomnolence, ophthalmoplegia, diplopia, ptosis; moderate recovery after 2 months
9. Flu symptoms, hypersomnolence, ptosis, ophthalmoplegia, strabismus; virtually complete recovery after 3 weeks
10. Flu symptoms, delirium, dysphagia, hyperkinesias of lower limbs; died after 3 weeks (same day as hyperkinesias evident)
11. Delirium, restlessness, ophthalmoplegia, unresponsive; died within 8 days.

From this rather divergent collection of signs and symptoms (note that hypersomnolence was not evident in three of the cases), a major disease complex developed, characterized by an immensely diverse array of symptoms, stages, and types. Furthermore, eight of the cases showed flu-like symptoms, and case 5 showed pulmonary edema at autopsy. So, why did von Economo consider these cases to compose a separate disease entity, and why did he not consider it to be part of the influenza epidemic?

Von Economo's initial cases of the disease were admitted to the Vienna Neurologic Clinic at University Hospital at the beginning of 1917, when most of the clinic's patients were injured soldiers. When von Economo was called in to examine these cases, he deduced the common denominator among them from their symptoms and, by May, he had written a paper on the disease (van Bogaert & Théodoridès, 1979). He stated, "[these cases] do not fit our usual diagnoses. Nevertheless, they show a similarity in type of onset and symptomatology that forces one to group them into one clinical picture. We are dealing with a kind of sleeping sickness, so to speak, having a usually prolonged course" (van Bogaert

& Théodoridès, 1979; p. 79). In November, he wrote a second paper on EL (1917b). In this second paper, he observed that sleepiness and torpor may occur independently, but this dissociation is variable.

Von Economo's original deduction, that these cases represent a distinct disease syndrome, was probably based not only on his patients' clinical symptoms and signs, but also on the experimental work that "confirmed" the cause of the disease and on the neuropathology of the patients who died. In his first article, von Economo stated that, in examining stained tissue from the meninges of deceased patients, he saw "coccus-like formations." And he stated that further bacterial investigations were being conducted by Professor von Wiesner at the Pathological Institute. In his second 1917 article, von Economo wrote that Professor von Wiesner "confirmed" that a specific infectious virus is the responsible agent, and that it was possible to isolate the virus. This conclusion was based on von Wiesner's experiments in which a monkey was inoculated with brain substance from case 10. The monkey then became ill with encephalitis within 24 hours, and died after 48 hours. Postmortem examination of the animal revealed acute hemorrhagic encephalitis, with both the cortex and basal ganglia being hyperemic and edematous. In a controlled experiment, another monkey was injected with filtrate of case 10's brain substance; this animal showed no effects, leading von Economo to conclude that the disease was caused by a living virus that could not pass through the Berkefeld filter, as the poliovirus did. However, a more reasonable conclusion based on this experiment would be that the disease was caused by bacteria, which are too large to pass through the filter. Clearly, some confusion existed at this time as to the differences between viruses and bacteria. Von Wiesner also isolated a gram-positive diplostreptococcus from a culture grown from case 10's brain substance. Later reports could not confirm the presence of this diplostreptococcus in the brains of EL victims, and, in his 1929 monograph, von Economo updated his findings noting that, contrary to von Wiesner's original results, the disease is transmittable via a filtrate.

Von Economo's views of both the etiology and neuropathology of his cases clearly reinforced his ideas that these cases represented a distinct disease entity. It is now clear, however, that the microbiological analysis that he relied upon was flawed. And, the neuropathology indicated a polioencephalitis, a gray matter disease, but without consistent localization (see Chapter 10). Thus, the questions that remain are whether the clinical signs alone are consistent and distinct enough to justify designation of a new disease, and whether this disease is the same as that diagnosed later throughout the world. Relative to these issues, von Economo's cases certainly were less diverse, compared to the spectrum of EL signs and symptoms that were identified during the next few years. Based on this analysis, then, the designation of EL as a distinct and unitary disease entity may be questioned and some of the mystery of EL may result from the fact that it is actually not a single disorder. We repeatedly address this issue in this volume and suggest that EL, as well as postencephalitic parkinsonism, may have been multifactorial, at least pertaining to etiology (see Chapter 12).

Although von Economo is commonly considered to have originally defined EL, two others believed that they were entitled to primacy in description. In 1921, C. I. Urechia authored a description of ten putative EL cases from Romania. All cases had pathological confirmation of inflammatory processes consistent with EL, but only 25%–30% of the patients had been lethargic; the author suggested that these latter patients had different types of EL, such as "mental" and parkinsonian. In five of the cases, a diplococcus was found that was considered the same as that identified by von Economo in 1917, and Urechia suggested that this was the agent of EL. Accordingly, he proposed that his prior (1916) description of two patients who were examined in 1915, one lethargic and one myoclonic, also should be considered EL, presumably its first description (Obregia et al., 1916). The title of their 1916 article was, however, *Encéphalite hemorragique avec un diplocoque encapsulé* (Hemorrhagic encephalitis with an encapsulated diplococcus), and, at the time, the authors did not indicate that this was a new disorder.

In 1917, René Cruchet, while serving in the neuropsychiatric services at various French military hospitals (first at Verdun, then at Commercy, and finally at Bar-le-duc), authored an article, *Quarante cas d'encephéphalomyélite subaiguë* (Forty cases of subacute encephalitis), which described 40 cases of encephalomyelitis that he believed differed from forms seen previously. At the onset, the patients were lethargic, with a physical and mental asthenia; they had severe headaches, and complained of a "feeling of heaviness." All of the patients were between 25 and 45 years of age, showed inert facies, emotional indifference, loss of weight, and had an earthy appearance (subjaundiced). Following a similar onset, the patients progressed to one of nine different types of the disease: mental, convulsive, meningic, hemiplegic, pontocerebellar, bulbopontine, mild, ataxic, and anterior poliomyelitic. Whereas two of the patients died, all the others slowly recovered (Cruchet, 1920). A detailed description of these patients, as well as of 24 more with some neuropathology, is provided in Cruchet's 1928 monograph, *Encéphalite Epidémique*. Cruchet insisted that these cases, which were technically described in an article published on April 27, 1917, preceded von Economo's May 1917 published description of what he believed to be the identical syndrome. Cruchet did not believe "encephalitis lethargica" to be an appropriate name for the condition and suggested instead, "epidemic encephalomyelitis" or "the disease of Cruchet."

In his 1929 monograph, von Economo evaluated Cruchet's claim and considered it meritless. Von Economo stated that only one of Cruchet's original 40 cases was fully consistent with the symptomatology of EL, whereas two cases were marginally consistent. He considered the remaining cases to be war-time psychoses, epilepsies, hemiplegias, or cases of myelitis or neuritis. Von Economo further stated that, if these cases represent a disease entity, it is not EL; he also stated that the neuropathology of the two cases who died was not consistent with findings in EL.

Although von Economo in his 1929 monograph denied Cruchet's contention of primacy and undoubtedly would have denied Urechia's primacy as well, he stated the following in his second 1917 article on EL (1917b):

> In a brilliant presentation to the Vienna Society of Physicians in the year 1890, Mauthner expressed the opinion that "Nona" must be polioencephalitis superior acuta epidemica, which he compared to meningitis epidemica. Today, on the basis of our findings, we can say that Mauthner, with a prophetic vision 27 years ago, made the true diagnosis. Encephalitis epidemica lethargica, which we are facing now, is probably identical with "Nona," and also with the old "sleeping sickness," and shows the anatomical picture of a polioencephalitis superior acuta. Perhaps the other sporadic cases of encephalitis also belong to this category. (van Bogaert & Théodoridés; p. 94; see also Chapter 4 for details on the late 19th-century EL-like disease, nona)

Similarly, in the same 1929 monograph in which he denied Cruchet's primacy, von Economo stated, "Today, we can with some certainty maintain that nona and encephalitis lethargica are identical diseases" (1931; p. 6). Thus, von Economo believed that EL was not a new disease and apparently that, depending on conditions, it waxed between sporadic and epidemic conditions. If true, it certainly is reasonable that the massive movements of troops during World War I and/or the Spanish influenza of the time may have contributed to the epidemic nature of the disease during this period. This view would also be consistent with the continued sporadic cases of the disease that occur in the present day (see Chapter 5) and may explain some of the young-onset cases of parkinsonism that were identified prior to the 1920s (see Chapter 7). Furthermore, this view also suggests that neither von Economo, Urechia, or Cruchet first characterized the disease, and primacy cannot be attributed to any one of them. And, there is no reason to try to determine the first cases of EL because sporadic cases probably were occurring for decades, if not centuries, before 1917. More likely, von Economo's, Cruchet's, and Urechia's reports simply reflect an endemic disease slowly increasing in incidence and assuming epidemic dimensions. And, finally, this view also would be consistent with a very varied expression of the disease, with spatial and temporal changes in the genetic composition of the pathological agent (presumably a virus). On the other hand, we again emphasize the possibility that EL was not a unitary condition and therefore may not have been the same as nona.

OTHER EARLY DESCRIPTIONS

In the early spring of 1918, an epidemic of encephalitis occurred in England, with Arthur Hall summarizing the clinical issues in October of that year and describing 16 cases that he had seen (Hall, 1918). Hall noted that the three cardinal signs were lethargy, general asthenia, and cranial nerve palsies. However, not all patients showed all three, and one sign may have predominated in specific patients. Hall also added that the patient's attitude in bed suggested "an effigy on a tomb" and that they had a mask-like face, without facial paralysis. None of Hall's patients died, with seven showing complete recovery, six moderate recoveries, and three incomplete recoveries. Hall did not associate these cases with those of von Economo, presumably because he was unaware of von Economo's description.

A later 1918 British report (Newsholme et. al., 1918) stated, "For identification and description, it was decided to follow von Economo in terming the illness encephalitis lethargica, a name which has the right of priority and indicates a characteristic clinical feature" (p. 3). In that report, one of the contributors, A. Salusbury MacNalty, divided EL patients into six groups:

1. Cases with general symptoms and without localizing signs
2. Cases with oculomotor nerve paralysis and general disturbances in the function of the central nervous system (CNS)
3. Cases with facial paralysis and general disturbances in the function of the CNS
4. Cases with spinal manifestations and general disturbances of the CNS
5. Cases with polyneuritis manifestations and general disturbances in the function of the CNS
6. Cases with mild or transient manifestations ("abortive" cases)

Also in the British 1918 report is a detailed description of the symptomatology of the disease. This description is not often cited, but is quite specific, and we suggest it is probably one of the most important because it was developed before the manifestations of the disease became so variable as almost to defy diagnosis. It was based on 126 cases that had been carefully evaluated to eliminate other disease entities. The symptoms, as described in this volume during the acute or prodromal phase, are summarized below (also see Fig 2.1–2.3).

Lethargy–progressive lethargy is the salient feature; it occurred in 80% of cases. The patient becomes apathetic and dull, with heaviness of the eyelids, blurred vision, photophobia. Lethargy typically merges into stupor; in a few cases, lethargy is replaced by insomnia or early delirium. The other important features are:

- Headache occurred in 70%
- Vertigo (30%)
- Diplopia (20%)
- Asthenia: Lassitude and general muscle weakness
- Muscular tremors: Tremors or fibrillar twitches sometimes seen in prodromal stage
- Pains: Aches and pains are not infrequent
- Mental state: Patient is "strange in manner," laughs and weeps without apparent cause; some patients are restless

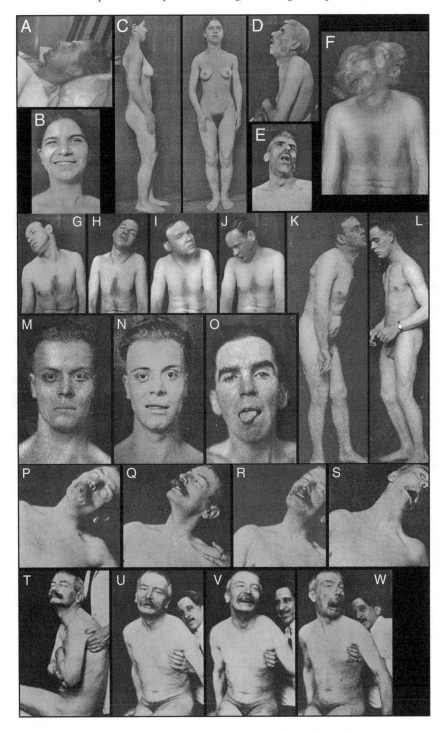

Figure 2.1 A. A 29-year-old man whose primary complaint is insomnia.
B–C. A 16-year-old girl who initially complained of excessive drowsiness and who now

(Continued)

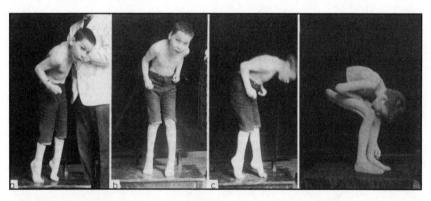

Figure 2.2 Photographs of two postencephalitic boys to show postural instability; in a-c (*original labels*) a boy with rigidity is standing on a stool; the sequential images show loss of postural control with flexion dystonia, a manifestation of the postencephalitic parkinsonian syndrome (see Chapter 10). The equinus posture is part of the manifestation of his flexion dystonia. In the remaining image, an older boy shows extreme flexion dystonia, which is also found in idiopathic parkinsonism, although not to this degree. Images from Martin (1983).

- Speech changes: May be aphonic or have difficulties in articulation
- Gastrointestinal symptoms: Vomiting is not common (10% of cases)

Later symptoms include:

- Attitude and face: Patient cannot make any voluntary movements; face is mask-like and expressionless (superficial resemblance to paralysis agitans); often there is a facial flush with bilateral twitching of facial muscles
- Stupor: Patient is semiconscious or unconscious, or, typically, patients can be roused and can answer questions
- Insomnia

Figure 2.1 continued
shows left-sided facial weakness; parkinsonian facies; stiff, slightly flexed posture, and tremor of right hand. **D–E.** A 53-year-old man who is unable to move his jaw or swallow and can barely speak. **F–K.** A 40-year-old man who has involuntary movements of his head. F shows five exposures on a single plate, whereas G–J show the sequential movements; K shows flexed standing posture. **L–N.** A 21-year-old man with flexion posture, flexed upper limbs, and who has slight tremor of lower limbs, masked facies, and right facial weakness. **O.** A 28-year-old man with weakness of right hypoglossal nerve. **P–W.** A 43-year-old man who shows almost continuous spasmodic movements of the head and left upper and lower limbs, left lower limb drags during gait (P–S are sequential, and T–W are sequential). Images from Tilney and Howe (1920).

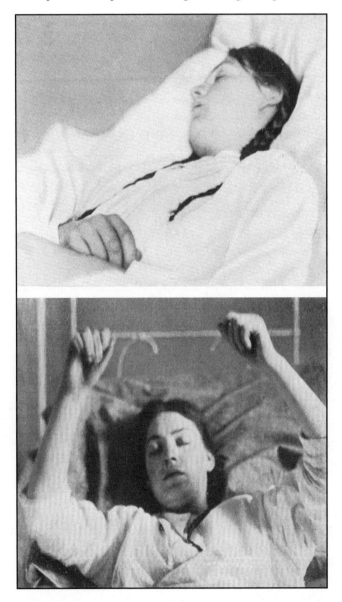

Figure 2.3 Top. Encephalitic sleeping condition with relaxed posture. **Bottom.** The same patient, with soft catalepsy in hypersomnatic state. From Stern, 1928.

- Delirium: Rambling speech, inarticulate mutterings; delirium is usually nocturnal
- Asthenia
- Rigidity: Typically of a "plastic" type
- Speech: Changes in speech are almost pathognomonic; either the voice becomes nasal and monotonous, or speech is initially hesitant,

but once started is rapid, but then relapses into slow, hesitating
speech
- Choreiform movements: Irregular, nonrhythmical, spontaneous
movements of the face, trunk, and limbs; appear late in the disease
- Pain and hyperesthesia: Muscular pains may persist throughout
illness; marked hyperesthesia may also be present
- Sweating: Moderate to profuse
- Skin eruptions: Rash-type eruptions on various parts of the body

Similar to the initial descriptions of EL in England, Netter (1918) provided
the first complete description of EL in France. He stated that the disease had
never been seen there before, but he knew that others had called it EL. Headache,
somnolence, and vomiting were the initial symptoms (note that in the British
report, vomiting was not considered to be common). Similar to the British
and Austrian reports, Netter stated that the patients could definitely respond to
questions and commands but then would fall back asleep. Eventually, a comatose
state develops from which it is impossible to wake the patient, but sleep was interrupted with delirious speech and convulsions. In addition to excessive sleep,
patients showed various other manifestations, typically eye muscle paralysis.
Nystagmus was common, and paralysis could spread to the face, pharynx, and
larynx. Most patients had fever, which could be of short duration. Netter stated
that normal cerebrospinal fluid (CSF) was very important for diagnosis. Typically,
the disease lasted for weeks or months.

Numerical data pertaining to symptom and sign frequency are relatively rare
among the early EL reports. However, two instructive graphs of signs and symptoms were presented in reports by Smith for the United States in 1921, and by
Parsons et al. in 1922 for England (Fig. 2.4).

Smith (1921) had previously been an Assistant Surgeon within the U.S.
Surgeon General's Office and had conducted a study of EL in the United
States for the Surgeon General. The graph (Fig. 2.4 top; based on 122 cases) suggests all forms of paralysis are the most common sign. Constipation is remarkably
high on this list, and insomnia is surprisingly not even listed. It is unclear why
"paralysis" is noted to include "all forms" but yet "facial paralysis" is listed
separately.

Smith (1921) divided the symptoms and signs of acute EL into a "general"
category and those attributable to disturbances of the CNS. General symptoms
and signs were headache, lassitude, fever, asthenia, vomiting, constipation, diarrhea,
skin eruptions, excessive sweating, vertigo, muscular pains, and urinary
disturbances.

Figure 2.4 (bottom) is part of a British Public Health and Medical Subjects
report that was published in 1922. The data are based on 1,174 cases, represent
only initial symptoms, and therefore are not entirely comparable to Smith's 1921
graph. Some of the differences, however, are striking (e.g., paralysis is virtually

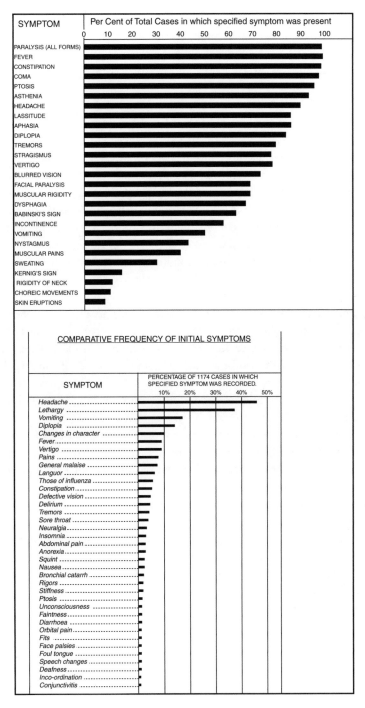

Figure 2.4 Charts from Smith (1921) (*top*) and Parsons et al. (1922) *bottom* showing the frequencies of signs and symptoms in encephalitis lethargica.

nonexistent in the British report, whereas it has the highest frequency in Smith's report). Similarly, diplopia is surprisingly low in the British report, but was reported to occur at a frequency of about 90% in the American report. These findings again suggest that EL may not be a unitary entity and/or was grossly overdiagnosed (see below).

The following is a list of signs and symptoms reported to be present in patients during the acute phase of EL, based on EL reports from that period. The purpose of the listing is to convey the incredible range in EL symptomatology; the signs and symptoms include sleep disturbances (more commonly, drowsiness, but also insomnia that was refractory to large doses of hypnotics); sleep inversion (believed to be pathognomonic in children); pyrexia (usually slight); headache; disturbances of cranial nerves III–VI, resulting in extraocular/masticatory muscle paralyses or palsies (diplopia and ptosis); pupillary disturbances of any form (myosis, mydriasis, anisocoria, sluggish responses to light and/or accommodation); Arygll-Robertson pupil; shivering; vertigo; vomiting; swallowing disturbances; facial nerve weakness (loss of facial lines); Babinski sign; Kernig sign; Romberg sign; aphasia, myoclonic twitches; chorea; ceaseless motor activity; mental disturbances (delirium, hallucinations); emotional disturbances; intellectual impairment; demoralization (primarily in children); facial swelling; dysarthria; nystagmus; strabismus; epileptic seizures; bradykinesia; catatonia; tremors, masked facies; parkinsonian posture; festination; loss of associated movements during gait; hypotonia; hypertonia; ankle clonus; trismus; facial herpes outbreak; greasy face; sialorrhea; limb palsies or paresis; rapid weight loss; dry and furred tongue; halitosis; erythema; increased CSF pressure, pleocytosis; slight increase in protein content in CSF; slight increase in glucose in CSF; decerebrate posture; absence of abdominal reflexes; stocking-and-glove type of sensory loss; acute diarrhea; constipation; cerebellar signs; peripheral neuritis; hiccups; disturbances of taste; bradycardia; tachycardia; and urinary difficulties.

Although the constellation of signs and symptoms within specific epidemics might be limited relative to the above listing, the constellation was still usually polymorphic. Rarely, however, epidemics were monosymptomatic, with the most well-known involving hiccup epidemics that occurred in Europe and North America (MacNalty, 1929; see Chapter 6). Interestingly, diagnosis of EL was further complicated because the signs and symptoms would typically change within an individual, so that a patient could rapidly move from mild sleepiness to stupor to coma, or to insomnia. A peculiar aspect of the sleepiness of these patients during the acute phase was that, even when apparently asleep, they could typically be awakened and readily answer questions about activities that occurred during their apparent slumber (see above; Crafts, 1927; Stern, 1928; Wilson, 1940). Crafts (1927) stated that EL patients had a strange mixture of alert mental action and lethargy (see Case 2 above). This characteristic was sometimes referred to as "pseudosomnolence" or "false sleep."

No sign or symptoms were pathognomonic for acute EL. For example, fever was considered a relatively constant sign by some investigators (e.g., Hall, 1918) but von Economo (1929) specifically noted that it should not be depended upon and that there was no relationship between the presence of fever and the severity of the disease. Von Economo suggested that rhythmical contractions of the abdominal muscles toward one side or the other, with umbilical deviation laterally, superiorly, or inferiorly, was a very typical sign of EL that could be used for differentiating the hyperkinetic form from general chorea and athetosis, but Hall, in his 1924 monograph, stated that changes in the abdominal reflexes were not constant (and von Economo did not note this feature in any of his original cases; see above). Similarly, Neal (1942) suggested that the absence of abdominal reflexes was an important sign from the standpoint of diagnosis. Hall, however, thought that a thick white coating on the tongue was a diagnostic sign. He also thought that foul-smelling breath was important, representing the fact that the mouth and nasopharynx were the primary sites of infection. But few others recorded either as being important.

Because of the absence of a pathognomonic sign, symptom, or serological or bacterial test, EL was diagnosed by exclusion of other conditions, as determined by the patient history, and typically by the unusual combination of signs and symptoms found in each individual case, which suggested an illness involving more than one body system. Netter (1920) noted that diagnosis could not be done in the same manner as that used for meningitis, tuberculosis, or syphilis. Netter also noted that EL was easy to confuse with meningitis, syphilis, typhoid fever, chorea, epilepsy, poliomyelitis, multiple sclerosis, mania, gastric crises, and tabes dorsalis. He indicated that ocular signs were present in 75% of cases.

Von Ecomono stated that, initially, EL might be difficult to distinguish from meningitis, but that meningeal symptoms tended to fade, and large numbers of cells in the CSF suggested meningitis. Also, a slight increase in glucose in the CSF indicated EL rather than meningitis.

Walshe (1920) suggested that reducing symptoms to their anatomical basis could help diagnose the disease. Accordingly, he viewed the signs and symptoms of EL in the manner of Hughlings Jackson, based on positive and negative, and general and focal signs and symptoms. Positive general signs included delirium, mania, restlessness, and hallucinations, whereas positive focal symptoms included convulsions, muscular contractions, rigidity, and pain. Negative general signs were lethargy and coma, whereas negative focal signs were those of paralysis.

Neal (1942) developed specific criteria to help differentiate EL from other conditions (Table 2.1).

According to von Economo, about 15% of acute cases die (40% of those who are bedridden). Death typically occurs because the disease progresses to the medulla or because of cachexia. Only a small minority shows complete recovery.

Table 2.1 Neal's (1942) Differential Diagnosis Criteria for Specific Diseases

Disease	Differential Diagnosis
St. Louis encephalitis	Not distinguishable from encephalitis lethargica (EL) unless in epidemic form
Eastern or Western equine virus	Presence of associated epidemics among horses or mules; symptoms typically more severe than EL; (Eastern) typically shows high cerebrospinal fluid (CSF) cell count; virus found in blood and CSF in Western type
Encephalitis from rabies or smallpox	Both are suggested by patient history
Disseminated encephalomyelitis	Impossible to make complete distinction; usually gray masses not involved in encephalomyelitis
Nonparalytic poliomyelitis	Difficult, if not impossible, to distinguish consistently from meningeal forms of EL
Syphilis	Positive Wasserman in syphilis but not always reliable
Guillain-Barré	More extensive paralyses and more sensory changes than in EL; high protein level in CSF in Guillain-Barré
Bacterial meningitis	Demonstration of organisms in CSF by culture; CSF spinal fluid sugar is low compared to EL
Brain abscess	Abscess suggested if patient has sinusitis, otitis media, or mastoiditis
Brain tumor	Usually progresses more slowly than EL; papilledema more common in tumor
Stroke	Hypertension, cerebral arteriosclerosis
Chorea	EL is not usually monosymptomatic
Functional disorders	EL usually has some fever, changes in reflexes; cranial nerve and other palsies/paralyses
Influenza	CSF typically shows increase in cells and protein in EL; isolation of virus from nasopharyngeal washings in influenza

The prognosis of clinically well-marked cases is therefore 40% mortality, 14% complete recovery, 26% recovery with defect, and 20% remaining invalid. Twenty-one percent of Neal's (1942) cases had mortality during the acute stage. Wilson (1940) stated that, of 100 cases 3 years after the acute phase, 25 will have survived without serious consequences, 35 will have died, and 40 will have chronic sequelae.

This discussion reveals why some clinicians of the period developed typo-logical classifications of the disease (see below). In 1920, the well-known British neurologist, F. M. R. Walshe, addressed the varieties of EL by stating that, in reality, the types were grouping of cases that, within one phase of the disease, showed similar symptoms. He stated that pure cases were extremely rare and that, in most

cases, all of the EL symptoms were superimposed upon, precede, follow, or alternate with one of the numerous symptoms complexes of the disease.

STAGES AND TYPES OF ENCEPHALITIS LETHARGICA

Encephalitis lethargica was typically divided into acute and chronic phases (von
Economo, 1929; Neal, 1942). Most of the signs and symptoms discussed above
have primarily pertained to the acute phase, although in some cases they probably
applied to both (e.g., Smith, 1921). Neal suggested that the term "chronic encephalitis" should be reserved to a condition in which the disease process is usually
progressive and that develops either immediately following the acute stage, or
after an interval of months or many years of apparent recovery (Neal, 1942).
However, she also commented on the virtual impossibility of making this division
in many cases, and other authors also indicated that the signs and symptoms of the
acute and chronic stages are often indistinguishable, and that some patients appear
to pass directly into a chronic stage without showing an obvious acute stage (Hall,
1924; von Economo, 1929). In fact, Hall commented that it was impossible to
recognize definite stages.

Raimist, based on the EL outbreak in the Ukraine in 1918, described prodromal and four subsequent stages during the acute phase that spanned a total of
8 weeks, and then a chronic stage (cited in Hall, 1924). Smith (1921) referred to a
prodromal stage with fatigue, lethargy, headache, giddiness, and disturbance of
vision; a stage of acute manifestations characterized by vomiting, fever, paralysis of
certain cranial nerves, changes in tendon reflexes, alterations of speech, marked
general weakness, and, in the majority of cases, coma of varying intensity; and, a
variable period of convalescence. Von Economo considered the "prodromal" stage
to be characterized by slight fever and mild pharyngitis. Neal (1942) stated that
she was impressed that the symptoms of EL followed directly or shortly after a
more or less severe respiratory or "grippe-like" infection." Wilson (1940) also suggested that a prodromal phase existed, characterized by headache, malaise, slight
fever, aches, and pains. Other authors inserted a subacute ("light") phase between
the acute and chronic stages (Ulitovsky, 1961).

Table 2.2 presents stage data for 377 EL cases from Neal (1942). It is noteworthy
that 149 of the cases did not show an acute phase, and the longest interval between
acute and chronic stages for a patient with a definitive acute phase was 14 years.

More details on the chronic stage of EL are presented in Chapter 7.

Table 2.2 Interval in Years Between Acute and Chronic Stages (from Neal, 1942)

	0	0–1	1	2	3	4	5	6	7	8	9	10	>10	Total
Acute EL	69	18	5	22	24	14	14	13	12	11	5	17	4	228
No acute EL														149

TYPES OF ENCEPHALITIS LETHARGICA

Table 2.3 presents information on 28 types of acute EL that were described during the epidemic period. These classifications were based on the clinical signs and symptoms, the presumed anatomical loci of the lesions, or some combination of the two. The purpose of classifying EL into types was to assist clinicians with diagnosis. However, some authorities of the time questioned the value of such

Table 2.3 Encephalitis Lethargica Types

Type	Signs/Symptoms	Presumed Anatomical Loci	Sources
1. Somnolent-ophthalmoplegic (sometimes together, sometimes as separate types)	Profound somnolence (but sometimes insomnia); diplopia, strabismus, ptosis; facial paralysis, speech/swallowing disturbances	Cranial nerve III, sometimes other cranial nerves especially IV,V,VI; midbrain	Wilson (1940); Newsholme et al. (1918); Hall (1924); Rietta (1935); von Economo (1929); Bramwell and Miller (1920); Dunn and Heagey (1920); Russel (1920); von Dreyfus (1920); Barker (1921); House (1929)
2. Paralysis agitans (amyostatic, pallidal)	Parkinsonism with bradykinesia, rigidity, tremor, festination, loss of associated movements during gait, masked face	Striatum, globus pallidus	Wilson (1940); Timme et al. (1921); Tilney and Howe (1920); Wimmer (1929); Rietta (1935); von Economo (1929); Bramwell and Miller(1920); Dunn and Heagey (1920); Russel (1920); Barker (1921); House (1929)
3. Psychiatric	Hallucinations, illusions, delirium, depression, incontinence	Multiple foci in telencephalon	Wilson (1940); Tilney and Howe (1920); Rietta (1935); von Economo (1929); Dunn and Heagey (1920); Russel (1920); von Dreyfus (1920); Barker (1921); House (1929)

Table 2.3 continued

Type	Signs/Symptoms	Presumed Anatomical Loci	Sources
4. Abortive (mild, transient)	Tightness in muscles; mild fixity of expression; slight tremors; patient typically recovers completely after brief period		Wilson (1940); Newsholme et al. (1918); Hall (1924); Timme et al. (1921); Bramwell and Miller (1920); Barker (1921); House (1929)
5. Cerebellar	Ataxia of gait and speech; patients generally recover	Cerebellum	Hall 1924); Timme et al. (1921); Rietta (1935); von Economo(1929); Bramwell and Miller (1920); Cruchet (1920); Barker (1921)
6. Hyperkinetic (sometimes differentiated by type of movement disorder)	Chorea, athetosis, seizures, restlessness		Wilson (1940; Timme et al. (1921); Wimmer (1929); Hall (1924); Rietta (1935); von Economo (1929); von Dreyfus (1920); Barker (1921)
7. Hemiplegic (hemiparetic)	Hemiplegic signs and symptoms		Timme et al. (1921); Russel (1920); Cruchet (1920); Von Dreyfus (1920); House (1929)
8. Cortical (cerebral cortical)	Convulsions, amnesia, disorientation, dysarthria, lethargy	Cerebral cortex	Wilson (1940); Hall (1924); Timme et al. (1921); Bramwell and Miller (1920); Cruchet (1920)
9. Spinal (radicular–spinal)	Paresis, loss of knee jerks, myoclonic movements and fasciculations	Spinal cord	Wilson (1940); Newsholme et al. (1918); Hall (1924); Timme et al. (1921); Rietta (1935)
10. Polyneuritic	Peripheral nerve lesions	Peripheral nerves	Newsholme et al. (1918); Hall (1924); Timme et al. (1921); Rietta (1935); House (1929)

(Continued)

Table 2.3 Encephalitis Lethargica Types (continued)

Type	Signs/Symptoms	Presumed Anatomical Loci	Sources
11. Cataleptic	Catalepsy, vertigo, nystagmus, ataxia		Dunn and Heagey (1920); Tilney and Howe (1920); Timme et al. (1921)
12. Meningeal	Dull pounding headache; stiff neck	Meninges	Rietta (1935); Dunn and Heagey (1920); Von Dreyfus (1920); House (1929)
13. Anterior polymyelitic	Lower motor neuron weakness similar to infantile paralysis; affects lower limbs	Lower motor neurons	Wilson (1940); Peng (1993); Hall (1924)
14. Hyperalgesic (posterior poliomyelitic)	Segmental pain similar to postherpetic neuralgia	Dorsal root ganglion or posterior horns of spinal cord	Tilney and Howe (1920); Cruchet (1920); House (1929)
15. General symptoms without localizing signs	Headache, confusion, sleep disorders	Brainstem	Newsholme et al. (1918); Hall (1924); Bramwell and Miller (1920)
16. Infantile	Infants with identical EL symptoms as adults		Tilney and Howe (1920); House (1929)
17. Progressive	Progressive symptoms	Renewal of inflammatory process	Timme et al. (1921); Bramwell and Miller (1920)
18. Aberrant/ autonomic	Intestinal, cutaneous, vagal symptoms		von Economo (1929); Barker (1921)
19. Monosymptomatic	Single symptom, usually hiccups		Wilson (1940); von Economo (1929)
20. Tabetic	Arygll–Robertson pupils, loss of deep tendon reflexes, lancinating pain	Posterior columns, dorsal roots	Barker (1921)
21. Insomnia	Insomnia		Russel (1920)

Table 2.3 continued

Type	Signs/Symptoms	Presumed Anatomical Loci	Sources
22. Paralytic	Akinesia, hypokinesia	Nuclei of corresponding motor nerves	Barker (1921)
23. Myelitic	Urinary incontinence, Babinski sign, disturbed reflexes, clonus		Dunn and Heagey (1920)
24. Pallido-pyramidal	Combination of spastic paralysis and parkinsonism (more complete paralysis); clonus, Babinski sign	Pyramidal and pallidal system involvement	Timme et al. (1921)
25. Mixed striatal	Bizarre combinations uniting elements of chorea and paralysis agitans		Timme et al. (1921)
26. Myoclonic	Rare; rhythmical movements of distal parts of extremities	Striatum	Timme et al. (1921)
27. Thalamic	Spontaneous pain of intolerable intensity; ataxia		Timme et al. (1921)
28. Juvenile pseudopsychopathia	Only in juveniles; lack of inhibitions (morals) but no intellectual defect		von Economo (1929)

schemes because of the changing characteristics of the disease across time, even within individuals (see above; Symonds, 1921; Wilson, 1940; Neal, 1942). Nevertheless, Kaneko (1925) specifically noted that he was able to use classifications to differentiate EL from the Japanese encephalitis that was occurring contemporaneously because the Japanese cases had a very simple course compared to EL. The "abortive" type of EL could, of course, have a simple course, but it would be unusual to have only this single type of EL in such a large population.

Table 2.3 was based on the work of clinicians (20 sources) who diagnosed EL cases and developed their classifications independently, based on their own observations. However, most reviewed the literature as well as their own cases, and therefore almost none of these classification schemes was developed completely de novo, but was based to some degree on earlier descriptions.

The 28 separate types are depicted in order of frequency of listing: 13 were listed in only one or two of the typological classification schemes. The two most frequent types, each cited by 11 of the 20 sources, were a somnolent-ophthalmoplegic type (although in some schemes the two signs were separated) and a parkinsonian type.

Although only mentioned as a specific type by one source, the juvenile pseudopsychopathia type (No. 28) is significant because of its diagnostic value. In children, in addition to the somatic effects on the patients, which could be similar to those in adults, EL typically had a profound psychiatric component. The application of the term "Apache" (as in Apache Indians) to refer to EL in children best conveys their behavioral problems (Thorpe, 1946). Von Economo (1929), as well as many others, described how, in previously normal children, the disease resulted in dramatic alterations in personality, which he referred to as a kind of moral insanity or irritating imbecility. The change in behavior occurred very acutely, sometimes almost instantaneously. The children lacked inhibitions, becoming troublesome and antisocial. They begged, lied, stole, even killed; often they ran away from home repeatedly and had to be institutionalized or placed in special schools that were developed for them in many countries, including the United Kingdom, Germany, and the United States (Vilensky et al., 2007). Perhaps most significant was that these children recognized that their behavior was abnormal and were typically apologetic for their misdeeds. They would commonly state, "I cannot help it, I have got to do it; I know that I am impertinent and do not want to be" (von Economo, 1929, Fig. 2.5). This self-awareness differentiated these children from other children with antisocial behavior.

There are hundreds of descriptive case reports of such children. One example is from a monograph by Bond and Appel (1931) that detailed the treatment of these children at a special school for them in Pennsylvania. "Blanche was a normal girl up to the age of eight. She had an IQ of 120. Her attack of encephalitis came on suddenly; the symptoms were temporary paralysis, crossing of the eyes, double vision, and sleepiness. A change in behaviour manifested itself in tantrums, jealously, overactivity, over-affectionateness, and sexual misdemeanors. Brought to the

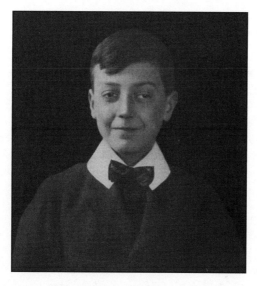

Figure 2.5 Angelic-looking boy with encephalitis lethargica showing masked face. Plate IX, from Hall (1924).

hospital and placed with adult patients, she was wild, stole, broke the water coolers, upset trays and dishes, and 'lied out of everything.' In the continuous bath, she pinched and pushed a ward maid and laughed to see her fall; she soaked a nurse who came to rescue, then she jumped out of the tub and kicked the ward maid viciously as the latter leaned over; then she got back in the tub and assumed an expression of angelic innocence. Four weeks in the hospital did her no good. At home, she was put in a cage. She was sent to a reformatory and to a state mental hospital" (Bond and Appel, 1931, p. 10–11).

CONCLUSION

Even a thorough analysis of epidemic-period EL cases does not bring finality on how this disease should best be diagnosed. There is little doubt, that during the epidemic period and probably still today, incorrect diagnoses have been made. In 1930 Riley wrote:

> There can be no question, however, that the diagnosis of epidemic encephalitis has offered a refuge which serves in many cases as a cloak under which one often attempts to hide ignorance or inability to reconcile the results of examinations. The facile ability of this disease to ape any of the well-known syndromes of nervous involvement is so omnipresent that the temptation is well nigh irresistible to call any puzzling combination of signs of neural involvement by this name. Therefore, in the name of diagnostic honesty, every effort should be made

to exhaust all means of diagnosis and to invoke every other possible etiologic
factor before resort is made to this diagnosis. (p. 600)

Similarly, in 1937, Ford wrote:

It is a matter of great difficulty to offer a satisfactory discussion of the clinical
features of this disease because of its manifestations, its tendency to variation and
fluctuations, and especially because of the unfortunate habit of many medical
writers to include in this diagnosis almost all unusual nervous conditions, thereby
encumbering the literature with a hundred absurd [our italics] syndromes.
As a result, many articles on this subject are more misleading than informative.
(p. 341)

This tendency was further revealed in a report on 30 postmortems done on
putative EL victims: 20% proved to have tubercular meningitis; 17% cerebral
tumors, 7% cerebral thrombosis, and 3% meningismus. The remaining 53% presumably had true EL (Williamson-Noble, 1928) but, as indicated in Chapter 10,
the neuropathology of EL is also quite variable, so that a postmortem diagnosis
cannot always be confirmatory.

These evaluations by Riley (1930) and Ford (1937), both written during the
epidemic period, clearly expressed a sentiment that readily surfaces when contemporary clinicians review the EL material from the epidemic period. Diagnosis
is further clouded by the recent hypothesis advanced by Kroker (2004) that neurologists, especially in New York City, wished to use EL to increase the standing
of the discipline of neurology (both publically and professionally) and therefore
had a possible political motive for diagnosing EL.

But, even allowing for misdiagnoses, one cannot escape from the view that
some type of strange neurologic illness or illnesses were pervasive during the epidemic period. We hypothesize that perhaps there were actually multiple conditions, some perhaps related to influenza or poliomyelitis, and others perhaps new
viral variants. Thus, the EL of 1917 may not have been caused by the same agent
as the EL of 1921.

Accordingly, as delineated in Chapter 5, we believe that diagnosis of any putative
modern cases of EL should not be based on the great variability in symptomatology
seen during the epidemic period. Rather, these cases should, in our view, conform
closely to the signs and symptoms exhibited by von Economo's original cases, and
thus be consistent with the somnolent-ophthalmoplegic type of the disease.

REFERENCES CITED

Barker, L. F. (1921). Diagnostic criteria in epidemic encephalitis and encephalomyelitis.
    Archives of Neurology and Psychiatry, 5, 173–196.
Bond, E. D., & Appel, K. E. (1931). *The treatment of behavior disorders following encephalitis.*
    New York: The Commonwealth Fund.

Bramwell, E., & Miller, J. (1920). Encephalitis lethargic (epidemic encephalitis) with a note on post-mortem findings in a series of cases. *Lancet, 1*, 1152–1158.

Crafts, L. M. (1927). *Epidemic Encephalitis (Encephalo-Myelitis).* Boston: Richard G. Badger.

Cruchet, R. (1917). Quarante cas d'encephalomyelite subaigue. *Bulletins et Me'moires de la Société médicale des hopitaux* de Paris, *3*, 614–616.

Cruchet, R. (1920). The Bordelaise conception of encephalitis lethargica. *New York Medical Journal, 112*, 173–174.

Cruchet, R. (1928). *Encéphalite Épidémique.* Paris: Gaston Doin & Cie.

Dunn, A. D., & Heagey, F. W. (1920). Epidemic encephalitis: Including a review of 115 American cases. *American Journal of the Medical Science*, clx, 568–582.

Ford, F R. (1937). *Diseases of the Nervous System in Infancy, Childhood, and Adolescence.* Baltimore: Charles C. Thomas.

Hall, A. J. (1918). Epidemic encephalitis. *British Medical Journal, 2*, 461–463.

Hall, A. J. (1924). *Epidemic encephalitis (encephalitis lethargica).* Bristol: John Wright & Sons.

House, W. B. (1929). Epidemic encephalitis. *The Journal of the American Institute of Homeopathy, 5*, 139–149.

Kaneko, R. (1925). On the epidemic encephalitis, which occurred in Japan. *The Japan Medical World, 5*, 237–241.

Kroker, K. (2004). Epidemic encephalitis and American neurology, 1919–1940. *Bulletin of Medical History, 78*, 108–147.

MacNalty, A. S. (1929). Epidemic hiccup. *Lancet 5*, 62–63.

Martin, J.P. (1983). Old photographs: postencephalitic parkinsonism in two small boys. *Journal of Neurology, Neurosurgery, and Psychiatry, 46*, 953–955.

Neal, J. B. (1942). *Encephalitis: A Clinical Study.* New York: Grune & Stratton.

Netter, A. (1918). Encephalite lethargique epidemique. *Bulletin de l'Academie nationale de medecine*, lxxix, 337–347.

Netter, A. (1920). Diagnostic et tratement de l'encephalite lethargique. *Medecine, 1*, 668–670.

Newsholme, A., James, S. P., MacNalty, A. S., Marinesco, G., McIntosh, J., & Draper, G. (1918). *Report of an enquiry into an obscure disease, encephalitis lethargica.* Reports to the Local Government Board on public health and medical subjects, new ser., no. 121. London: Printed under the authority of His Majesty's Stationery Office by Jas. Truscott & Son.

Obregia, Urechia, & Carniol. (1916). Encéphalite hemoragique avec un diplocoque encapsulé. *Spiatul*, 15–18(347), 307.

Parsons, A. C., MacNalty, A. S., & Perdrau, J. R. (1922). *Report on Encephalitis Lethargica: being an account of further enquiries into the epidemiology and clinical features of the disease; including the analysis of over 1,250 reports on cases notified in England and Wales during 1919 and 1920, together with comprehensive bibliography of the subject.* London: His Majesty's Stationery Office.

Peng, S. L. (1993). Reductionism and encephalitis lethargica, 1916–1939. *New Jersey Medicine, 6*, 459–462.

Rietta, F. (1935). *Encefalite Letargica Acuta and Cronica.* Milano: Tip Soiceta Editrice Libraia.

Riley, H. A. (1930). Epidemic encephalitis. *Archives of Neurology, 24*, 574–604.

Russel, C. K. (1920). A study of epidemic encephalitis based on the study of seventeen cases with two autopsies. *Journal of Canada Medical Association, 10*, 696–704.

Smith, H. F. (1921). Epidemic encephalitis (encephalitis lethargica, Nona): Report of studies conducted in the United States. *Public Health Reports, 6*, 207–242.

Stern, F. (1928). *Die Epidemische Encephalitis.* Berlin: Springer.

Symonds, C. P. (1921). Critical review: Encephalitis lethargica. *Quarterly Journal of Medicine, 14*, 283–308.

Thorpe, F. T. (1946). Prefrontal leucotomy in treatment of post-encephalitic conduct disorder. *British Medical Journal, 1*, 312–314.

Tilney, F., & Howe, H. S. (1920). *Epidemic Encephalitis [Encephalitis Lethargica].* New York: Paul B. Hoeber.

Timme, W. (ed.). (1921). *Acute Epidemic Encephalitis [Lethargic Encephalitis]: An Investigation by The Association for Research in Nervous and Mental Diseases.* Report of the Papers and Discussions at the Meeting of the Association. New York: Paul B. Hoeber.

Ulitovsky, D.A. (1961). Encephalitis Lethargica. In Kh. G. Khodos (Ed.), *Infektsionnye i toksicheskie zabolevaniia nervnoj sistemy (infectious and toxic diseases of nervous system)* (pp. 62–73). Irkutsk: Irkutsk Book Publishers.

Urechia, C. I. (1921). Dix cas d'encephalite epidemique avec autopsie. *Archives internationales de neurologie, 2*, 65–78.

Van Bogaert, L., & Théodoridès, J. (1979). *Constantin von Economo (1876–1931): The Man and the Scientist.* Wien: Ernst Becvar.

Vilensky, J. A., Foley, P., & Gilman S. (2007). Children and encephalitis lethargica: A historical review. *Pediatric Neurology, 37*, 79–84.

von Dreyfus, G. L. (1920). Die gegenwärtige Enzephalitisepidemie. *Munchener Medizinische Wochenschrift*, lxvii, 538–541.

von Economo, C. (1917a). Encephalitis lethargica. *Wiener klinische Wochenschrift, 30*, 581–585.

von Economo, C. (1917b). Neue Beitrage zur Encephalitis lethargica. *Neurologisches Centralblatt, 5*, 866–878.

von Economo, C. (1929). *Die Encephalitis lethargica, ihre Nachkrankheiten und ihre Behardlung.* Berlin: Urban and Schwarzenberg. (Published in English in 1931: Translated by K. O. Newman; London: Oxford University Press).

Walshe, F. M. R. (1920). On the symptom-complexes of lethargic encephalitis with special reference to involuntary muscular contractions. *Brain, 43*, 197–219.

Wilkins, R. H., & Brody, I. A. (1968). Encephalitis lethargica. [Translation of von Economo, 1917). *Archives of Neurology, 18*, 325–328.

Wilson, S. A. K. (1940). *Neurology.* Baltimore: Williams & Wilkins.

Williamson-Noble, F. (1928). Ocular complications of encephalitis lethargic. *Proceedings of the Royal Society of Medicine, 21*, 985–996.

Wimmer, A. (1929). *Further Studies Upon Chronic Epidemic Encephalitis.* Copenhagen: Levin & Munksgaard Publishers.

3

EPIDEMIOLOGY OF ENCEPHALITIS LETHARGICA

Dana Marlowe, Hope E. Owens, Jennifer A. Cook, and Joel A. Vilensky

In 1929, the first and largest of the three Matheson Commission literature surveys of encephalitis lethargica (EL) was published under the leadership of Dr. Josephine Neal (Matheson Commission; see below). Dr. Neal (Fig. 3.1) was a noted researcher in the area of infectious diseases of the nervous system, including encephalitis, meningitis, and poliomyelitis. Her contributions to the Matheson Reports, and her subsequent 1942 monograph, "Encephalitis: A clinical study," provide a worldwide perspective on the epidemiology of EL.

The epidemiology of EL up until 1929 was well described in the first Matheson Commission report, and much of the information in this chapter is derived from that volume. (William Matheson was a noted chemist and philanthropist who supported research into EL; see Kroker, 2004.) Unless otherwise stated, all references in this chapter to the Matheson Commission report refer to that survey and not to those published in 1932 and 1939 (Fig. 3.2).

In addition to the Matheson Report, we also in subsequent sections of this chapter highlight the epidemiological conclusions about EL that were published in 1921 by Raymond Pearl. Dr. Pearl, who was a renowned biologist and Chief Statistician of the School of Hygiene and Public Health at Johns Hopkins University, statistically analyzed 549 EL cases reported in New York City in 1920, using techniques that are still used today. This approach was quite unique for the time in that the vast majority of descriptions of EL were purely qualitative,

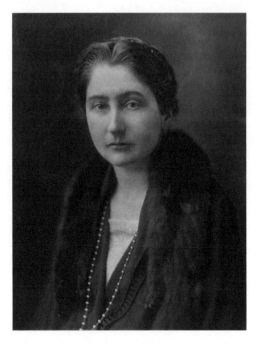

Figure 3.1 Photograph of Dr. Josephine Bicknell Neal (1880–1955; circa 1925).

without any statistical analysis. As far as we know, Pearl's significant contribution to the epidemiology of EL has not been cited since the epidemic period.

INCIDENCE

The number of people worldwide who contracted EL during the epidemic period is unknown, with the highest estimate being more than one million (Ravenholt & Foege, 1982). The Matheson Report suggested that, between 1919 and 1928, there were about 52,781 EL cases based upon official notifications. However, the report also highlighted that EL was not officially notifiable (i.e., physicians were not required to report cases of EL to government health agencies) in every country. In some countries, it was only made notifiable after the epidemic had passed, and even then not every case of EL was reported. Accordingly, Parsons (1928) suggested that 50% to 75% of EL cases were unreported. Brincker (1927) similarly suggested that the total number of EL cases reported in London from 1919 to 1926 was inaccurate because of all the mild cases that "escape notification." Brincker estimated that the number of cases that occurred was "considerably more than double" the number officially notified. Riley (1930) stated that "[s]uch figures as are available at the present time are not only grossly inadequate but actually misleading" (p. 574). He continued that even the "most ambitious"

EPIDEMIC ENCEPHALITIS

ETIOLOGY ⸱ EPIDEMIOLOGY
TREATMENT

REPORT OF A SURVEY BY THE
MATHESON COMMISSION

WILLIAM DARRACH, Chairman

HAVEN EMERSON	CHARLES R. STOCKARD
FREDERICK P. GAY	FREDERICK TILNEY
WILLIAM H. PARK	WILLIS D. WOOD

HUBERT S. HOWE, Secretary

JOSEPHINE B. NEAL, Director of Survey
HELEN HARRINGTON, Epidemiologist

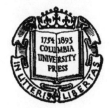

NEW YORK
COLUMBIA UNIVERSITY PRESS
1929

Figure 3.2   Cover page of the 1929 Matheson Commission Report.

study being conducted at that time, the Matheson Report, gathered data only from the 14 countries reporting such data, and then included only data from those cases that were formally diagnosed. He added that "only a small proportion of the total morbidity receives official cognizance" (p. 575). Riley believed that approximately 25% of actual cases were reported.

SEASONALITY

Initially, EL was primarily a disease of the winter months, with some extensions into the spring (Newsholme, James, MacNalty, et al., 1918; Butt, 1921; MacNalty, 1925; Robb, 1927; Matheson Commission). However, after the end of the major epidem-

Table 3.1 Encephalitis Lethargica Outbreaks Not Confined to Winter Months

Country	Years	Seasonality Source
Ireland	1918–1923: April–June; peak in May	Matheson Commission
Western Samoa	1919: Two peaks in May and December; 1920: Peak in May; 1921: No peaks	Ravenholt and Foege (1982)
England (Derby outbreak)	1919: August	MacNalty (1925)
Poland	1920: April–June, highest number in April with 730/1,462 cases; 1922: Highest in September, 1922, with 108/407 cases	Matheson Commission
Sweden	1920: Winter months, but second peak in summer	Matheson Commission
European summary	1920: Continuous outbreaks, no declines during spring and summer; 1921: Outbreak occurred in spring	von Economo (1929)
Ireland (Belfast only)	1924: April–June	Robb (1927)
Ireland	1924: May–July	Matheson Commission
South Africa	1924–1926: Both winter and summer (little difference seen by author)	Berry (1927)

ics in the early 1920s, a seasonal trend was no longer apparent in the smaller epidemics and sporadic cases that continued to occur (Hurst, 1934; Neal, 1942). There were also reports of outbreaks during the earlier period that did not occur during the winter and spring (Table 3.1).

AGES AFFECTED

Although EL affected all ages, individuals in early adulthood (i.e., aged 20–30 years) were considered to have the greatest susceptibility. Based upon 7,584 worldwide cases, the Matheson Report stated that 25.3% were within the 20–30 year age range. Other reports, for specific years and/or from specific regions, conflict with this generalization, however. For example, Newsholme, et al. (1918) stated that 20.6% of the English cases they reviewed were under 10 years of age, whereas Netter, as cited in the Matheson Report, observed that most cases in France were in the 30–40 age group. Pearl (1921) found a peak of 23.1% of the cases occurring between the ages of 20 and 30 years. However, he determined that there was no statistically significant difference in age distribution overall for affected cases, although the same could not be said for mortality (see below).

The high prevalence in young adults led to the hypothesis that the onset of puberty may increase the likelihood of contracting EL (Chasanow, 1930). In accordance with this idea, Brincker (1927) revealed a large prevalence in males during the onset of puberty in his study of EL cases in England from 1919–1926. Descriptions of cessation or irregularities of menses, as well as findings of hypothyroidism, led to suggestions by Russian clinicians that the endocrine system played a role in the etiology of EL (Raimist, 1921; Chasanow, 1930).

MORTALITY

Most studies reported that the highest fatality rates were in the very young and the elderly throughout the world (Matheson Commission). However, a few notable exceptions existed. Newsholme, et al. (1918), chronicling the first EL cases reported in England, stated that the highest mortality occurred at ages 30–39. Similarly, Pearl (1921) reported a statistically significant tendency for an increased fatality rate after age 35, in both males and females, for those affected in New York City in 1920. Additionally, the U.S. Public Health Report (Anonymous, 1922) noted that the highest mortality rates were within the 20–29 age group. Denmark reported the highest mortality in the 25–35 age group (Matheson Commission; see Fig. 3.3).

SEX

The Matheson Report indicated that 57.8% of their cases were male and 42.2% were female. However, the sex ratio varied in specific epidemics and city reports. For example, Pfister (1929) reported that 80% of the 100 patients seen at Peking Union Medical Hospital were male, and the Medical Research Council (1926) noted that about 1.5 times more males were affected with EL than females in their report on cases from Sheffield, England. Pearl's analysis (1921) of New York City cases in 1920 also found that males were statistically more likely to be susceptible to EL than were females (see Fig. 3.3). Pearl's data agree closely with those of the Matheson Report, with a distribution of 57.6% male and 42.4% female. The data collected by John and Stockebrand (1922) for Mülheim, Germany, showed that the majority of cases were female. In still other reports, sex appeared to have no influence on susceptibility. Van Boeckel (1923), reporting on cases from Belgium, and Parsons, et al.,1922), reporting on cases from England and Wales, both stated that there was no significant difference between the sexes in incidence. Hall (1918) stated that both sexes were "about equally represented" among the 16 cases under his care. Smith (1921) also found similar incidences, reporting a 1:1 ratio in his

Ages	Cases			Deaths		
	Male	Female	Total	Male	Female	Total
Under 5 years	23	24	47	10	8	18
5–9 years	26	14	40	10	2	12
10–14 "	26	14	40	10	2	12
15–19 "	23	24	47	5	5	10
20–24 "	37	34	71	13	11	24
25–29 "	29	27	56	11	14	25
30–34 "	35	18	53	8	8	16
35–39 "	30	18	48	14	11	25
40–44 "	19	14	33	7	10	17
45–49 "	24	16	40	13	7	20
50–54 "	15	8	23	8	3	11
55–59 "	8	3	11	6	1	7
60–64 "	7	7	14	3	5	8
65–69 "	4	4	8	2	1	3
70–74 "	3	2	5	2	1	3
75–79 "	0	1	1	0	1	1
80–84 "	1	1	2	0	0	0
85 years and over .	. .	. .	. .	. .	. .	. .
Totals	316	233	549	118	93	211

Figure 3.3 Data from Pearl, 1921.

review of cases in the United States. He noted, however, that male cases outnumbered female cases in certain contexts; male EL patients who had a history of influenza showed a 2.5:1 ratio compared to females with a similar history. Parsons et al. (1922) reported that a higher incidence of EL was found among females of child-bearing age than in males of corresponding age. Roques (1928) concluded that a first pregnancy occurring between the ages of 25 and 35 increased susceptibility to EL.

SEXUAL TRENDS IN MORTALITY

The Medical Research Council (1926) in their review of the EL outbreak in Sheffield showed that, whereas there were more male cases of EL (176 out of 301), females had a higher incidence of death, except between the ages of 15 and 30 years. In this age group, ten male deaths occurred whereas only one female death occurred. In a review of the epidemic in Switzerland and Sweden, the Matheson Report noted that a "marked excess of male deaths" from EL was observed after the age of 40–50 years. This was also seen in the review of cases from England and Wales. Citing the *League of Nations Monthly Epidemiological Reports,* the Matheson Report stated that, after the age of 45 years, more male deaths were reported, and that only between the ages of 20 and 24 were there more deaths among females. In Warsaw, Poland, 11 of 14 deaths during 1920 were male. However, Brincker (1927) noted a higher mortality among females in the 0–5 and 10–15 age groups in London.

Finally, some authors reported that there was no difference in mortality between the sexes when age is not a factor. Pearl (1921) found no statistically significant difference between males and females in his analysis of fatalities in New York City in 1920, when compared to the distribution of the sexes in the population. Borthwick (1931), in his review of EL in England and Wales between the years 1919 and 1929, reported that death rates were almost equal for males and females. Van Rooyen and Rhodes (1948) also observed that there was no trend of EL deaths in favor of one sex or the other. And, both the Public Health Report (Anonymous, 1922) and the Matheson Report stated that, in the United States, the mortality rates were distributed evenly among the sexes regardless of age.

RACE/ETHNICITY

Some reports suggested a higher prevalence of EL among Jews, as well as in a "high percentage of natives" who contracted EL in South Africa, India, and the Philippines (Table 3.2).

In the United States, blacks and whites were similarly affected; however, mortality was lower among blacks (Fig. 3.4). Data based on the *League of Nations Reports* suggest that older whites had the highest mortality rate (Matheson Commission).

MILITARY FACTORS

Pfister (1929) hypothesized that the movement of troops during World War I accounted for the spread of EL worldwide, and suggested that EL in China was a result of Indo-Chinese troops traveling back from France, carrying it with them. Johnson (1998), citing P. Yakovlev, said that EL's first appearance "coincided with the movement of Mongolian troops into the Balkans during the unrest preceding World War I" (p. 373). MacNalty (1925), although not mentioning EL, did state that the "transportation of troops" helped to spread influenza and cerebrospinal meningitis. However, van Bogaert and Théodoridès (1979) did not support a link

Table 3.2 Ethnic and Racial Trends Observed in Encephalitis Lethargica Patients

Ethnic Group/Race	Observation	Region	Source
Jewish	"Graver outbreak of Jews"; proportion of Jewish race affected was relatively high,	Poland	Jorge, 1920 Sterling, 1922, cited in Matheson Report
	12.3 per 100,000 of Jewish population 1918–1928 affected, compared with 4 per 100,000 of "White Russian population."	White Russia (modern-day Belarus)	Chasanow, 1930
	12/301 cases dating 1923–1956 were Jewish.	Eastern Siberia and Irkutsk Region of Russia	Ulitovsky, 1961
Black	All 13 cases in 1920 were "natives;" 5/13 were from same tribe; 25/31 cases dating 1925–1926 were "natives."	South Africa	Butt, 1921 Berry, 1927
	52/1,505 EL deaths in 1920.	United States	Anonymous, 1922
	Observed that Caucasians "more persistently attacked than the coloured"; however, stated that blacks "suffered no less than the white, but with a lower rate of mortality."	Worldwide	Wilson, 1940
Indian	"High percentage of natives"	India	Wilson, 1940
Filipino	"High percentage of natives"	Philippines	Wilson, 1940

between the movements of soldiers and EL. They stated that, because of the war, troops were given more medical attention than civilians, and this may have resulted in a higher notification rate of EL among soldiers. Furthermore, the Matheson Report, in its discussion of the communicability of EL, stated that whereas some authors support this "soldier" contribution, "epidemics in armies have been rare." On the other hand, Watson (1928) attributed the spread of EL to the "most unusual contact between the dwellers of all five continents" during World War I.

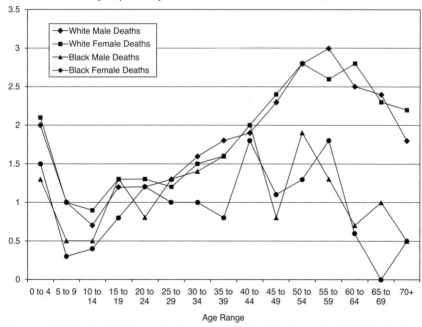

Figure 3.4 Graph depicting white and "coloured" EL mortality in the United States by race and sex (*League of Nations Monthly Epidemiological Reports,* cited in Matheson Report, 1929).

Similarly, MacNalty (1925) stated that "modern methods of transportation" aided in sending a person from one country to the next, thus facilitating the distribution of EL. The British Local Government Board Report (1919), although mentioning the wounded troops that were brought into Great Britain for treatment, also suggested that the movements of citizens to other countries because of the war contributed to the spread of the disease. For example, about 200,000 Belgians were moved to Great Britain because of the German occupation of their country at that time. Then, because of the language barrier, many relocated to France. Finally, after the war, the majority of these displaced people moved back to their own country.

OCCUPATION, SOCIOECONOMIC LEVEL, AND URBAN VERSUS RURAL SUSCEPTIBILITY

Parsons, et al (1922), in their discussion of cases reviewed from England and Wales, reported that those who spent a majority of their time inside were more affected than others. The Medical Research Council (1926) found that the occupations most affected among the cases from the Sheffield outbreak were "domestic servants" and "married women employed in household duties," followed by metal workers. Metal-working was also the occupation with the highest incidence in Vienna (Matheson Commission). Newsholme, et al. (1918) found that, among female cases, the occupation of "housework" was often seen; however, there was no preponderance of any occupation among male cases. The highest prevalence in Eastern Siberia and the Irkutsk region in Russia occurred in manual workers, whereas the lowest prevalence was among students (Ulitovsky, 1961). Strauss and Wechsler (1921) noted that 17 out of 200 of their cases seen at New York Mount Sinai Hospital were physicians. Crafts (1927) also referred to a high reported incidence among physicians, as did Newsholme et al., who reported that five of 126 cases were medical staff. However, Parsons et al. (1922) stated that, compared to all other occupations mentioned, medical staff personnel were little affected.

In regard to socioeconomic level and incidence of EL, no link was reported. Brincker (1927) failed to find any connection between poverty and incidence of the disease when examining the London and Sheffield data. He also found that overcrowding did not correlate with an increased incidence of the disease. Similarly, the Medical Research Council (1926) did not find that overcrowding or unsanitary conditions were a factor in the onset of EL. Bramwell (1920), as well, found that the British middle class was as much affected as the lower class. In regard to both occupation and social condition, the Matheson Report concluded that neither "bears any relationship to the susceptibility to epidemic encephalitis" (p. 212).

Patients with encephalitis lethargica were typically reported to live in urban populations (Table 3.3). Berry (1927), for example, proposed that the stress due to living in a "town" environment versus a rural one may "render [some] more vulnerable" to EL. However, Parsons, et al (1922) noted that the higher incidences of EL in "large cities" and "industrial centres" were due only to these areas having larger populations and better diagnostic facilities than the rural areas. They concluded that the poorer and more congested areas had these higher incidences because of the population factor and not the state of sanitation. Still, data collected from Peking, China, and the surrounding regions from 1923–1925 by Pfister (1929) showed that farmers had a lower incidence of EL than did sedentary workers (Table 3.3). Yew and Watson (1937), in their study of Yunnan Province, China, found that most of the male patients had traveled 18 days or more to the nearest hospital, implying that the majority of them were from rural areas. Pertaining to the Eastern Siberia and Irkutsk regions of Russia, Ulitovsky (1961) suggested that many of the cases that were considered to be "urban" were actually residents of towns close to a city. He considered, accordingly, that the apparent prevalence of urban cases was deceptive, especially because the living conditions of people in the towns closely resembled those of people in the country.

Table 3.3 Incidence of Encephalitis Lethargica in Urban Versus Rural Populations

Nation	Observation	Years	Source
England	Highest incidence noted in Sheffield, London, and Glasgow.	1924	Anonymous, 1926
	Greater prevalence noted in urban areas.	1926	Matheson Commission, citing *League of Nations Monthly Epidemiological Reports*
	Larger number of cases in urban areas; number of cases correlated with population size.	1926	Van Rooyen and Rhodes, 1948
	Suggests increased number of large towns and crowding increases "opportunity for personal infection" to EL.		MacNalty, 1937
Ireland	Most patients did business in Belfast or visited recently; most reported cases occurred "in, and around, the chief industrial center of Ireland (Belfast)."	1921	Parsons, et al., 1922
United States	Majority of deaths were from urban areas (1,129/1,505).	1920	Anonymous, 1922
White Russia (modern-day Belarus)	55% of 919 cases were from urban areas, especially in Minsk and Bobruisk; overall in 7.2 per 100,000 inhabitants.	1918–1928	Chasanow, 1930
Russia	Higher prevalence noted in Irkutsk city and near railroads.	1932–1956	Ulitovsky, 1961
Spain	More than half of 120 cases lived in Madrid, Barcelona, and Valencia.	1918–1936	Corral-Corral and Rodríguez-Navarro, 2007
France	Number of EL cases was proportional to population number, and EL did not affect one specific region over another.	1920	Bernard, 1920; Anonymous, 1921
Bloemfontein, South Africa	Higher prevalence noted in urban areas as opposed to rural areas, due to stress caused by "town life."	1922–1926	Berry, 1927
Peking, and surrounding areas, China	Farmers were less affected than sedentary workers.	1923–1925	Pfister, 1929
Worldwide	More prevalent in large cities.		Ford, 1937

GEOGRAPHICAL SPREAD

As discussed in Chapter 2, it is difficult to pinpoint the earliest cases of EL, with various sources considering them to have occurred in Romania, France, or Austria between 1915 and 1917 (Matheson Commission). More interestingly, because EL is believed to have spread from east to west across the world (Riley, 1930), a few sporadic cases were seen in the United States as early as 1910. For example, the Matheson Report described a U.S. case, in New York City, of a 2-year-old who, in 1912, appeared to have acute EL that resulted in his being diagnosed with chronic EL in 1928. A possible caveat here is that the diagnosis of EL was post hoc and therefore possibly incorrect (see Chapter 7). In addition to the small 1917 outbreak in Vienna that von Economo (1929) described, the Matheson Report stated that there were also reported cases from Italy and Morocco that same year. In 1918, cases from France were starting to be reported in epidemic proportions, and Ireland, Scotland, the Netherlands, England, Belgium, Germany, Sweden, Yugoslavia, Algeria, South Africa, and the United States also reported cases of EL. Cases from Switzerland, Norway, Portugal, Spain, Bulgaria, Russia, South America, India, China, and Japan then followed in 1919 (Smith, 1921; Pfister, 1929; von Economo, 1929; Riley, 1930; Hurst, 1934; van Bogaert & Théodoridès, 1979; Vilensky, Mukhamedzyanov, & Gilman, 2008; Matheson Commission). The first reported case from Greece was in 1920 (van Bogaert & Théodoridès), as were the first cases from Denmark and Finland (Matheson Commission) (Fig. 3.5). In that same year, Italy experienced a "violent outbreak" of EL, and, according to von Economo (1929), the disease spread out from Verona to the rest of Northern Italy, then spread from there to Southern Tyrol and the Adriatic coast. The following week, EL appeared with "particular violence" in Vienna, and subsequently spread "with an unparalleled rapidity over the face of Europe." Crafts (1927), however, wrote that by the winter of 1919, EL was already "rapidly" extending to the "far corners of the earth," based on reports appearing in medical journals at that time.

The distribution of EL in the United States was characterized as "radiating outward from the debarkation ports of New York City, Boston, Philadelphia, and southern cities… [to] the Pacific coast" (Riley, 1930, p. 577). Although some believed the first well-recognized case of EL was seen in New York City in September of 1918 (Smith, 1921; Hurst, 1934), followed by three more cases, also in New York, in October of that same year (Smith, 1921), others reported different dates and locations. For example, Crafts (1927) stated in his book on EL that the first case in the United States occurred in December 1918, in the central northwest.

YEAR OF COMPULSORY NOTIFICATION

Encephalitis lethargica became a reportable disease in most of the industrialized countries around the world during the epidemic period (Table 3.4).

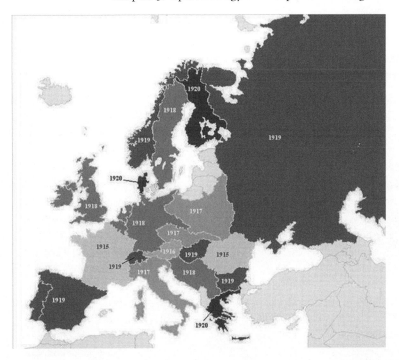

Figure 3.5 Map of Europe, Scandinavia, and Russia with dates corresponding to year of first reported cases of EL.

POLITICAL ISSUES

Kroker (2004) published a major analysis of EL in the United States and concluded that the disease was overdiagnosed, especially in New York, because New York neurologists had chosen to focus on the treatment and curing of this disease. He postulated that these neurologists were concerned by the increasing capabilities of some of the other medical specialties, and they believed that, unless neurologists could identify a disease to cure, neurology might not persist as a medical specialty. Kroker's data are convincing and suggest that at least some of the EL diagnoses by neurologists may have consciously or unconsciously reflected political considerations.

CONCLUSION

Many reasons exist for the multitude of inconsistencies in the reported data on the epidemiology of EL: poor medical record-keeping at the time, the polymorphism of the disease, disruptions caused by World War I, the roughly contemporaneous Spanish influenza epidemic, and perhaps even political considerations (Kroker, 2004). Although the Matheson Report reflected data from a worldwide

Table 3.4 Summary of Dates When It Became Required by Law to Report Encephalitis Lethargica Cases

Date of Compulsory Notification	Nation	Source
1919, January 1	England and Wales	Brincker, 1927; Matheson Commission
1920, February	France	Netter, 1921; Bernard and Renault, 1920
1920, February 17	Switzerland	Matheson Commission
1920, March	Poland	Matheson Commission
1920, June 1	Portugal	Matheson Commission
1920, July 1	Sweden	Matheson Commission
1920, August	Union of South Africa	Berry, 1927
1920, Unknown month	Spain	Corral-Corral and Rodríguez-Navarro, 2007
1921, March	United States, but not all states were required to report EL	Holt, 1937; Hurst, 1934
1924, January	Holland	Matheson Commission
1927, January	Austria	Matheson Commission
Compulsory notification not instituted	Germany	Matheson Commission

dataset, and Pearl's statistical analysis was based solely on cases in New York City, their separate findings were remarkably consistent and, in our opinion, as factual as one can discern. In this chapter, we have tried to summarize the most complete epidemiological analyses of the disease that were published; nevertheless, much ambiguity remains and this uncertainty is unlikely ever to be resolved.

REFERENCES CITED

Anonymous. (1919). *Forty-eighth Annual Report of the Local Government Board: 1918–1919.* London: His Majesty's Stationery Office.

Anonymous. (1921). World-wide prevalence of encephalitis lethargica. *Public Health Reports, 36,* 602–607.

Anonymous. (1922). Deaths from lethargic encephalitis in the United States registration area, 1920. *Public Health Reports, 37,* 644–647.

Anonymous. (1926). *The Sheffield Outbreak of Epidemic Encephalitis in 1924: The Report of a Sub-committee Appointed by the Medical Advisory Committee of the Local Division of the British Medical Association.* London: His Majesty's Stationery Office.

Bernard, L., & Renault, J. (1920). L'enquête épidémiologique du ministère de l'Hygiène sur l'encéphalite léthargique en France. *Bulletin de l'Académie Nationale de Medicine, 18,* 470–474.

Berry, W. A. (1927). Encephalitis lethargica and its occurrence in South Africa. *Journal of the Medical Association of South Africa, 1*, 33–36.

Borthwick, G. A. (1931). *Encephalitis lethargica.* London: London County Council.

Bramwell, E. (1920). Encephalitis lethargica (epidemic encephalitis). *Lancet, 1*, 1152–1158.

Brincker, J. A. (1927). Notifiable infectious diseases of the nervous system as they affect children of school age. *Journal of the Royal Sanitary Institute, 48*, 92–112.

Butt, H. T. H. (1921). Epidemic encephalitis: An account of an outbreak amongst native South African labourers. *The Medical Journal of South Africa, 16*, 146–151.

Chasanow, M. (1930). Einige Zahlen und Beobachtungen über die epidemische encephalitis in Weißrußland. *Archiv für Psychiatrie und Nervenkrankheiten, 93*, 116–129.

Corral-Corral, I., & Rodríguez-Navarro, C. Q. (2007). ¿Cómo fue la encefalitis letárgica en España? Análisis de los casos publicados entre 1918 y 1936. *Revista de Neurologia, 44*, 245–253.

Crafts, L. M. (1927). *Epidemic Encephalitis (Encephalo-myelitis).* Boston: Richard G. Badger.

Ford, F. R. (1937). *Diseases of the Nervous System in Infancy, Childhood, and Adolescence.* Springfield, IL: Charles C. Thomas.

Hall, A. J. (1918). Epidemic encephalitis. *British Medical Journal, 2*, 461–463.

Holt, W. L. (1937). Epidemic encephalitis: A follow-up study of two hundred and sixty-six cases. *Archives of Neurology and Psychiatry, 38*, 1135–1144.

Hurst, J. H. (1934). The relationship of influenza and epidemic encephalitis. *Medical Bulletin of the Veterans' Administration, 11*, 110–134.

John & Stockebrand. (1922). Ueber eine eigenartige, unter dem Bilde einer epidemischen Bulbärlähmung auftretende Massenerkrankung in einem Mülheimer Fürsorgehause. *Münchener Medizinische Wochenschrift, 69*, 1500–1503.

Johnson, R. T. (1998). *Viral Infections of the Nervous System.* Philadelphia: Lippincott-Raven.

Jorge, R. (1920). L'encéphalite léthargique: Épidémiologie, nosologie, histoire. *Buletin Mensuel de l'Office International d'Hygiène Publique, 12*, 1275–1325.

Kroker, K. (2004). Epidemic encephalitis and American neurology, 1919–1940. *Bulletin of Medical History, 78*, 108–147.

MacNalty, A. S. (1925). Milroy lectures on epidemic diseases of the central nervous system: lecture 1. *Lancet, 1*, 475–480.

MacNalty, A. S. (1937). The epidemiology of encephalitis lethargica. *Proceedings of the Royal Society of Medicine, 31*, 1–8.

Matheson Commission Report. (1929). *Epidemic Encephalitis: Etiology, Epidemiology, Treatment.* New York: Columbia University Press.

Matheson Commission Report. (1932). *Epidemic Encephalitis: Etiology, Epidemiology, Treatment.* Second Report by the Matheson Commission. New York: Columbia University Press.

Matheson Commission Report. (1939). *Epidemic Encephalitis: Etiology, Epidemiology, Treatment.* Third Report by the Matheson Commission. New York: Columbia University Press.

Neal, J. B. (1942). *Encephalitis: A Clinical Study.* New York: Grune & Stratton.

Netter, A. (1921). Sur l'étiologie et la prophylaxie de l'encéphalite léthargique; sa déclaration obligatoire. *Buletin Academie de Medicin, 85*, 278–298.

Newsholme, A., James, S. P., MacNalty, A. S., Marinesco, G., McIntosh, J., & Draper, G., (1918). *Report of an Enquiry into an Obscure Disease, Encephalitis Lethargica.* Reports to the Local Government Board on public health and medical subjects, new ser., no. 121. London: Printed under the authority of His Majesty's Stationery Office by Jas. Truscott and Son.

Parsons, A. C. (1928). *Report of an Inquiry into the After-histories of Persons Attacked by Encephalitis Lethargica.* Reports on public health and medical subjects, no. 49. London: His Majesty's Stationery Office.

Parsons, A. C., MacNalty, A. S., & Perdrau, J. R. (1922). *Report on EL: Being an Account of Further Enquiries into the Epidemiology and Clinical Features of the Disease; Including the Analysis of over 1,250 Reports on Cases Notified in England and Wales During 1919 and 1920, Together with Comprehensive Bibliography of the Subject.* London: His Majesty's Stationery Office.

Pearl, R. (1921). A statistical note on epidemic encephalitis. *Johns Hopkins Hospital Bulletin, 32*, 1–12.

Pfister, M. O. (1929). Prevalence of encephalitis epidemica in China: A contribution to the history of the disease in the Far East. *The British Medical Journal, 5*, 1156–1157.

Raimist, Y. M. (1921). Chronic period of epidemic encephalitis (in Russian). *Modern Medicine, 1*, 36–59.

Ravenholt, R. T., & Foege, W. H. (1982). 1918 influenza, encephalitis lethargica, parkinsonism. *Lancet, 2*, 860–864.

Riley, H. A. (1930). Epidemic encephalitis. *Archives of Neurology and Psychiatry, 24*, 574–604.

Robb, A. G. (1927). Epidemic encephalitis: The proportion of permanent recoveries. *British Medical Journal, 1*, 615–616.

Roques, F. (1928). Epidemic encephalitis in association with pregnancy, labour, and the puerperium: A review and report of twenty-one cases. *The Journal of Obstetrics and Gynæcology of the British Empire, 35*, 1–113.

Smith, H. F. (1921). Epidemic encephalitis (encephalitis lethargica, nona): Report of studies conducted in the United States. *Public Health Reports, 36*, 207–242.

Strauss, I., & Wechsler, I. S. (1921). Epidemic encephalitis (encephalitis lethargica). *International Journal of Public Health, 11*, 449–464.

Ulitovsky, D. A. (1961). Epidemic (lethargic) encephalitis. In Kh. G. Khodos (Ed.), *Infectious and Toxic Diseases of the Nervous System.* Irkutsk: Irkutsk Book Publishers.

van Boeckel, L., Bessemans, A., & Nelis, C. (1923). *L'encéphalite léthargique: ses particularités en Belgique: la clinique–l'expérimentation.* Bruxelles: Imprimerie Ch. Nossent and Cie.

van Bogaert, L., & Théodoridès, J. (1979). *Constantin von Economo (1876–1931): The Man and the Scientist.* Vienna: Verlag Der Österreichischen Akademie Der Wissenschaften.

van Rooyen, C. E., & Rhodes, A. J. (1948). *Virus Diseases of Man.* New York: Thomas Nelson and Sons.

Vilensky, J. A., Mukhamedzyanov, R., & Gilman, S. (2008). Encephalitis lethargica in the Soviet Union. *European Neurology, 60*, 113–121.

von Economo, C. (1929). *Die Encephalitis lethargica, ihre Nachkrankheiten und ihre Behardlung.* Berlin: Urban and Schwarzenberg. (Published in English in 1931: Translated by K. O. Newman; London: Oxford University Press.)

Watson, A. J. (1928). The origin of encephalitis lethargica. *China Medical Journal, 42*, 427–432.

Wilson, S. A. K. (1940). *Neurology.* Baltimore: Williams and Wilkins.

Yew, H. P., & Watson, A. J. (1937). Diseases of the central nervous system in Yunnan. *Chinese Medical Journal, 52*, 843–856.

4

ENCEPHALITIS LETHARGICA–LIKE
DISORDERS PRIOR TO VON ECONOMO

Paul B. Foley

Arthur J. Hall, author of the most comprehensive volume on encephalitis lethargica (EL) published in the United Kingdom, noted that "… no condition exactly comparable with this outbreak of 1917 was familiar to the present generation, either from personal experience or from current medical literature" (Hall, 1924; p. 3). However, many authors during the 1920s confidently determined that the onset of EL in some patients lay as far back as 1915 (e.g., Gutmann & Kudelski, 1921; Maillard & Godet, 1921). Hall (1924) cited a number of cases that had been described by various authors in the early 20th century, cases characterized by lethargy, somnolence, or parkinsonian symptoms, and that had defied exact nosological classification; he regarded them as sporadic cases of EL.

Also complicating the question of whether EL was a novel disease was that it overlapped in time with the Spanish influenza pandemic. And, as discussed in Chapter 2, not only did no test at the time confirm a diagnosis of EL, neither was one available to confirm an influenza diagnosis; indeed, no agreement existed as to what constituted the pathological basis of influenza, with a number of bacterial and infra-visible pathogens drawing attention from investigators. Influenza, as was the case with EL, was therefore diagnosed on the basis of its clinical presentation alone, and physicians were aware that this made absolute certainty nigh impossible. After the influenza virus was discovered in the early 1930s, and then accepted as the pathogen underlying both seasonal and pandemic influenza, it became evident that many presumed "influenza" cases were actually other respiratory diseases (including pneumonia, bronchitis, sinusitis. and chronic rhinitis), pulmonary tuberculosis, typhus, or malaria (reviewed in Foley, 2009a-c). And, we would similarly expect that many EL cases were probably influenza or brain tumors (see Chapter 12).

Whether EL was caused by the influenza "virus" was vigorously debated during the 1920s (see Chapter 9), but another question was inevitably posed by both the "unitarian" camp and those who considered EL as a disease *sui generis*: Was it really a new disease, or was it an old malady returned? This question could be approached in a number of ways. One, favored by the unitarians, was to scour the records of past influenza epidemics for evidence of EL-like symptoms; this clearly begged the question of whether the two infections were related, but nevertheless disclosed much valuable information pertaining to the issue. The second was to seek past instances of one of the hallmark symptoms of EL. But, the problem here was the nature of EL itself. Not only were there no unambiguous instances of epidemic EL apart from the 1920s (see Chapter 5), but the descriptions from that period include a number of quite different if overlapping clinical forms, with many different signs and symptoms (Chapter 2). Most contemporary observers chose as the defining feature of EL, not unreasonably, the curious lethargy that had earned the disease its initial designation, and they looked for accounts of unusual somnolence in the historical records. Others, however, sought descriptions of ocular symptoms similar to those seen in EL, as such problems were thought to be a more consistent feature of EL throughout the 1920s.

The search for these conditions in the pre-1917 literature is fraught with difficulties in terminology, language translations, and validity of the observations. Here, we have used three tables to summarize the most pertinent data pertaining to pre-1917 EL-like conditions based on influenza, sleep disorders, and ocular problems to investigate which, if any, were likely to have been EL. As delineated in our conclusion, our analysis certainly suggests that EL did occur prior to 1917. Furthermore, before beginning our analyses using these three tables, we discuss the potential relationship between EL and African sleeping sickness.

AFRICAN SLEEPING SICKNESS

African sleeping sickness or *nélevan* is an EL-like disorder that attracted great attention at the end of the 19th century. African sleeping sickness is characterized by an afebrile course, loss of muscle tonus and insecurity of gait, ptosis, apathy, and great somnolence. The patient is ultimately bedridden, although no true paralysis or muscular wasting occurs; if death occurs (and it does in 95% of cases), it ensues after only a period of months. The disease inspired fear in and posed a serious challenge for colonialist authorities, and it was the focus of intensive research from the late 19th century until its etiology (transmission of *Trypanosoma* parasites by the tsetse fly) had been clarified and the rudiments of effective management of the disorder had been initiated. Early studies of EL neuropathology recognized similarities to that of African sleeping sickness (see Chapter 10), but no evidence of parasitic infection was found in EL patients. Nevertheless, among local lay persons in western Germany in 1918 and 1919, one of the explanations for the emergence of EL was that the dreaded "Negro disorder" had been introduced by French African occupation troops in the Rhineland (Anonymous, 1920). Mauthner (1890) postulated that similar disorders were endemic to Europe.

ENCEPHALITIS LETHARGICA–LIKE SYMPTOMS ASSOCIATED WITH PREVIOUS INFLUENZA EPIDEMICS

The most prominent authors who considered EL to be a historical disease were British epidemiologist Francis Crookshank and German internist and tuberculosis specialist Julius Kayser-Petersen; each published several papers on the subject, as did Leipzig physician Erich Ebstein, who, in 1921, published a detailed paper on the history of EL-like disorders. These authors shared the view that EL was, in principle, directly linked with influenza, and their search through historical records therefore focused on identifying EL-like phenomena during past "influenza" epidemics (Table 4.1). Crookshank argued that, not only EL and influenza, but also encephalitis acuta hemorrhagica, polioencephalitis, poliomyelitis, and a collection of historical disorders including the English sweats and ergotism were all manifestations of a single disorder, "epidemic encephalomyelitis" (Crookshank, 1918, 1922).

The first major disease episode to which attention was drawn by EL historical reviewers in the 1920s was the 1673–1675 "continued fever" described by Thomas Sydenham as a *febris soporosa* (Table 4.1; the table lists some earlier, relatively minor episodes as well). Sydenham remarked that, in addition to fever, sweats, and general aches in joints and limbs, profound somnolence was notable.

Sydenham had seen similar sopor before, particularly in children and youth, but not to the same degree. Recovery from the continuous fever of the 1670s was generally achieved within a month; sooner, if the described somnolence was absent. Other cases, however, did present an agitated delirium, and the prognosis for full restoration was then less favorable. Kayser-Petersen (1923) and Ebstein (1921) were convinced that Sydenham's disorder was none other than EL, despite the latter's caution with regard to subsequent historical epidemics of "soporous," "comatose," or "apoplectic fevers." Nevertheless, even Sydenham's epidemic must be regarded with reservation, given his emphasis upon the fever and pleurisy that characterized the disorder and that were notably absent in EL.

Following febris soporosa, the next significant EL-like disease episode mentioned by 1920s authorities occurred in Tübingen, Germany, in 1712 (Table 4.1). Von Economo himself had early identified it as a possible forerunner of EL (1917).

Table 4.1 Pre-1917 Influenza-related Disorders Thought to Resemble Encephalitis Lethargica

Condition	Reference	Characteristics	Comment
Cephalalgia catarrhalis or simply the "new disease," and later designated *cephalitis epidemica* (1510/Europe)	Short (1749)	Severe headache, respiratory difficulties, hoarseness, severe cough; loss of strength and appetite; restlessness, insomnia	Primarily respiratory fever; no somnolence
European influenza epidemic (1580)	Corradi (1866); other citations in Kayser-Petersen (1923)	Contagious headache, delirium and confused speech; neuralgia; perhaps hiccough, disturbed sleep, some sufferers twisting in tortured insomnia, others succumbing to irresistible slumber; limb tremor	Kayser-Petersen (1923) suggested it was the same as EL.
Copenhagen fever (Mid-1600s)	Bartholin (1661, p. 11f.)	"In what was certainly a cold winter, but without much snow, an affliction has brought about cases of deep sleep in our city, tormenting with its precise attacks. With our care, many have evaded the continuous deep sleep. The soporous disorder crept in from the south within the space of a month, and when awoken by their caretakers they fell back into sleep." Also accompanied by headache and ended with the summer.	The limited available information suggests an EL-like condition.

"Epidemic fever chiefly infestous to the brain and nervous stock"; Sydenham's disease; *febris soporosa* (Great Britain/1673–1675)	Willis (1684); Sydenham (1848)	Afflicted mostly children and youth; persisted more than an acute disorder; initial fever was rather gradual and low-grade, but elicited "a languishing of the spirits and a turpitude or numbness of the animal function"; vertigo and tinnitus	Crookshank (1918), Bates (1965), Ebstein (1921), and Kayser-Petersen (1923) identified this fever with EL, although others suggested typhoid fever or ergotism; Willis (1684) makes no mention of ocular problems, while discussing in detail a violent, chesty cough; most patients recovered completely, but only after a period of several months; possibly EL.
Influenza (Germany/circa 1695)	Albrecht (1705/10)	In 1695, woman (20 years) developed continuous fever, with an extremely severe headache and dryness of the mouth that were added to the other cold-like symptoms; however, the most prominent feature was the excessive inclination to sleep, which relieved the head pain; after 11 days of treatment, the distortion of her eyes was such that the only the lower white part of the eyeball was visible.	Often cited during the 1920s as an example of pre-1917 EL; possible early descriptions of oculogyric crises.
Schlafkrankheit ("sleeping disease") (Tübingen/1712)	Von Economo (1929)	Sleeplessness and others with heavy somnolence	Although originally suggested by von Economo as being EL, he later corrected himself because the original reference (Camerarius, 1715) only saw such cases in those who had used opiates.
1768 influenza epidemic (Normandy)	(Lépecq de La Cloture 1778)	*Coma somnolentum* with a "putrid miliary fever," which succeeded it	

(Continued)

Table 4.1 Pre-1917 Influenza-related Disorders Thought to Resemble Encephalitis Lethargica (continued)

Condition	Reference	Characteristics	Comment
1780s and 1830s European influenza epidemics	Malcorps (1874)	Soporose state, whereas others tormented by continuous wakefulness, or their sleep was anxious, agitated, often interrupted; trembling of the lips; anxiety; syncope; spasms; convulsions frequently in children; cramps in the lower extremities	Both physical and mental conditions resemble EL somewhat, although cramps are not common in EL.
Influenza pandemic (Europe/1889–1890)	André (1908, p. 343ff)	"[E]xtraordinary prostration, this singular neuralgic pain, these astounding neurasthenic states, these violent cerebral disturbances which at that time were commonplace," sometimes confused with narcolepsy	Mainly chronic neuropathies of a bewildering array of types, most of which Blocq (1890) classified as "neuroses"; he concluded that cases did not differ substantially in presentation from other hysterias, and that influenza probably played the role of an *agent provocateur*; EL–like states are conspicuously absent in available case histories.
La Nona (Northern Italy/circa 1890)	Longuet (1892), Ladame (1890a), Amadei (1890)	Deep somnolence, usually commencing well into recovery from influenza, often with minimal fever; most cases were children, but the age range spanned 2– to 40-year-olds, with a marked absence in 20- to 40-year-olds; stiffness of the neck, rigid jaw, dilated or unequal pupils, constipation, and occasionally amnesia; hysterical sleep, catalepsy, narcolepsy, catatonia, or soporose symptoms common	*British Medical Journal* concluded that information was too contradictory to conclude "new disorder" (Anonymous 1890b); investigations by the Italian and Austrian governments concluded that *nona* was simply a somnolent form of meningoencephalitis associated with influenza or typhus, and thereby nothing new; von Economo (1929) believed EL and

Description	Reference	Clinical features	Comments
			nona were identical; in the U.K. and U.S., *nona* was sometimes a synonym for EL (Dragotti, 1918; Anonymous, 1919; Bassoe, 1919; Smith, 1921), but victims of *la nona* either returned to full health or died, and there were no reports of neuropsychiatric sequelae, although no cases were followed for more than a few weeks
Acute hemorrhagic polioencephalitis following influenza (Turin/circa 1900)	Bozzolo (1900)	Two cases who recovered completed; exaggerated sleepiness, ocular and facial palsies and stiffness of the neck in absence of other meningeal signs	Cited by Hall (1924) as evidence of pre-1917 EL; good example of sporadic cases, but no epidemic was reported.
Parkinsonism following influenza in child (1908/Bristol)	Nixon & Sweetser (1921)	Male (7 years) following a 4-week period of lethargy and mild fever, was discharged with typical parkinsonian signs and symptoms	Cited by Hall (1924) as evidence of pre-1917 EL; good example of sporadic case, but no epidemic was reported.
Psychomotor disorders (circa 1908/Germany)	Kleist (1908) Germany	Psychomotor motor disturbances reported in mental patients	Considered by von Economo (1929) as early EL but apparently rejected by Kleist (von Economo, 1929).

The 1712 influenza epidemic in this German city was described by Rudolf Jakob Camerarius (1712/1715; volume dated to 1715, but observation was first written in 1712) as the *Schlafkrankheit* ("sleeping disease"). This identification was repeated by a number of subsequent authors, but later von Economo discovered that the reported cases that resembled EL had involved the use of opiates.

On the other hand, Camerarius did mention the impact of the disease—the French called it *coqueluche*, which at that time could refer to influenza or pertussis (whooping cough)—upon the eyes: "The nights certainly grave, disturbed by fantasies, often also during the day the complaint of grievously troubled eyes, not at all inflamed, yet only opened with great effort, nor admitting light" (Camerarius, 1715, p. 137).

There is thus an intriguing possibility that a combination of a respiratory disease, ocular symptoms and, perhaps, sleep disturbance had occurred in the autumn of 1712 in Tübingen. The disorder was discussed *en passant* in a 1717 report on an unrelated epidemic in Holstein, but here no mention was made of excessive sleep or ocular symptoms, but rather an emphasis on both the violent coughing that marked its attack, as well as upon its otherwise benign course. According to the author of this account, medical professor Christian Stephan Scheffel (1717), the 1712 *Flubfieber* (denoting at this point a catarrhal fever, not the streptococcal rheumatic fever that it later indicated) had not been restricted to Tübingen, but rather visited all of Europe; it reminded observers of accounts of the 1580 catarrhal fever (influenza?) epidemic.

Crookshank (1918) particularly noted that the similarities between the 1712 epidemic in Tübingen and EL might be further supported by what was also described in Turin that year:

> Towards January, the hitherto stubborn mists condensed into thin rain, where-upon, amongst diverse catarrhal illnesses, such as coughs, hoarseness, and excessive salivation, the soporous fevers often crept in, as dangerous for the old as for the young, with cold towards the head of the bed-ridden patient, which a somewhat diminished fever followed. The ill were meanwhile slowly dying, either comatose or cataleptic or aphonic. Most were wracked by convulsions before their deaths. (Bianchi, 1725, p. 718)

Crookshank (1818) appropriately noted that this was not unlike the EL situation in London, in 1918. On the other hand, the Tübingen report is the only one of many "influenza" accounts available for the years 1711–1712 that placed any emphasis upon neurologic symptoms, so that it was at best a highly localized epidemic.

A major influenza epidemic swept Europe in 1889–1890, and it was reported to have numerous neurologic and psychiatric signs and symptoms. These episodes were extensively reviewed by Ruhemann (1891), Althaus (1892), Ripperger (1892), Bossers (1894), Schürmayer (1896), Marty (1898), and André (1908). Even in the first modern history of influenza, that of Georg Heinrich Most, published with the aim of alerting Europe to the danger posed by what he considered to be the inevitable next pandemic, the first symptom listed was neither cough nor fever, but rather oppressive headache (Most, 1820). Some equivocation also existed in the hypothesized linkage of influenza and nervous symptoms. The prominent French neuropathologist and Charcot protégé Paul Blocq, for instance, curiously attributed some cases of chorea, neuralgia, and paralysis to the foregoing influenza, but other nervous forms of the disorder, when unaccompanied by marked fever, to "auto-suggestion" (Blocq, 1890). Similarly, Le Joubioux (1890) reported as a case of postinfluenzal hysteria a soldier for whom influenza was quickly followed by visual troubles, a fall with loss of consciousness, painful limb contractures, anaesthesia, analgesia, and eyelid tic. André (1908) described the case of an old woman who experienced dizzy spells in the wake of a mood disturbance subsequent to influenza. She presented with hearing a buzzing noise in her head, feeling jolts in her arms and legs, Cheyne-Stokes breathing irregularities, nausea, and vomiting, but with conservation of consciousness. "Was it hysteria?" wondered André (p. 341), "was it the vertigo of Ménière?"

Blocq (1890) suggested that the nervous symptoms associated with influenza may have been recognized more readily in 1890 than previously because physicians had become more aware of their existence; he concluded that such phenomena were far from rare. André stated: "There is no practitioner who did not observe at that time the profound attack mounted by influenza upon the nervous system, and we have already stressed this point. Since then, we have never again encountered in seasonal, undoubtedly influenzal constitutions this deep shock, this extraordinary prostration, this singular neuralgic pain, these astounding neurasthenic states, these violent cerebral disturbances which at that time were commonplace" (p. 343f).

Immediate nervous consequences included headache, prostration, neuralgias, and a variety of ocular paralyses, all of which, in most cases, resolved themselves with time, regardless of therapy. "Secondary influenzal neuropathies," mostly affecting the visual and auditory senses but also including neurasthenia, hemiplegias, and some paralyses, were attributed to secondary infections rather than to influenza itself. The bulk of postinfluenzal nervous phenomena, however, consisted of chronic neuropathies of a bewildering array of types, most of which Blocq classified as "neuroses." In particular, he discussed postinfluenzal hysteria at length, concluding—on the basis that such cases did not differ substantially in presentation from other hysterias—that influenza probably played the role of an *agent provocateur*, activating a predisposition that may otherwise have gone undetected. He emphasized that the degree of hysteria could far exceed what might have been expected on the basis of the influenza attack itself. In this colorful collection of postinfluenza complaints, however, EL-like states are conspicuously absent (Blocq, 1890).

André emphasized lethargy in his discussion of postinfluenzal neurological complications: "This postinfluenzal lethargic state could be confused with narcolepsy, sometimes observed in the obese, neuropaths, persons with heart conditions, etc.; or with hysterical sleep, the paralyzing vertigo of Gerlier, or with the sleeping sickness of Negros" (André, 1908, p. 343).

André was referring specifically referring to *la nona* (Table 4.1). This was one of the more curious phenomena that accompanied the beginning of the 1889–1892 influenza pandemic:

> It is doubtful that the name "nona" elicits in the majority of readers an accurate memory or an animated echo of the very real excitement that it caused in the general public towards the end of the epidemic of influenza of 1889–1890. Influenza, indeed, was only just in decline, and public opinion had not yet recovered from the grave disappointments inflicted by the brutality of reality upon our presumptions of prophylaxis, when the threat of a new and mysterious epidemic associated with grippe suddenly appeared, they said, in Italy: "nona" carried in a few days, in a few hours even, many inhabitants of the province of Mantua in a lethargic or delirious state. (Longuet, 1892)

The mysterious illness was initially most prominent in northern Italy and adjacent areas of central Europe in the winter of 1889–1890, although cases (albeit dubious) were also subsequently reported as far away as England (where it was called "trance," a 19th-century term for pathological somnolence; Raw, 1890) and the United States (Anonymous, 1890a). The disorder was characterized by deep somnolence, to the point at which the patient could not be roused, usually commencing well into recovery from influenza, often with minimal fever. Most cases in the medical literature were children, but the age range spanned 2 to 50 years, with a marked absence in the 20- to 40-year-old group. Stiffness of the neck, rigid jaw, dilated or unequal pupils, constipation, and occasionally amnesia following recovery were also reported in various cases; Longuet suggested that rudimentary forms of the disorder were characterized by a period of preternatural sleep that was soon succeeded by complete recovery (Longuet, 1892).

The origin of the term *nona* itself is obscure: the word is Italian for "nine," and it may have referred to the number of days its victims might hope to survive. Some writers traced its origin from the (unlikely) vulgar corruption of "coma," while others sought its derivation from *nonna* ("grandmother"; Anonymous, 1890b; Ebstein, 1891; Longuet, 1892). *Nona* may simply refer to the year 1890 (*nonagesimo* = 90th) or to the fact that the ninth hour of the day (3 P.M.) was associated with afternoon rest in central Europe; it is perhaps even relevant that in south German dialects *nauneln* is used for "doze" or "slumber."

Whatever the truth pertaining to its name, *nona* caused anxious excitement in affected regions and in the popular press, where it was described as extreme somnolence that often terminated in death, or in "apparent death," in which some patients came perilously close to internment before recovering consciousness. In one particular town (Zozzoi di Sovramoutane), ten persons were said to have died from *nona* in the space of a few hours. An immediate medical investigation concluded that *nona* was a "fever of the exanthematous, miliariform type, with a contagious character," which could be interpreted as any of influenza, dengue, or typhoid fever, and that death ensued not in the space of hours, but rather after a minimum of 2 days (Anonymous, 1890c). Interestingly, an increased number of fatal stroke (*Schlagfluß*) cases occurred in nearby Switzerland in January 1890 (Schmid, 1895), which could conceivably have been related to or confused with *nona*, whereas the rate did not increase elsewhere during the influenza pandemic (Leichtenstern, 1896). Viennese authorities considered *nona* attributable to the lack of resistance of some patients to the prostration of influenza, an "asthenic psychosis" culminating in lethargy and coma (Ladame, 1890).

Few cases of *nona* were actually reported in the medical literature (daily newspapers showed greater interest), and some leading journals, such as *The Lancet*, published only second-hand reports (e.g., Anonymous 1890d). As noted in Table 4.1, *The British Medical Journal* (based on the reports from their Rome correspondent) concluded that the information on the disease was contradictory. In 1890, Viennese ophthalmologist Ludwig Mauthner published an influential series of papers in the *Wiener medizinische Wochenschrift* on the physiological basis and pathology of sleep, and prefaced his discussion with the comment that public fears regarding *nona* were unjustified: "As far as I know, there is no pathological evidence for the existence of nona: on the contrary, that which has been described as 'nona' has turned out to be deep alcoholic intoxication or... as the long known comatose (comatöse) condition which accompanies well known brain disorders, above all meningitis" (Mauthner, 1890, p. 891).

Amadei (1890) was even more ruthless in his demolition of the "legend of la nona," suggesting that the newspaper reports concerned not a new and mysterious disease, but rather: "Hysterical problems, hysterical sleep, catalepsy, or narcolepsy, or catatonia, or soporose symptoms of common illnesses, such as typhus. They weren't even similar to those epidemic diseases with predominant symptoms of drowsiness, that were apparently not infrequent, and that passed under many and varied names, such as apoplectic fever, carotic fever, soporose-tetanic fever, nervous adynamic fever, comatose typhus, apoplectic typhus, etc." (p. 89).

La nona was subsequently forgotten by the medical community, but it survived in the memories of those who had experienced it; von Economo, for example, was reminded by his initial EL cases of his grandmother's tales of the *nona*, and assertively stated in 1931 that "today we can declare with almost total confidence that the *nona* and EL were identical disorders" (1931, p. 12). In the United Kingdom and United States, *nona* was even briefly employed as a synonym for EL (Dragotti, 1918; Anonymous, 1919; Bassoe, 1919; Smith, 1921).

The major specific link between this curiosity and EL was the profound somnolence that attracted puzzled and fearful attention, and even this similarity may have been more misleading than enlightening. It was very difficult—and in some cases impossible—to rouse a patient from sleep in *nona*, whereas this was often remarkably easy in EL (at least initially). The sleep of *nona* was certainly calm, and the depiction by Isidor Priester of a 45-year-old patient in Lower Austria was not unlike that of EL:

> The patient lay mostly asleep with closed eyelids, did not react if people entered. However, he was able to lift his eyelids; the eyeballs in all directions moveable. Vertigo, however no double vision, reflexes conserved. During this state, which lasted about four weeks, P. lay completely apathetically and slept day and night. He had to be awakened for a little nourishment; he himself demanded neither food nor drink. One also woke him to urinate. His sleep was absolutely calm, only now and then he pulled at the covers, he never spoke in his sleep… . Old friends, whom he had not seen for years and who had come from great distance to see him, received only a curt greeting. If woken, however, he was in possession of his full intelligence, and was even been able to express his last will. When he woke spontaneously, he yawned several times and soon fell asleep again. (p. 1160)

Most *nona* victims, however, were more intransigent sleepers, in contrast to EL. Whereas the sleep in acute EL resembled normal sleep, patients often reported that they were aware of their surroundings while asleep (pseudosomnolence; see Chapter 2). The sleep of EL may have been less a loss or reduction of consciousness than a lack of willpower to actively participate in external events, consistent with the bradyphrenia (slowness of thought) and bradykinesia (slowness of movement) that characterized the chronic stage of the disorder.

The chronic stage of EL also distinguished it from *nona*: victims of the latter either returned to full health or died, and there were no reports of neuropsychiatric sequelae, although it must be conceded that none of the reported cases was followed for more than a few weeks. The other features associated with EL—choreiform or athetotic movements during the acute phase, paralysis of ocular accommodation, parkinsonism—were similarly absent from the scant literature devoted to *la nona*. The brain of only one patient whose death was attributed to *nona* was examined postmortem: Tranjen (1980) reported from Bulgaria that a soldier who had died after 10 days presented "hyperemia of the cerebral meninges, without exudate, and edema of the brain." Apart from this case, nothing is known pertaining to the neuropathology of the disorder, although this description is consistent with acute encephalitis.

There is thus no question that at least some of the pre-1917 "influenza epidemics" had frequently been accompanied by neurological symptoms, ranging from the merely irritating to the life-threatening. However, although respecting appreciation of historical antecedents for understanding current medical problems, descriptions of past epidemics of "influenza" should be viewed with great caution, and the interpretation of combinations of influenza-like symptoms combined with excessive somnolence as constituting EL-like disorders is problematic. Encephalitis lethargica was a much more complex disease than simple sleepiness, and influenza-like symptoms were in many—and perhaps most—cases unremarkable. In his detailed review of the available information concerning influenza,

Jordan (1927) dismissed even the postinfluenzal somnolent disorders of 1889–1890, including *nona*, as being relevant to EL.

DISORDERS OF EXCESSIVE SLEEP PRIOR TO ENCEPHALITIS LETHARGICA

Attempts were made by several authors during the EL period to establish continuity among EL, *lethargos,* and related disorders of consciousness or sleep (Table 4.2). Unfortunately, however, until the early 19th century, "sleep disorders" had been subject to a bewilderingly chaotic variety of classifications, using schemes ostensibly drawn from Greek and Latin predecessors, but deployed in an inconsistent and linguistically illogical manner, as exhaustively demonstrated by Kayser-Petersen in his paper on "The nomenclature of depressive disturbances of consciousness" (1924). *Lethargos* (λήθαργος) was originally employed in Hippocratic texts to designate a specific disease in which fever, somnolence, and forgetfulness were prominent, whereas *coma* (κῶμα) and *caros* (κάρος), among a plethora of further terms, were symptomatic stages in the course of this disorder. *Lethargos*, regarded as hardly less serious than apoplexy, in that death within 7 days could be expected, was especially associated with major delirium and post-waking amnesia, from which it derived its name.

The prominent 20th-century Portuguese public hygienist Ricardo Jorge was initially skeptical of the relevance of ancient *lethargos* to EL until he noted several references that emphasized that it was an unnatural somnolence that occurred *without* marked fever (presumably referring to the discussion of *lethargia* by Caelius Aurelianus (*Celerum passionum* II, 1–32; edition published in 1990 but original publication dates to fifth century AD). The recognition that the Hippocratic authors spoke of transitions between *lethargus* and *phrenitis* in some patients also reminded Jorge of EL cases in which somnolence alternated with agitation, especially in children (Jorge 1920, 1921). There are, however, details pertaining to Hippocratic *lethargos* that are as alien to acute EL as the somnolence is familiar. Some aspects of *lethargos* are reminiscent of chronic EL, such as, for example, abundant, watery expectoration; tremor of the hands; and tension in the bowels, but others are not recognizable in either stage of EL, such as its association with coughing and purulent pneumonia, poor skin color, loss of voluntary control of bladder and bowels, and malodorous, bilious stools (*Morb.* II, 65; III, 5 [Littré 1839–1861:VII, 100; 122]; *Coac.* II, 136 [ibid.,V, xxx]; these references are standard citations for Hippocrates; the book, volume, and page numbers are from Littré).

Lisbon had been visited by the *mal de modorro* disorder (Table 4.2) in 1521, which claimed, among many noble victims, King Manuel himself. Witnesses described it as a "feverish sleepy disease," and mourned the 200 nobles "wasted away by drowsiness."The eminent period Portuguese physician and author Gomez Pereira identified the disorder with the Greek *cataphora* in his *Novae, veraeque*

Table 4.2 Pre-1917 Sleep-related Disorders Thought to Resemble Encephalitis Lethargica

Condition	Reference	Characteristics	Comment
Mal de mazucho; mal de modorra or *madorrilha* (Europe/mid–1500s)	Jorge (1920, 1921); Pereira 1558 (1749); Fontoura (2009)	Patients had fever, heavy sleep, but it was possible to rouse them; some victims died, others recovered; ptosis was noted.	Jorge (1920, 1921) recognized sleepiness and ptosis; he considered it to be EL.
Cataphora (by the early 19th century, the term was supplanted in most texts by *lethargus* (Europe/ late 1700s)	Schindler (1829); Boissier de Sauvages (1763)	Somnolence distinguished from normal sleep by greater length and depth (but patients alert if awakened); not accompanied by disturbances of most bodily functions; little fever or mental disorders; patients responsive if awakened; sleep reversal (*somnum inordinatus*)	Sleep reversal (Chapter 2) tends to be diagnostic for EL, especially in children.
Periodic remittent nervous fever (Germany/late 1700s)	Frank (1844)	Dimming of the eyes; severe headache, dulling of the senses; dizziness; reduced strength; frequently fainting; vomiting, diarrhea; dilute and pale or red, viscous, stinking urine; painful urination; spasms; loss of tone; cramps; cardiac palpitations; irregular, slow or weak pulse; notable change in facial expression	Except for changes in urine and diarrhea, the symptoms/signs resemble various types of EL.
Febbri perniciose encefaliche, encephalitis soporosa, or *lethargica, encephalitica, encephalitis delirante* (Turin/1824)	Bellingeri (1825)	Various forms, but common to all types were nausea, sleepiness, and, crushing headache; no delirium; patients could answer questions but then relapsed into sleep; sensitivity of the eyes to light; swollen glands in neck; mild abdominal pain; mild fever; *formes frustes* noted; most patients recovered completely by the 14th day, although some cases died early.	Virtually all symptoms/signs reminiscent of EL, especially the pseudosomnolence and the *formes frustes.*

Idiopathic chronic somnolence (Germany)	Schindler (1829)	Increased muscular tone during sleep and a tendency to stiffness; twisting or turning (*Verdrehen*) of the eyes; twitching of the eyelids; tight closure of the jaw; soft pulse; neuropathologic exam revealed only serous exudates.	Was a highly individual disease, with no confirmed reports of epidemic occurrences; thus, not EL-like.
Forms of somnolence as a disease recognized by Parisian pathologist August François Chomel (mid 1800s)	Chomel (1856)	Somnolence or drowsiness (*somnolentia*) is a state which, situated between sleep and wakefulness, allows neither; *sopor* or *cataphora* is a more intense sleep, from which it is difficult to rouse the patient; *coma* is a still deeper sleep, whence it is more difficult to rouse the patient. *Lethargy* (*lethargus, veternus*) is a still deeper sleep, but from which it is not impossible to arouse the patient; finally, *carus* consists of total insensitivity, from which nothing can arouse the patient, not even briefly.	The sleep of EL at different stages could resemble any of these conditions.
Hysterical sleep (France/mid-1800s)	(Löwenfeld 1889)	Characterized by Charcot in Paris and other French neurologists, particularly Pitres and Gilles de la Tourette; encompassed those conditions that had earlier been categorized as "hysterical lethargy, hysterical coma, hysterical syncope, hysterical apoplexy and, hysterical apparent death; most cases were associated with precedent cramp attacks and headache, followed by the development of irresistible sleepiness.	It is unlikely that most cases were closely related to EL; in most instances, the "sleep attacks" were periodic events unrelated to any apparent infectious or other physiological disease.
Narcolepsy (no specific location/late 1800s–early 1900s)	Redlich (1931; see also review by Schenck et al. 2007)	Redlich noted that narcolepsy appeared to have increased in frequency during the 1920s, and also commented that it was predominantly presented by males (80%) around the time of puberty (65%).	Redlich thought EL accounted for some cases.

medicinae, experimentis et evidentibus rationibus comprobatae; he described how the patient, 5 or 6 days into a continuous fever:

> Was taken by an impregnable sleep so heavy that could only be broken by raised voices and shaking, he may be unable to open his eyes because of this sleep, which, after responding when addressed, he soon closes again, sometimes 12 hours, others more than 15. (Pereira 1558/1749, p. 319; 1749 edition used, but originally published in 1558)

The inert sleeper sometimes resembled that of a patient in the terminal stage of apoplexy; the sleepiness could, however, also be associated with agitation. In any case, recovery could quickly follow this crisis.

Jorge (1920, 1921) emphasized the combination of sleepiness and ptosis, and recognized in these descriptions EL, with which he was all too familiar. The details are, however, insufficient to determine whether the 16th- and 20th-century disorders were identical; at best, it can be concluded that a fatal sleepy disease was current in the western Mediterranean in the 16th century.

The pre-EL sleep condition that most consistently approached EL symptomatology was *cataphora* (Table 4.2), although, by the early 19th century, the term was being supplanted in most texts by *lethargus*. *Cataphora* was subdivided into subforms according to its apparent immediate cause or accompanying symptoms (*arthritica, scorbutica, exanthematica,* etc.), so that it is not inconceivable that an EL-like version might have been included in this rubric, but no indubitable exemplar is identifiable. Interestingly, Sauvages cites as one species of the *cataphora* genus the *cataphora chronica* described by Wilhelm Homberg in Paris, in 1707, in which diurnal sleepiness was paired with nocturnal sleeplessness, "so that this condition is a type of disordered sleep" (sleep reversal [see Chapter 2]; *somnum inordinatus*; Boissier de Sauvages, 1763, II, 2, p. 435). Closer to the picture of EL was *cataphora coma*, which Sauvages identified with the *subeth asarim* of Avicenna, in which somnolence prevented an active life; "they can respond appropriately when awoken, but quickly fall asleep again. The aged, however, are most prone to this disorder, which can end fatally within days or extend peacefully over years" (ibid., p. 433).

The description by the German physician and public health advocate Johann Frank of the pernicious form of the "genuinely periodic remittent nervous fever" (1700s) is also suggestive of EL-like conditions (Table 4.2). Frank (1844) listed four variants of the disorder in which disturbance of sleep was prominent—comatose, lethargic, carotic, apoplectic—which simply related to the degree of somnolence involved. Infants, recent mothers, sensitive persons (but not hypochondriacs and hysterics), and the aged were most at risk for such conditions, which culminated in major fever waves of life-threatening magnitude.

Carlo Bellingeri, on the other hand, distinguished three forms of the *febbri perniciose encefaliche* that were encountered in epidemic form in Turin in 1824 (Table 4.2): the *encephalitis soporosa* or *lethargica*, which was the most frequent form; the *encephalitis delirante*, in which agitation was present; and the *encephalitis cephalalgica*, the most benign form, in which headache was the major symptom. As listed in Table 4.2, the symptomatology of *febbri perniciose encefaliche* was very reminiscent of EL and, at least based on Bellingeri's description, it is hard to argue that this was not EL (Bellingeri, 1825).

The Paris pathologist August François Chomel summarized the recognized forms of lethargy in his *Eléments de pathologie* (second edition, 1840; but unchanged in the cited fourth edition, 1856; Table 4.2). This framework, largely consistent with that of Pinel's student Léon Rostan, in his *Traité élémentaire de diagnostic* (1826, 1830), was widely cited in and outside France (e.g., Fosbroke, 1835). Accordingly, curious case reports on sleeping disorders were not uncommon toward the end of the 19th century (e.g., Eberman, 1884). These cases were, almost without exception, sporadic instances of unclear etiology and treated by a battery of heroic pharmacological and physical interventions. Some cases were associated with phenomena providing a tenuous link with EL, such as the 16-year-old French girl whose ultimately fatal somnolence was accompanied by respiratory phenomena including hiccup (Haime, 1866). Fascination with the "sleeper" extended to the general public, with exhibitions of "sleeping beauties" and somnambulists being popular attractions at fairs around the world. Memories of such exhibits, combined with more recent experiences of EL and the psychological nihilism of much of Weimar Republic culture, were incorporated into the 1920 German expressionist film *Das Cabinet des Dr. Caligari* (see also Hoffmann, 2006).

A final phenomenon of relevance to the present discussion was *hysterical sleep* (Table 4.2). In a review lecture on the theme in Munich, in late 1889, Leopold Löwenfeld commented that: "The symptom complex described by recent French authors as *hysterical sleep* is indubitably one of the most interesting aspects in the area of hysteria" (Löwenfeld, 1889, p. 922).

The outward form of hysterical sleep was not markedly different from that of normal sleep, and many of the features described are consistent with those previously documented for *lethargy* or *cataphora*: fluttering of the eyelids, fixation of the jaw to such a degree that feeding was often only possible by forcing fluid through a straw into the sleeper's mouth, relaxation of most of the other muscles, although tonic cramps ranging to total corporeal rigidity were also typical. The attacks observed by Löwenfeld lasted from 10 minutes to 16 hours, but he was aware of reports in the literature that indicated that the symptoms lasted for years.

The phenomenon of hysterical sleep was well-known during the 19th century, but it cannot be certain whether these cases began with hysteria, or rather with genuine somnolence that was then extended by conscious malingering (Table 4.2). It is interesting, however, that Gairdner (1884) mentioned a case in which a girl, after a period of muttering in her sleep and being fed by tube and then by mouth, gradually regained her strength: "Ultimately she perfectly recovered both in body and mind, continuing well for many years. During her attack, she was taken up daily and dressed, just as a corpse might have been; then put on a chair, and there she remained" (Gairdner, 1884, p. 6).

This was not dissimilar to the course of some cases of EL, particularly the akinesia unaccompanied by mental deterioration that sometimes characterized recovery, but the scant details are insufficient for an unambiguous interpretation. The young woman died in 1881 or 1882 (that is, while in her mid-20s), probably of tubercular disease (Gairdner, 1884).

"Hysterical sleep" became an increasingly rare diagnosis at the end of the 19th century, as some symptoms were gradually separated from "hysteria"—partly into the category of narcolepsy and related disorders, and also because the incidence of sleeping disorders appears to have declined. Their appearance in the medical literature was certainly unusual by the time EL first emerged, and they were no longer even reported as curiosities in the major daily newspapers. They had not, however, completely vanished; Claude and Baruk (1928) discussed at length the nature of "cataleptic crises," which they distinguished from EL and epilepsy, and divided into two classes, hysteric and catatonic crises. The major distinctive features of these "crises" was the absence of vegetative changes accompanying the incidents, which on the contrary were typical of EL, and the constant fluttering of the eyelids, which suggested to the authors that the sleep was only "apparent."

Another phenomenon of the 19th century was the fear of "apparent death" or, more specifically, the fear of being buried alive (taphephobia), as immortalized in the 1854 painting by Antoine Joseph Wiertz, *L'inhumation précipitée*, and in several of Edgar Allan Poe's stories. There were numerous accounts of patients apparently passing away and even being prepared for burial. There were also gruesome tales of those who were actually buried, and a number of measures were undertaken to avoid this fate, including the installation of signaling systems in coffins, and the opening of the carotid arteries or the puncturing of the heart prior to death. An investigation by Thouret in Paris discovered 181 cases of persons prematurely buried in the Cemetery of the Innocents, of whom 72 were discovered too late. Whether these figures are indicative of the number of such errors is hard to ascertain, but it certainly underscores the then-current concern with this frightening possibility (Pfendler, 1833). This morbid fear may have been encouraged by a combination of the number of high-fatality epidemics that visited Europe in the early part of the century (including influenza, typhus, and the initial appearance in Europe of Asian cholera) and the then prevailing technical difficulties in discriminating between comatose states and death. In any case, such states cannot be compared with the sleep of EL, in which patients rarely if ever even soiled their beds, rising as the occasion demanded.

Encephalitis lethargica was clearly distinguished from narcolepsy (Table 4.2) during the 1920s, although there were some reports of typical narcolepsy presenting during the chronic phase of EL, the first in 1921 (Bénard & Rouquier 1921; Delater & Rouquier 1921). Redlich (1931), nevertheless, remained unconvinced that EL or EL-like disorders could be held responsible for all cases.

OCULAR AND OTHER MOTOR SIGNS/SYMPTOMS

Ocular signs and symptoms, particularly diplopia and paralyses of accommodation, were often considered harbingers of EL. Such symptoms were, however, not pathognomic for EL, and were particularly common in diphtheria, as well as in influenza. During the 1890s pandemic, ocular symptoms, as well as facial nerve pareses, were reported particularly often in the German literature, but these descriptions usually referred to direct impact upon the eye or to neuronitis (Pflüger, 1890; Horstmann, 1892). Oculomotor nerve paralyses were relatively uncommon in influenza encephalitis, whereas they were characteristic of EL (Cords, 1921). More typical for influenza, and also reported during the 1918–1919 pandemic, was loss of abducent function, leading to paralysis of the lateral rectus muscle and of the facial nerve; further, these paralyses were usually combined with significant cerebral symptoms (Stricker, 1892; Böhmig, 1919; Pichler, 1919; Marcus, 1920). Ocular muscle problems in general appear to have been less prominent during the 1918–1919 influenza pandemic than in the previous pandemic (Eversbusch, 1890; Galezowski, 1890; Uhthoff, 1890; Zimmermann, 1919).

Cases of accommodation paralysis associated with the 1890 influenza pandemic included three cases by Uhthoff (1890) and two cases of "polioencephalitis superior, inferior, and poliomyelitis anterior," one following influenza and ending in death, the other of unclear etiology and ending more happily (Goldflam, 1890; Table 4.3). The two cases detailed in Table 4.3 are typical of similar cases cited by later authors as providing examples of EL prior to 1917. The fact is that a number of similar cases were reported during the 1880s and 1890s, only some of which were associated with influenza, and their resemblance to EL was limited. These cases and EL both involved the brainstem (although autopsy failed to reveal significant nervous lesions in most cases), leading to respiratory problems of various types in both disorders, and ptosis and diplopia were also common to both. But this is where the similarities ended, at least as far as the documented cases are concerned. Most notably, sleepiness was never an issue in the 1890s cases, even where ptosis was extreme.

Ocular symptoms, including oculomotor paralyses, were also specifically recorded in the official report on the 1890 influenza epidemic in the German Army. Acute ophthalmoplegia was, however, quite rare; Baquis wrote in 1892 that only seven subacute (course of between 3 and 8 months) and six acute (and ultimately fatal) cases (course of 3 weeks or less) were recorded in detail in the literature, and he described a case of his own (Table 4.3).

The myoclonic form of EL reminded French and Italian writers, in particular, of *Dubini's electric chorea*, first described in Lombardy in the middle of the 19th century by Milanese physician Angelo Dubini (1846; Table 4.3). Dubini noted that that the disorder was not associated with other infectious diseases or with a particular time of year; and, although he had seen cases from all age groups,

Table 4.3. Pre-1917 Ocular and Other Related Motor Disorders Thought to Resemble Encephalitis Lethargica

Condition	Reference	Characteristics	Comment
Ocular problems (Poland/ late 1800s)	Goldflam (1890)	60-year-old man with ptosis and diplopia during recovery from influenza; subsequently anesthesia and paralysis, particularly of the arms, followed by increased difficulties with breathing and swallowing and death (6 months); 30-year-old woman with severe headache, quickly followed by ptosis, diplopia, and general fatigue; after 3 months total paralysis and respiratory difficulties; at 8 months excessive salivation, muscular atrophy, impaired swallowing and speech, and superficial respiration punctuated by severe dyspneic attacks; recovery after 2 more months.	Both presented cases have some EL-like features, but the absence of sleep problems is noteworthy.
Acute ophthalmoplegia (Germany/late 1800s)	Baquis (1892)	Seven subacute (3–8 months) and six acute (and ultimately fatal) cases (3 weeks or less) were recorded; one case was a 65-year-old woman with influenza 6 months prior who showed a sudden change in character from active and busy to morose; her gait slowed and became unsteady, she spoke chiefly in response to questions; followed by deepening somnolence and diplopia over 3 months; a few weeks later, flaccid tendon reflexes extinguished, a few days after which total paralysis occurred and the patient died.	Consistent with EL, especially both fatal and nonfatal cases.
Dubini's electric chorea; later known as atypical jacksonian epilepsy or epileptic encephalitis (Italy/1800s–early 1900s)	Dubini (1846); Sicard & Litvak (1920); Roch (1932)	Prodrome consisted of pain in the head and neck, but no opisthotonos or vomiting; characterized by jolts similar to an electric shock, always identical in form and always in the same muscles; the "jolts" could be observed in the face, tongue, arm, leg; following the spasms, fever, consecutive paralyses; "sopor" occurred after muscular tiredness, but never preceded it; illness terminated in coma and death.	Myoclonic form of EL reminded French and Italian writers of Dubini's electric chorea; but EL did not consistently cause death.

Poliomyelitis (*childhood paralysis, Heine-Medin disease*), and particularly with the form designated Strümpell's disease (acute polioencephalomyelitis in children) (Europe, especially Germany/late 1800s and early 1900s)	Strümpell (1885); Gerlach (1920); Wickman (1913)	Muscle weakness and flaccid paralysis; paralysis of one or more of the extraocular muscles was not uncommon.	Preference of both poliomyelitis and EL for the gray matter linked them pathoanatomically, with EL, perhaps representing an atypically anterior localization of the poliomyelitis "virus" (Häuptli 1921; see also Chapter 9).
Acute polioencephalitis superior (Germany/Mid-1800s)	Wernicke (1882)	Described three cases, two associated with alcohol abuse, one following an industrial accident, who exhibited ocular muscle paralysis, apathy, general muscular weakness with a staggering gait in the absence of motor and sensory deficits, combined with a deep somnolence that progressed with time; Wernicke located the lesion to the region between the infundibulum and the abducens nucleus on the floor of the IV ventricle, and distinguished it from an inferior form that he identified with bulbar paralysis.	Neither somnolence or insomnia was mentioned by Wernicke, but were noted in subsequent cases of this disorder.

it favored "the robust and well nourished youth, aged 7 to 20 years" (Dubini, 1846). The neuropathology in cases of Dubini's chorea consisted merely of mild inflammation; postmortem cerebrospinal fluid was normal, and there was little evidence of transmissibility of the disorder, with no instance of two members of the same family being affected. Dubini considered the differential diagnosis in great detail, demarcating it from a variety of similar conditions including epilepsy, eclampsia, lead encephalopathy, ergotism, tubercular and cerebrospinal meningitis, syphilis, malacia, and brain tumors (Dubini, 1846). A colleague of Dubini, Frua, identified stupor as an integral symptom, whereas another colleague, Pignacca, listed muscular spasms, muscular contractions, epileptiform attacks, and nervous symptoms, including headache and somnolence, as hallmarks of the disorder (cited in Litvak, 1920).

During a discussion of Sicard and Litvak's 1920 paper at the Société Médicale des Hôpitaux de Paris, the physician and medical biologist Arnold Netter, one of the foremost EL experts in France (see Chapter 2), commented that EL's diaphragmatic spasms were not mentioned by Dubini but were included in descriptions of a similar condition, medieval epidemic dancing or chorea major, a phenomenon variously attributed to "mass hysteria," ergotism, and, indeed, EL; the *Trommelsucht* (tympanitis), for instance, was interpreted as the action of the Devil.

There was some suggestion during the early 1920s that EL might be linked with poliomyelitis (childhood paralysis, Heine-Medin disease; Table 4.3), particularly with the form designated Strümpell's disease (acute polioencephalomyelitis in children). Swedish physician Ivar Wickmann included in his authoritative account of the various clinical forms of poliomyelitis a variation, "bulbar or pontine poliomyelitis," which referred to lesions in the brainstem and mesencephalon (Wickman, 1913; see also Oppenheim 1899a, b; Batten 1916).

CONCLUSION

The investigations into pre-1917 EL were not impartial. Most of those who searched the early literature had the preconception that EL was essentially a form of influenza, or at best was a closely allied condition that occurred only as a "rider" of epidemic influenza. This approach was most exemplified by Crookshank and his attempts to provide a unified explanation for all forms of epidemic neurological disease under the title "epidemic encephalomyelitis." It is doubtful that all the phenomena that, since the early 19th century, have retrospectively been labeled "influenza" were, in fact, of common etiology, let alone identical with viral influenza. This makes the conjugation of influenza and EL-like disorders even more difficult, as it involves looking for evidence of an admittedly rare disease in the history of an apparently all too familiar disorder that may, when more closely examined, be less than singular itself. Similarly, it should be borne in mind that investigators with immediate experience of EL were not unanimous in their opinions of its relationship with *la nona* of 1889–1890, only a generation prior to their own observations. Comparisons with even earlier phenomena must, in this light, be seen as even more tentative. As Winkle expressed it: "What we often find in such cases, as with Plato's cave metaphor, are only the shadows of reality, which allow no certainty, but only supposition" (Winkle, 2000; p. 240).

Having expressed this caution, I believe that, just as it appears that there have been sporadic cases of EL occurring since 1940 (see Chapter 5), it seems very reasonable that some of the descriptions I have provided were indeed sporadic cases of EL (see Tables 4.1–4.3). To me, the most important question is not whether EL occurred prior to 1917 and after 1940, but rather what caused it to become epidemic during that period. Influenza seems the most logical explanation, but our historical analysis provides evidence for and against this view, leading us to question whether EL will be return in epidemic form with the next influenza pandemic.

REFERENCES CITED

Albrecht (von Hildesheim), P. J. (1705/10). De febre lethargica in strabismum utriusque oculi desinente. *Ephemeridum medico-physicarum Germanicarum Academiae Caesareo-Leopoldinae Naturae Curiosorum*, Dec. III, Ann. 9/10, 1–3.

Althaus, J. (1892). *Influenza: Its pathology, symptoms, complications, and Sequelae; Its Origin and Mode of Spreading; and Its Diagnosis, Prognosis, and Treatment,* 2nd ed. London: Longmans & Co.

Amadei, G. (1890). La leggenda della nona. *Bullettino medico cremonese, 10,* 88–91.

André, G. (1908). *La grippe ou influenza.* Paris: Masson.

Anonymous. (1890a). Painful epidemic at Muncie, Ind.; Doctors think it is "la Nona"—500 people suffering. *Chicago Daily Tribune,* April 27, 1890, p. 1.

Anonymous. (1890b). Rome. La Nona, the so-called new disease. *British Medical Journal, 1,* 748.

Anonymous. (1890c). Unclassified disease. *Lancet, 1,* 869.

Anonymous. (1890d). The alleged "new disease." *Lancet, 1,* 669.

Anonymous. (1919). Epidemic or lethargic encephalitis (nona). *Journal of the American Medical Association, 72,* 794–795.

Anonymous. (1920). Die schwarzen Truppen als Verbreiter der Schlafkrankheit. *Hamburger Nachrichten* Nr. 226, May 7, 1920 (included in: *Preußisches Geheimstaatsarchiv* (GStA, Berlin) Rep. 76 VIIIB, Nr. 3835).

Baquis, E. (1892). Della oftalmoplegia subacuta soporosa. Studio clinico. *Annali di ottalmologia, 21,* 369–376.

Bartholin, T. (1661). *Historiarum anatomicarum medicarum rariorum, centuria V. & VI. Hafniae.* Copenhagen: Typis Henrici Goüdiani, sumptibus Petri Hauboldi.

Bassoe, P. (1919). Epidemic encephalitis (nona). *Journal of the American Medical Association, 72,* 971–977.

Bates, D. G. (1965). Thomas Willis and the epidemic fever of 1661: A commentary. *Bulletin of the History of Medicine, 39,* 393–414.

Batten, F. E. (1916). Acute poliomyelitis. *Brain, 39,* 115–211.

Bellingeri, C. F. J. (1825). *Storia delle encefalitidi che furono epidemiche in Torino nell'anno* 1824 *con considerazioni sopra di esse e sulla encefalitide in generale.* Torino: Marietti.

Bénard, R., & Rouquier, A. (1921). Les modifications humorales au cours du pithiatisme grave; narcolepsie pithiatique et encéphalite léthargique. *Paris médical, 11,* 217–220.

Bianchi, G. B. (1725). *Historia hepatica: in hâc tertiâ editione, numeris tandem omnibus absoluta; seu, Theoria ac praxis omnium morborum hepatis, & bilis, cum ejusdem visceris anatome pluribus in partibus novâ: adjectis dissertationibus aliquot; Aeneis tabulis, accuratis earum explicationibus. Tomus primus. Theoriam, praxim, & anatomen complectens.* Geneva: Gabriel de Tournes et Filii.

Blocq, P. (1890). Grippe et maladies du système nerveux. *Gazette Hebdomadaire de Médecine et de Chirurgie, 37,* 267–270.

Böhmig, A. (1919). Über abducenslähmung nach Grippe. *Klinische Monatsblätter für Augenheilkunde, 63,* 741–743.

Boissier de Sauvages, F. (1763). *Nosologica methodica sistems morborum classes, genera et species, juxta Sydenhami mentem & botanicorum ordinem.* Amsterdam: Fratrum de Tournes.

Bossers, A. J. (1894). *Die Geschichte der Influenza und ihre nervösen und psychischen Nachkrankheiten.* Thesis, Freiburg im Breisgau. Leiden: Eduard Ijdo.

Bozzolo, C. (1900). Polioencefaliti emorragiche acuta da influenza. *Rivista critica di clinica medica (Firenze), 1,* 69–73.

Caelius Aurelianus. (1990). Celerum passionum libri III/Tardarum passionum libri V. Teil I. Akute Krankheiten I-III; Chronische Krankheiten I-II. Corpus Medicorum Latinorum VI/1. Ed. G Bendz; transl. I Pape. Berlin: Akademie Verlag.

Camerarius, R.J. (1715). De febre catarrhali epidemia (Observatio LVIII). *Academiae Caesareo-Leopoldinae Naturae Curiosorum Ephemerides, Cent.*

Chomel, A. F. (1856). *Éléments de pathologie générale,* 4th ed. Paris: Victor Masson.

Claude, H. & Baruk, H. (1928). Les crises de catalepsie. Leur diagnostic avec le sommeil pathologique. Leurs rapports avec l'hysterie et la catatonie. *L'Encéphale, 23,* 374–402.

Cords, R. (1921). Die Augensymptome bei der Encephalitis epidemica. Sammelreferat unter Verwertung von neuen eigenen Erfahrungen. *Zentralblatt für die gesamte Ophthalmologie und ihre Grenzgebiete, 5,* 225–258.

Corradi, A. (1866). L'influenza od epidemia di febbre catarrale dell'anno 1580 in Italia con nuovi documenti illustrata. Saggio di epidemiologia storica. *Annali universali di medicina, 197,* 515–544; *198,* 3–78.

Crookshank, F. G. (1918). A note on the history of epidemic encephalitis. *Proceedings of the Royal Society of Medicine,* 12 (Section of the History of Medicine), 1–21.

Crookshank, F. G. (1922). The history of epidemic encephalomyelitis in relation to influenza. In F. G. Crookshank (Ed)., *Influenza: Essays by Several Authors* (pp. 81–101). London: William Heinemann.

Crookshank, F. G. (1931). *Epidemiological Essays.* New York: Macmillan.

Delater, G.A., & Rouquier, A. (1921). Un cas d'encéphalite épidémique aiguë à localisation corticale (forme mentale pure avec narcolepsie). *Bulletins et Mémoires de la Société Médicale des Hôpitaux de Paris, 37,* 1483–1486.

Dragotti, G. (1918). Il nona o encefalite letargica epidemica. *Policlinico (Sezione pratica), 25,* 952–954.

Dubini, A. (1846). Primi cenni sulla Corea elettrica. *Annali universali di medicina, Ser. 3, 21,* 5–50.

Eberman, A.L. (1884). Случае пйатимещачнаго сна (Lethargia, Schlafsucht, somnus catalepticus или hypnosis prolongator). Протоколы и сообщения С.-Петербургского медицинского общества, *1,* 190–198.

Ebstein, E. (1921). Beiträge zur Geschichte der Schlafsucht, mit besonderer Berücksichtigung der Encephalitis epidemica. *Deutsche Zeitschrift für Nervenheilkunde, 72*, 225–235.

Ebstein, W. (1891). Einige Bemerkungen über die sogenannte Nona. *Berliner Klinische Wochenschrift, 28*, 1005–1008.

Eversbusch, O. (1890). Über die bei Influenza vorkommenden Augenstörungen. *Münchener medicinische Wochenschrift, 37*, 89–90.

Foley, P. B. (2009a). Encephalitis lethargica and influenza. I. The role of the influenza virus in the influenza pandemic of 1918/1919. *Journal of Neural Transmission, 116*, 143–150.

Foley, P. B. (2009b). Encephalitis lethargica and influenza. II. The influenza pandemic of 1918/1919 and encephalitis lethargic: epidemiology and symptoms. *Journal of Neural Transmission, 116*, 1275–1308.

Foley, P. B. (2009c). Encephalitis lethargica and influenza. III. The influenza pandemic of 1918/1919 and encephalitis lethargica: neuropathology and discussion. *Journal of Neural Transmission, 116*, 1309–1321.

Fontoura, P. (2009). Neurological practice in the *Centuriae* of Amatus Lusitanus. *Brain, 132*, 296–308.

Fosbroke, J. (1835). Reply… to Dr. Cox respecting coma somnolentum and the causes of lethargy (letter). *Lancet, 24*, 603–605.

Frank, J. P. (1844). *Grundsätze über die Behandlung der Krankheiten des Menschen; zu akademischen Vorlesungen bestimmt*, 4th ed. Mannheim: Götz.

Gacek, R. R. (2008). Evidence for a viral neuropathy in recurrent vertigo. *Journal for oto-rhino-laryngology and its related specialties, 70*, 6–14; discussion 14–15.

Gairdner, W. T. (1884). Case of lethargic stupor, or "trance," extending continuously over more than twenty-three weeks, during which life was preserved mainly by feeding with the stomach-tube. *Lancet, 123*, 5–6, 56–58.

Galezowski. (1890). Des accidents oculaires dans l'influenza. *Recueil d'Ophthalmologie, 12*, 69–79.

Gerlach, K. W. (1920). *Über Encephalitis lethargica im Kindesalter.* Thesis, Jena.

Goldflam, S. (1890). Ein Fall von Polioencephalitis superior, inferior und Poliomyelitis anterior nach Influenza mit tödlichem Ausgang, ein anderer aus unbekannter Ursache mit Übergang in Genesung. *Neurologisches Centralblatt, 9*, 162–167, 204–214.

Gutmann, R.-A., & Kudelski, C. (1921). Encéphalite léthargique datant de cinq ans avec séquelles myopathiques à type Landouzy-Déjerine. *Bulletins et Mémoires de la Société Médicale des Hôpitaux de Paris, 37*, 24–27.

Haime. (1866). Sur le sommeil léthargique, sans trouble apparent des fonctions, à l'occasion d'un cas très remarquable de ce genre, récemment observé à Tours. *Recueil des Travaux de la Société Médicale du Département d'Indre-et-Loire, 65*, 22–31.

Hall, A. J. (1924). *Epidemic Encephalitis (Encephalitis Lethargica).* Bristol: John Wright.

Hoffmann, K. A. (2006). Sleeping beauties in the fairground. The Spitzner, Pedley and Chemisé exhibits. *Early Popular Visual Culture, 4*, 139–159.

Horstmann, K. (1892). Affectionen der Augen. In E Leyden & S Guttmann (Eds.), *Die Influenza-Epidemie 1889/90. Im Auftrage des Vereins für Innere Medicin in Berlin* (pp. 126–128). Wiesbaden: J. F. Bergmann.

Jordan, E. O. (1927). *Epidemic Influenza: A Survey.* Chicago: American Medical Association.

Jorge, R. (1920). L'encéphalite léthargique. Épidémiologie, nosologie, histoire. *Bulletin Mensuel de l'Office International d'Hygiène Publique, 12*, 1275–1325.

Jorge, R. (1921). A encefalite letarga e a epidemiologia dos quinhentos em Portugal e Hespanha. *Medicina contemporânea, 24* (Serie II), 65–70, 73–77.

Le Joubioux, É. (1890). *De l'hystérie consécutive à la grippe.* Thesis, Paris: Henri Jouve.

Kayser-Petersen, J. E. (1924). Wandlungen in der Nomenklatur der depressiven Bewußtseinsstörungen durch zwei Jahrtausende. *Deutsche Zeitschrift für Nervenheilkunde,* *80,* 277–290.

Kayser-Petersen J. E. (1923). Zur Geschichte der Gehirngrippe. *Deutsche Zeitschrift für Nervenheilkunde, 78,* 272–292.

Kleist, K. (1908). *Untersuchungen zur Kenntnis der psychomotorischen Bewegungsstörungen bei Geisteskranken.* Bibliothek medizinischer Monographien., Vol. VIII. Leipzig: Dr. Werner Klinkhardt.

Ladame, P. (1890). Des psychoses après l'influenza. *Annales médico-psychologiques, 12,* 20–44.

Leichtenstern, O. (1896). *Influenza und Dengue.* Specielle Pathologie und Therapie, 1st ed. Vienna, Leipzig: Alfred Hölder.

Lépecq de la Cloture, L. (1778). *Collection d'observations sur les maladies et constitutions épidémiques.* Rouen: Didot & Méquignon.

Littré, É. (ed.) (1839–1861). *Œuvres complètes d'Hippocrate. Traduction nouvelle, avec le texte grec en regard, collationné sur les manuscrits et toutes les éditions.* Paris: J. B. Baillière.

Litvak, A. (1920). Encefalite acuta mioclonica e la malattia di Dubini. *Riforma Medica, 36,* 322–324.

Longuet, R. (1892). La nona. *Semaine médicale, 12,* 275–278.

Löwenfeld, L. (1889). Über hysterische Schlafzustände (Referat). *Münchener medicinische Wochenschrift, 36,* 922–924.

Maillard, G., & Codet. (1921). Diagnostic rétrospectif d'encéphalite épidémique avec séquelles psychiques. *Journal de psychologie normale et pathologique,* 341–345.

Malcorps, F. J. (1874). La grippe et ses épidémies, ou, recherches historiques, théoriques et pratiques sur cette maladie; ou, Recherches historiques, théoriques et pratiques sur cette maladie. *Mémoires couronnés et autres mémoires. Académie royale de médecine de Belgique, 2,* 85–191.

Marcus, H. (1920). Die Influenza und das Nervensystem. Studie während der Epidemie in Schweden 1918—1919. *Zeitschrift für die gesamte Neurologie und Psychiatrie, 54,* 166–224.

Marty, J. (1898). Contribution a l'étude des accidents cérébro-spinaux dans le grippe. *Archives générales de médecine, Sér. 8, no 9,* 517–543.

Mauthner, L. (1890). Zur Pathologie und Physiologie des Schlafes nebst Bemerkungen über die "Nona." *Wiener medizinische Wochenschrift,* 40, 961–964; 1001–1004; 1049–1052; 1092–1095; 1144–1146; 1185–1188.

Most, G. H. (1820). *Influenza Europaea, oder die größeste Krankheits-Epidemie der neuern Zeit.* Hamburg: Perthes und Beffer.

Nixon, C. E., & Sweetser, T. H. (1921). A report of an epidemic with certain cases presenting the picture of meningo-encephalitis. *American Journal of the Medical Sciences, 161,* 845–859.

Oppenheim, H. (1899a). Weiterer Beitrag zur Lehre von der acuten, nicht-eitrigen Encephalitis und der Poliencephalomyelitis. *Deutsche Zeitschrift für Nervenheilkunde, 15,* 1–27.

Oppenheim, H. (1899b). Zur Encephalitis pontis des Kindesalters, zugleich ein Beitrag zur Symptomatologie der Facialis- und Hypoglossuslähmung. *Berliner Klinische Wochenschrift, 36,* 405–409.

Pereira, G. (1749). *Novae, veraeque medicinae, experimentis et evidentibus rationibus comprobatae. Tomus secundus* (pp. 452). Matriti (Madrid): Antonius Marin.

Pfendler, G.-F. (1833). *Quelques observations pour servir a l'histoire de la léthargie (Schlafsucht des Allemands).* Thesis, Paris: Didot le Jeune.

Pflüger, E-F. (1890). Die Erkrankungen des Sehorgans im Gefolge der Influenza. *Berliner Klinische Wochenschrift, 45,* 637–639.

Pichler, A. (1919). Fälle von akuter, rasch heilender beiderseitiger Abduzenslähmung, wahrscheinlich durch Influenza bedingt. *Zeitschrift für Augenheilkunde, 40,* 334–337.

Priester, I. (1891). Mittheilungen aus der Praxis. I. Ein Fall von "Nona" (?) nach Influenza. *Wiener medizinische Wochenschrift, 41,* 1159–1161.

Raw, N. (1890). Trance following influenza. *Lancet, 2,* 335–336.

Redlich, E. (1931). Epilegomena zur Narkolepsiefrage. *Zeitschrift für die gesamte Neurologie und Psychiatrie, 136,* 128–173.

Ripperger, A. (1892). *Die Influenza. Ihre Geschichte, Epidemiologie, Aetiologie, Symptomatologie und Therapie sowie ihre Complicationen und Nachkrankheiten.* Munich: J. F. Lehman.

Roch, M. (1932). De la maladie de Gerlier à l'encéphalite épidémique. *Presse Médicale, 40,* 323–324.

Rostan, L. (1826). *Traité élémentaire de diagnostic, de prognostic, d'indications thérapeutiques, on Curs de médecine clinque.* Paris: Béchet Jeune.

Rostan, L. (1830). *Cours de médecine clinique ou 'sont exposés les principes de la médecine organique; ou, Traité élémentaire de diagnostic, de pronostic, d'indications thérapeutiques, etc.* Paris: Béchet Jeune.

Ruhemann, J. (1891). *Die Influenza in dem Winter 1889/90 nebst einem Rückblick auf die früheren Influenzapandemien.* Leipzig: Georg Thieme.

Scheffel, C. S. (1717). *De morbo epidemio convulsivo, per Holsatiam grassante oppido raro.* Thesis, Kiliae (Kiel): Barthold Reuther.

Schenck, C. H., Bassetti, C. L., Arnulf, I., & Mignot, E. (2007). English translations of the first clinical reports on narcolepsy and cataplexy by Westphal and Gelineau in the late 19th century, with commentary. *Journal of Clinical Sleep Medicine, 3,* 301–311.

Schindler, H. B. (1829). *Die idiopathische, chronische Schlafsucht, beschrieben und durch Krankheitsfälle erläutert.* Hirschberg: C. W. L. Krahn.

Schmid, F. (1895). *Die Influenza in der Schweiz in den Jahren 1889-1894: auf Grund amtlicher Berichte und sonstigen Materials.* Bern: Schmid, Francke & Co.

Schürmayer, B. (1896). *Complicationen, Folgekrankheiten u. Folgeerscheinungen der Influenza.* Basel & Leipzig: Carl Sallmann.

Schweich H. (1836). *Die Influenza. Ein historischer und ätiologischer Versuch.* Berlin: Enslin.

Short, T. (1749). *A General Chronological History of the Air, Weather, Seasons, Meteors, &c. in Sundry Places and Different Times: More Particularly for the Space Of 250 Years: Together with Some of Their Most Remarkable Effects on Animal (Especially Human) Bodies and Vegetables, Vol.* 1. London: T. Longman and A. Millar.

Sicard, J., & Litvak, A. (1920). Encéphalite myoclonique et chorée électrique de Dubini. *Bulletins et Mémoires de la Société Médicale des Hôpitaux de Paris, 36,* 448–450.

Smith, H. F. (1921). Epidemic encephalitis (encephalitis lethargica, nona). Report of studies conducted in the United States. *Public Health Reports, 36,* 207–242.

Stricker, F. (1892). Mit- und Nachkrankheiten im Allgemeinen. In E. Leyden & S. Guttmann (Eds.), *Die Influenza-Epidemie 1889/90. Im Auftrage des Vereins für Innere Medicin in Berlin* (pp. 107–114). Wiesbaden: J. F. Bergmann.

Strümpell, A. (1885). Über die akute Encephalitis der Kinder (Polioencephalitis acuta, cerebrale Kinderlähmung). *Jahrbuch für Kinderheilkunde und physische Erziehung, 22,* 173–178.

Sydenham, T. (1848). *The Works of Thomas Sydenham, M.D.; With a Life of the Author by R. G. Latham. Vol.* 1. *Medical Observations Concerning the History and Cure of Acute Diseases* (trans. Greenhill). London: The Sydenham Society.

Tranjen. (1890). Die sogenannte "Nona." *Berliner Klinische Wochenschrift, 26,* 496.

Uhthoff, W. (1890). Über einige Fälle von doppelseitiger Accomodationslähmung infolge der Influenza, in dem einen dieser Fälle complicirt mit Ophthalmoplegia externa. *Münchener medicinische Wochenschrift*, *37*, 190–192.

von Economo, C. (1917). Encephalitis lethargica. *Wiener klinische Wochenschrift 30*, 581–585.

von Economo, C. (1929). *Die Encephalitis lethargica, ihre Nachkrankheiten und ihre Behardlung*. Berlin: Urban & Schwarzenberg. (Published in English in 1931: Translated by K. O. Newman; London: Oxford University Press.)

Wernicke, C. (1881). *Lehrbuch der Gehirnkrankheiten. Band II*. Kassel & Berlin: Theodor Fischer.

Wickman, I. (1913). *Acute Poliomyelitis: Heine-Medin's Disease*. Nervous and mental disease monograph series; 16. New York: The Journal of Nervous and Mental Disease.

Willis, T. (1684). *An Essay of the Pathology of the Brain and Nervous Stock: In Which Convulsive Diseases Are Treated of*. (trans. S. P.). London: T. Dring, J. Leigh and C. Harper.

Winkle, S. (2000). Die Tanzwut: Echte und scheinbare Enzephalitiden. Über das epidemieartige Auftreten von Nachahmungssyndromen. *Hamburger Ärzteblatt*, 240–245, 319–325, 374–380.

Zeviani, G.V. (1804). Sul catarro epidemico. *Memorie di matematica e di scienze fisiche e naturali della Società Italiana delle Scienze*, *11*, 476–530.

Zimmermann, W. (1919). Seltene Fälle von Augenkomplikationen nach Influenza. *Klinische Monatsblätter für Augenheilkunde*, *63*, 213–220.

5

POST–EPIDEMIC PERIOD ENCEPHALITIS
LETHARGICA

*Joel A. Vilensky, Sid Gilman, Roger C. Duvoisin, and
Ravil Z. Mukhamedzyanov*

A s described in Chapter 2, differential diagnosis of encephalitis lethargica (EL) during the epidemic period was based on "exclusion" and was therefore ambiguous, with the likelihood that the disorder was overdiagnosed (see quote from Ford, 1937; Chapter 2). Even immediately after the epidemic period, the renowned British neurologist S. A. Kinnier Wilson, in his neurology textbook (1940), could say only this pertaining to diagnosis:

> A disease whose symptoms range from cortex to periphery, from psychosis to neuritis, whose minor or atypical forms may be rather indescript [*sic*], will sometimes baffle even the most expert... . Diagnosis can thus become a matter of surmise rather than conviction; often we are required to rely more on the course pursued than on intrinsic factors (p. 139).

Since 1940, there have been approximately 80 reports worldwide describing cases of EL (cf. below). Although the earlier post-1940 reports tended to use von Economo's (1929) textbook as a basis for diagnosing EL, most of the reports since 1981 have relied on criteria proposed in one of two relatively recent articles (Rail et al., 1981; Howard & Lees, 1987). These criteria are listed and matched in Table 5.1.

A comparison of the two listings shows similarity in at least five of the criteria. Rail et al. had three criteria that were not among those listed by Howard and Lees (encephalitic illness, involuntary movements, and corticospinal tract signs),

Table 5.1 Recently Proposed Diagnostic Criteria for Encephalitis Lethargica (EL)

Rail et al. (1981)	Howard & Lees (1987)
1. Encephalitis illness	
2. Development of parkinsonian features	1. Signs of basal ganglia involvement
3. Oculogyric crises	2. Oculogyric crises
4. Alteration in sleep cycle	7. Somnolence and/or sleep inversion
5. Ocular or papillary changes	3. Ophthalmoplegia
6. Involuntary movements, e.g., torsion spasm, myoclonus	1. Signs of basal ganglia involvement
7. Mental changes	4. Obsessive-compulsive behavior
8. Corticospinal tract signs	
9. Respiratory disturbances	6. Central respiratory irregularities
	5. Akinetic mutism

whereas Howard and Lees had one (akinetic mutism) that was not listed by Rail et al. However, involuntary movements could be considered part of Howard and Lees' criterion 1, signs of basal ganglia involvement. Also, Howard and Lees noted that their criteria were applicable to cases of encephalitic illness where all known causes of encephalitis had been ruled out, and this additional un-numbered criterion corresponds to Rail et al.'s criterion 1. Howard and Lees suggested that three of their criteria would be sufficient for a diagnosis of EL; Rail et al. did not supply a specific number of criteria that would be necessary to make a diagnosis. Because the trend is to use these criteria (especially those of Howard and Lees) to diagnose recent cases of EL, it is important that they be evaluated relative to the signs and symptoms observed during the epidemic period.

Prior to that discussion, however, we wish to emphasize that the Rail et al. (1981) article is rather unclear pertaining to whether the signs listed are for EL and/or postencephalitic parkinsonism (PEP). The article is titled, "Post-encephalitic parkinsonism: Current experience," but the abstract states that the article presents criteria by which to diagnose EL. Furthermore, the table listing their criteria is titled, "Clinical features of encephalitis lethargica," but refers each listed criterion to at least two of the eight described cases, which were presumably PEP patients.

SPECIFIC CRITERIA

Criterion 1. Presence of an Encephalitis Illness

As emphasized previously, the diagnosis of an acute phase of EL during the epidemic period was very subjective; this was especially the case because the symptoms of encephalitis can be very general (i.e., "flu-like"). Accordingly, in 1920, Abrahamson stated that virtually every case of EL started with some catarrh of the mucous membranes. Similarly, von Economo (1929) stated that "almost without exception" EL begins with a few days of mild discomfort, mild pharyngitis, and slight fever. Von Economo believed that the precipitating illness was localized within the nasopharynx, thus providing access to the brain. (He thought this was also the case for meningitis and poliomyelitis, although polio is now known to initially infect the gastrointestinal tract.) Wilson (1940) noted that the premonitory symptoms were headache, malaise, slight fever, aches, and pains.

Neal (1942) reported that it was, "sometimes impossible to differentiate the appearance of the symptoms more suggestive of encephalitis from the rather mild headache and general feeling of malaise which might well have been a part of the upper respiratory infection frequently preceding it" (p. 147). Much more recently, Booss and Esiri (2003) stated that patients with encephalitis (nonspecific) have a short prodromal phase of fever, malaise, headache, and nausea. This may be followed by confusion and delirium, which may be followed by stupor and a decline of consciousness.

Based on these and other epidemic period reports, the initial occurrence of influenza-like symptoms is important and should be considered in building a diagnosis for a case of EL (see Chapter 12).

Criterion 2. Development of Parkinsonian Features

Von Economo considered the signs/symptoms of the amyostatic-akinetic acute form of EL to show a clinical picture of parkinsonism, but reserved the latter term itself for the chronic form of the disease. He described the movements of these patients as remarkably slow, and he considered some patients to be virtually catatonic. He also said that they typically have very poor speech and a coarse tremor, but are mentally intact and in that way are distinguishable from schizophrenics. When these patients walk, they assume a bent posture and use short steps, exhibiting a festinating gait without associated movements. Von Economo indicated that these patients have increased secretions, especially salivation, which is only minimally due to dysphagia. Von Economo reported that most of these cases pass into the chronic form because, once lodged in the basal ganglia, the virus is more difficult to remove than from other areas of the brain. Finally, he stated that this form was particularly prevalent in some EL epidemics, such as those in London in 1918 and Hamburg in 1919.

Cruchet, in a 1925 article specifically on the parkinsonian syndrome of EL, indicated that bradykinesia was the most important sign. He also stated that paradoxical kinesis was quite remarkable in the parkinsonian type of EL. Furthermore, Cruchet indicated that the onset of the parkinsonian type of EL was always easy to recognize because it begins rather acutely with somnolence, diplopia, agitation, and other symptoms suggestive of an infectious disease. Finally, Cruchet stated that the greatest number of patients with this type of EL were observed between November 1919 and April 1920.

Neal (1942) stated that occasionally during the acute period, clear signs of parkinsonism were present. She also stated that this was more prevalent during the earlier periods of the epidemic than during the later periods. Interestingly, however, she described these symptoms as typically being transient in character and consisting of masked facies, increased salivation, tremors, and rigidity of either the cogwheel or lead-pipe type.

Parkinsonian signs in relatively young patients are probably the diagnostic criteria most associated with EL since the end of the epidemic period. However, clinical investigations (most since 1940) have revealed numerous genetic and non-genetic conditions that can cause juvenile-onset or young-onset Parkinson disease (JOPD and YOPD, respectively; Table 5.2). This great increase in the number of disorders that are now known to cause JOPD or YOPD leads to the question of how many cases of EL/PEP during the epidemic period, and since, were one of these conditions. Most of the conditions listed in Table 5.2 are rather rare, so clearly the "epidemic" occurrence of parkinsonian signs in relatively young patients was not for the most part due to one of these syndromes. Similarly, some of the conditions have relatively pathognomonic signs that allow definitive diagnosis; so again, it is unlikely that many of the post-1940 cases are due to one of these disorders. Clearly, however, we cannot exclude the possibility that some of these conditions caused some of the described EL/PEP cases during and since the epidemic period. For example, the cerebellar type of EL may have included many patients with spinocerebellar ataxia or Niemann-Pick type C disease.

Based on this analysis, parkinsonian signs have probably been overused as a diagnostic tool for EL. We especially note that Neal (1942) considered them transitory, and also that they seem to have been confined to specific regional epidemics during the epidemic period (see Chapter 7).

Criterion 3. Oculogyric Crises

Although EL does not have a pathognomonic sign, for the recent cases, oculogyric crises (OCs) are very closely associated with the condition and perhaps can be considered a definitive sign of the disorder (Fig. 5.1). However, contrary to statements in some recent articles (see below), OCs were not part of the constellation of features observed in the acute phase of EL during the epidemic period and were not described by von Economo in his original characterization of EL (1917). Oeckinghaus (1921) was the first to putatively describe the sign in a German report. He related that, in October 1920, after sleeping uninterruptedly for 8 weeks because of EL, a farmer's 15-year-old daughter moved her muscles very stiffly and slowly, and salivated excessively. While in the hospital, she complained of her eyes rolling up.

Table 5.2 Conditions that May Cause Juvenile-onset or Young-onset Parkinson Disease*

Park mutations

Huntington disease (Westphal variant)

Spinocerebellar ataxia

Neuroacanthocytosis

Rapid-onset dystonia parkinsonism

Leigh disease and other mitochondrial diseases

Niemann-Pick type C

Juvenile neuronal ceroid lipofuscinosis

Hallervorden-Spatz syndrome/pantothenate kinase-associated

Neurodegeneration

HARP (hypo prebetalipoproteinemia, acanthocytosis, retinitis pigmentosa, and pallidal
    degeneration)

Neuroferritinopathy

Frontoparietal dementia and parkinsonism linked to chromosome 17 (FTDP17)

Cerebrotendinous xanthomatosis

Gaucher disease (type 2)

Fahr syndrome

Dopa-responsive dystonia parkinsonism

Wilson disease

Drug-induced parkinsonism

Japanese B encephalitis

Poliomyelitis

Coxsackie B

Measles

Varicella zoster (chicken pox)

Subacute sclerosing panencephalitis

HIV

Myoplasma pneumoniae

Epstein-Barr virus

Tick-borne encephalitis (chronic form)

Sydenham chorea

PANDAS (pediatric autoimmune neuropsychiatric disorders associated with streptococcal
    infections)

West Nile encephalitis

Western equine encephalitis

Structural lesions (stroke, space-occupying lesions, central extrapontine myelinolysis)

Hydrocephalus

Carbon monoxide poisoning and other toxins

Systemic lupus erythematosus

*Data from: Neal (1942); Mulder et al. (1951); Poser et al. (1969); Misra & Kalita (2002); Ben-Pazi et al. (2003); Booss & Esiri (2003); Paviour et al. (2004); McKee & Sussman (2005); Cardoso (2006); Schrag & Scott (2006); Roselli et al. (2006); Chinnery et al. (2007).

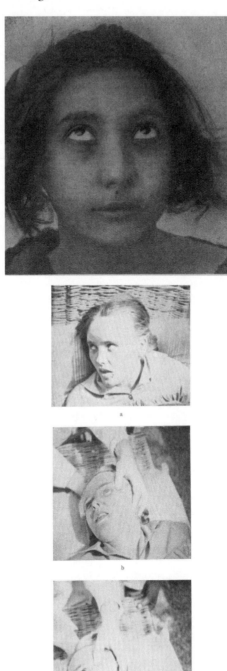

Figure 5.1 Oculogyric crises (OCs). *Top*: First published case of OCs in EL (from Rossi, 1922). Lower three images: OCs in a patient with lower jaw muscle spasms (from Stern, 1928).

We assume Oeckinghaus' patient was exhibiting OCs, although Oeckinghaus did not use those words. The term "oculogyric crisis" was first used in 1924, although it is unclear who actually coined it. It is noteworthy that OCs are not mentioned by Cords (1921) in his review of the ocular signs associated with EL. Similarly, a 1922 French doctoral thesis devoted to the ocular abnormalities associated with EL does not describe any phenomena that could be considered OCs (Houin, 1922). However, these phenomena were described in a thesis and general study on EL in 1922 in PEP patients in France (Jelliffe, 1927).

Hohman (1925) presented the first description of OCs in the United States (four cases). A year earlier, OCs had been described in publications in France and Germany by Fischer (1924), Meyer (1924), Ewald (1924), and Lemos (1924), and in Russia by Geimanowitsch et al. (1924). The earliest British account of OCs is that of Barkas in 1926, followed by two in 1928 (McCowan & Cook, 1928; Collier, in Bramwell, 1928a). Almost all of the occurrences were associated with chronic EL, almost always of the parkinsonian type, and both Fischer (1924) and Hohman (1925) noted that they could find no prior references to this type of ocular movement. Thus, it must be emphasized that OCs were not clearly apparent until at least 4 years after the first cases of epidemic EL were described (but see discussion of Jelliffe below).

Hohman's initial U.S. case (1925) was that of a street-car conductor who was discharged from his position because his eyes had "turned up" and he "could not get them down again." Hohman described the phenomenon as one in which the eyes involuntarily turn up and remain in that position. Although patients cannot depress their eyes, the spasm is not painful. There is no eye weakness or paralysis, and no eye imbalance. The attacks last from minutes to hours, occurring in some cases as often as twice a week or in others not more than once in several months. He considered OCs to be a late-onset sign of PEP, although in one case they occurred as early as 1 year after the onset of parkinsonian signs. Wimmer (1926) indicated that OCs occur 4 to 7 years after the development of chronic EL.

McCowan and Cook (1928) noted that the incidence of OCs was increasing; they reported an incidence of 17% among 136 institutionalized encephalitics. They also reported seeing their first OC in 1923 and stated that they bore no relationship to any specific epidemic: their patients had their initial EL episodes from 1919 until 1925. McCowan and Cook reported that the earliest occurrence of OCs was 6 months after EL onset, but they always appeared at least 1 month after the onset of parkinsonian signs.

Barkas (1926) described a British woman whose eyes, when she was emotionally stressed, "move up and to left, become fixed, can be brought down by volitional effort, but soon return to the position of spasm." Later, the patient developed parkinsonian signs, but the OCs were described as her first symptoms of disease. Another British patient was known to have had EL earlier, but showed no other parkinsonian signs other than OCs, although ankle clonus was noted; the OCs were associated with depression.

Bramwell (1928b), in a review of eye movements in EL, stated that there was no mention of OCs in the literature prior to 1923. He noted that in the 11 cases he had observed, OCs were always associated with manifestations of parkinsonism. He said the sign was "pathognomonic and is sometimes of diagnostic importance, since the accompanying indications of parkinsonism may be so slight" (p. 16) that they were unrecognizable.

In 1928, Critchley commented on the rarity of OCs, which occurred in 5.6% of his 72 EL cases. He noted that they were only found as part of the parkinsonian syndrome, and he suggested that they might have been occurring more frequently. Critchley observed that, during a crisis, the patient did not lose consciousness, but may have had hallucinations. He stated that the paroxysmal nature of the tonic eye spasms made one think they were of the same origin as the hyperkinesias (e.g., spasmodic torticollis, athetosis).

Renowned British neurologist Gordon Holmes also commented on OCs that same year (in Bramwell, 1928a). He said they were probably the most interesting feature of EL. (It is unclear whether he is referring to OCs in the acute or chronic phase.) Holmes also referred to Rudolf Magnus' findings on the relationship between head posture and eye position. (Magnus was a pioneer of early 20th-century neuroscience and is credited with first describing the tonic neck reflex in 1912; Shevell, 2009.) Holmes reported that, in one of his own cases, when the patient, who was lying flat while having a crisis, dropped her head over the end of the couch, the OCs became much less severe. He interpreted this to mean that a disturbance in the reflex mechanism concerned with posture (i.e., dropping the patient's head over the end of the couch) activated the oculocephalogyric reflex, driving the eyes downward; this is similar to the effects of activating neck and vestibular receptors in progressive supranuclear palsy, in which a reflex response can overcome a deficiency in the "voluntary" control of ocular movement.

Taylor and McDonald, also in 1928, reported that OCs only occurred in PEP, whereas Bennett and Patton (1930) reported that OCs, although a postencephalitic residual, may occur without any other parkinsonian sign, and they presented one case as an example.

Smith Ely Jelliffe was a very well-known neuropsychiatrist of the early 20th century. He published a monograph on OCs in 1932, *Psychopathology of Forced Movements and the Oculogyric Crises of Lethargic Encephalitis*, in which he maintained that OCs had been observed prior to the 1920 epidemic of EL, were not solely present in EL/PEP patients, were not isolated phenomena, and were typically associated with some affective disturbances (Jelliffe, 1932). In other words, although he recognized that there was an underlying organic basis to OCs, they represented how the remaining intact parts of the organism were responding, so that, in essence, they were secondary (functional) phenomena associated with psychiatric processes. Jelliffe also noted that OCs tended to occur rather late in the disease process; not during acute EL, but rather during the chronic phase. Although Jelliffe maintained that OCs had occurred earlier than the 1920s, the descriptions he presented from earlier centuries are not convincingly representative of OCs.

Four years earlier, McCowen and Cook (1928) had expressed a totally opposite view from that of Jelliffe (1932), suggesting that OCs were not at all functional or isolated phenomena, but rather reflected a lack of cortical inhibition on subcortical functions (release phenomena). Their theory was reliant on a belief that EL patients had diffuse cortical lesions, in addition to subcortical lesions (which is in agreement with the pathology data; see Chapter 10). Similarly, Shapiro (1935) rejected the idea that OCs were functional, but rather thought that they were similar to other hyperkinetic phenomena; he also rejected the idea that they represented inhibition of cortical function. Finally, from the epidemic period, Wilson in the EL chapter of his 1940 textbook, *Neurology*, and similar to almost all of the above-cited reports, only describes OCs as occurring in the chronic stage of EL and as being associated with parkinsonism.

Much more recently, Breggin (1993) suggested that nearly all the symptomatology associated with EL, including OCs, could be produced in neuroleptic malignant syndrome, suggesting that both neuroleptic drugs and EL have a common site of action in the basal ganglia. However, earlier, Onuaguluchi (1961) reported that the OCs produced by neuroleptic drugs were different from those found in EL/PEP in that, in the former, spasm of the neck muscles with head rotation—and even opisthoclonus—were common and typically preceded upward eye rotation by as much as 30 minutes. Onuaguluchi also found that the most severe forms of OCs in PEP patients occurred more commonly in women, required vestibular stimulation, and that increased cerumen might be a source of such stimulation. He also suggested that the lesion associated with OCs may somehow lower the threshold for the mechanism governing upward conjugate deviation of the eyes.

Roger Duvoisin (see Chapter 1) recalled that all the OCs he observed were in longstanding PEP patients and were quite different from ocular movements during grand mal seizures. Oculogyric crises were always accompanied by an increase in the parkinsonian features present in the particular patient (e.g., open mouth posture, anarthria, sialorrhea, dystonic posturing in one or both upper limbs, and tremor). Furthermore, the patient was conscious and often, at least momentarily, could overcome the episode, which could last minutes or hours. He indicated that nothing about an OC episode within PEP suggested cortical involvement: there was neither a "jacksonian march" nor loss of consciousness. Finally, he concluded that the ability of neuroleptic drugs to produce OCs (or a very similar phenomenon) probably resulted from blockage of the dopamine receptors in the striatum; thus, OCs would reflect a subcortical rather than a cortical release (personal communication, 2009).

The earliest report to describe OCs occurring during putative post-1940 acute EL is that of Rail et al. (1981), in which three cases were reported as exhibiting OCs, but only two showed OCs during the acute phase of EL. In case 7, OCs were exhibited by a 40-year-old woman, typically while emotionally stressed, and were associated with an acute manifestation of tremor of the hands, bradykinesia of the face, and lid retraction. She had no history of administration of neuroleptic drugs. In case 8, a 28-year-old man had fever, drowsiness, and eye movements characterized by upward deviation for a minute or more; 4 years later he was found to be parkinsonian.

Although not defined as OCs, Bojinov (1971) described a case of an 11-year-old girl who, in 1968, became ill with headache and fever, which was shortly followed by catatonia, wide-open eyes, and rare blinking. She was diagnosed with parkinsonian syndrome and was noted to have upward conjugate deviation of the eyes associated with brief tonic seizures in the right limbs, followed by somnolence.

Greenough and Davis (1983) reported a single episode of OCs that occurred in an 11-year-old boy with acute EL, but the episode was attributed to the prior administration of one dose of haloperidol.

Howard and Lees' (1987) four-case presentation and brief review of EL is undoubtedly the most cited post-epidemic EL report. On the first page of this article, the authors referred to von Economo's description of the somnolent-ophthalmoplegic form of EL and stated, "External ophthalmoplegia, often with pupillary involvement, *oculogyric crises* [our italics] and nystagmus were *early* [our italics] features... ." However, consistent with the other epidemic period reports, von Economo (1929) found OCs to occur only in the late, PEP stage of EL. Howard and Lees' first patient was a 17-year-old girl, who had had frequent OCs, but who also had been administered haloperidol previously. However, the OCs were still being observed 3 months after haloperidol treatment. Patients 2 and 3 were not reported to have OCs, whereas patient 4, a 31-year-old woman, had upward movements of her eyes that "were thought to be oculogyric crises." It is difficult from the presented clinical descriptions to be certain whether Howard and Lees are actually describing patients with acute EL who are showing OCs. Haloperidol may have been responsible for the OCs in case 1, even 3 months post treatment (see below), and the authors are hesitant about their characterization of OCs in patient 4.

Kapadia and Grant (1990) described a 19-year-old female patient who showed OCs in a putative acute stage of EL. Her drug treatment included acyclovir with phenytoin, benzodiazepine, midazolam, clomethiazole, chlorpromazine, and benztropine. These authors believed that their patient satisfied six of Howard and Lees' criteria, including criterion number 2 (OCs).

Dolan and Kamil (1992) described a 23-year-old man who was diagnosed with EL. The patient showed OCs and parkinsonian signs 9 months after an initial 1-week period characterized by extreme somnolence. Furthermore, relative to OCs, the patient had been administered neuroleptics and lithium, but the authors stated that, because the parkinsonian signs persisted even when medications were discontinued, it is unlikely that they caused the OCs. In this case, the OCs were not apparent during the acute stage of the disease.

Dekleva and Husain (1995) described a single case of a 34-year-old woman who, over several weeks, developed personality changes and restlessness for which she was treated with haloperidol, among other medications. Two weeks later, she exhibited catatonia and bizarre behavior and was treated with haloperidol and subsequently with dantrolene and bromocriptine for presumed neuroleptic malignant syndrome. Over the next 5 weeks, she had respiratory and oculogyric crises. Although the authors noted that the patient showed symptoms of EL prior to administration of neuroleptics, her OCs were apparently not seen prior to their administration. They considered this patient to have EL signs of basal ganglia involvement, catatonia, and respiratory and OCs.

Picard et al. (1996) described a 42-year-old man with PEP who, upon awakening from a coma when he was 5-years-old, showed OCs. Clearly, this was based on patient records, but it is one of the rare reports of OCs occurring during the putative acute phase of EL.

Blunt et al. (1997), similar to Howard and Lees (1987), incorrectly associated OCs with von Economo's description of the somnolent-ophthalmoplegic form of EL. They reported that their first patient's husband described an episode that was "compatible" with an OC and that she also exhibited an OC with opisthotonus during examination (as of that time, she had not received any neuroleptic drugs for 9 days). Patient 2 had two OCs during what seemed to be the acute phase of EL, without any features of parkinsonism.

Kiley and Esiri (2001) reported that their putative EL patient's husband had reported her eyes to "roll back and flicker," which the authors interpreted as possible OCs during her acute phase of EL. No further presumptive OCs were recorded, and this description does not seem consistent with OCs.

Three of Dale et al.'s (2004) putative EL cases exhibited OCs, all of whom also exhibited parkinsonian signs. A detailed description is provided for only one of these cases: a 15-year-old boy who showed OCs 1 week after developing acute personality changes. Dale and colleagues (2007) also described two EL patients in Australia, one of whom had OCs. However, these were attributed to the dopamine agonists being administered to the patient.

Raghav et al. (2007) described three putative acute EL patients, all of whom exhibited OCs. In case 1, a 23-year-old woman showed oculogyric posturing (which would last for several minutes) 3 weeks after an acute illness that was diagnosed as hypomania. Dystonic postures eventually developed, and she died 10 weeks after admission to the hospital. In case 2, a 36-year-old woman became psychotic with florid delusions, showed oculogyric posturing approximately 6 weeks after onset when most of her other involuntary movements had ceased, and had generalized hypertonia followed by death 4 months later. The third case was a 21-year-old woman who exhibited episodes of agitated behavior with extensor-like spasms and dyskinesia, and she also was observed to exhibit OCs, with eyes deviated upward or to the right with truncal spasms.

Four cases described by Lopez-Alberola et al. (2009) exhibited OCs during putative acute EL, and in three of these cases, the OCs occurred prior to any stated administration of neuroleptic drugs.

A final recent Western EL report (van Toorn & Schoeman, 2009) describes OCs in the acute stage in three of five childhood EL cases. There is no indication that the children were being administered any neuroleptic drug. Furthermore, although the children did exhibit some extrapyramidal features (e.g., generalized dystonia), none was parkinsonian.

Two Russian reports list OCs during the acute phase of EL. Davidenkova-Kulkova & Kostrova (1957) described one case of "spinal EL" with OCs. This EL type was observed during the epidemic period (Vilensky & Gilman, 2006; see Chapter 2), but OCs were not reported in these forms and do not seem consistent with a spinal localization of a viral agent. In a second Russian report, Strokina et al. (1976) reported OCs occurring during acute but not chronic EL, but it is not clear how many patients presented with this sign.

Today, OCs are usually associated with a thought or emotional disturbance, are preceded by a brief stare, and last for a few seconds to hours. In addition to EL/PEP and neuroleptic drugs, OCs have been associated with idiopathic Parkinson disease, familial-Parkinson-dementia syndrome, Wilson disease, neurosyphilis, multiple sclerosis, cerebellar disease, ataxia-telangiectasia, Rett syndrome, trauma, acute herpetic brainstem encephalitis, a third-ventricle cystic glioma, a juvenile with a striatocapsular infarction, and a JOPD patient who had complete loss of dopaminergic terminals upon administration of L-dopa or when smoking a cigarette. And, in addition to neuroleptic drugs, OCs have been observed after administration of Tegretol and tetrabenazine (Leigh et al., 1987; Liu et al., 1991; Kim et al., 1996; Hanagasi et al., 2007). Thus, OCs cannot be considered a pathognomic sign for EL/PEP, even when there is no administration of neuroleptic drugs.

The pathology associated with OCs is not well understood. Kakigi et al. (1986) described OCs in a 54-year-old man who, based on a computed tomography (CT) evaluation, had bilateral lesions in the paramedian region of the thalamus. The authors related the OCs to this lesion, although they could not rule out the involvement of upper midbrain structures. This paper is of interest in that it provides confirmation that a lesion—an infarct as well as EL—somewhere between the thalamus and the upper brainstem or midbrain can presumably provoke OCs. The lesion seen on CT scan was not small enough to pinpoint precisely which fiber tracts or nuclei were responsible for the observed OCs. The oculomotor nuclei were intact, or conjugate deviation of the eyes could not have occurred. The OCs were apparently due to an impaired supranuclear input, presumably from the thalamus, but possibly from higher levels. Not all supranuclear inputs were interrupted, however, because oculocephalic reflex eye movements (the "doll's-eye" phenomenon) were preserved. The fixation reflex was thus sufficiently intact to drive eyeball movement and therefore some corticobulbar input, presumably from the occipital lobes, was preserved. Some input from the frontal lobe eyefields, however, was reduced because voluntary gaze movements were similarly impaired.

Nangaku et al. (1990) described an 18-year-old with OCs, postural tremor, dystonic gait, pyramidal tract signs, and peripheral nerve damage. The patient showed radiographic (T2 magnetic resonance imaging [MRI]) abnormalities (hypodensity) in the globus pallidus. Shimpo et al. (1993) described a 50-year-old man with retrocollis, right hemiparesis, and OCs. MRI showed one small, old hematoma in the left posterior putamen and lesions in the right posterior puta- men and right globus pallidus. Kim et al. (1996) described a 16-year-old with OCs whose mother had ingested some toxic material at 3 months' gestation to induce an abortion but which had failed to do so. The patient showed OCs, but also showed choreic movements, dysarthria, mental retardation, right hemiparesis, and bilateral ankle clonus. The MRI revealed the presence of symmetrical high-signal- intensity lesions bilaterally in the posterior putamen. Finally, Lee et al. (1999) described OCs in an 11-year-old girl with Wilson disease. This patient also exhib- ited an expressionless face, stooped posture, and lack of arm swing, although she showed intact oculocephalic reflexes during OCs, thus suggesting to the authors that tonic firing of supranuclear neuronal structures caused the upward deviation of the eyes because vestibular neuronal inputs were strong enough to overcome the tonic supranuclear stimulation.

Leigh et al. (1987) suggested that, because the thought disorder and the ocular deviation can be eliminated by anticholinergic medications, OCs occur as a result of a pharmacological imbalance affecting two separate neural systems: mental symptoms and vertical gaze. Such disturbances might be caused by a temporary imbalance between increased cholinergic and reduced dopaminergic activity.

Aramideh et al. (1994) recorded eye movement and electromyographic activ- ity in the levator palpebrae superioris and orbicularis oculi during OCs. These authors noted that the term "oculogyric crises" is misleading and does not convey the actual ocular movement abnormalities. They preferred the term, *extraocular muscle dystonia* because:

1. The eye movements are never "gyric" (rotatory).
2. They rarely represent medical "crises."
3. They resemble other forms of focal dystonia.
4. They may be triggered or suppressed by various stimuli (voluntary or involuntary), in the same way as other dystonic disorders.
5. They probably involve the same anatomical structures as those in blepharospasm.

Aramideh et al. (1994) also suggested, based on their evidence and a review of previous reports on OCs and blepharospasm, that variations in the levels or properties of certain neurotransmitters or their relationship to one another are probably responsible for the generation of both OCs and blepharospasm. They suggested that the structures involved are most probably the basal ganglia—especially the substantia nigra pars reticularis—and brainstem structures, especially the paramedian pontine reticular formation.

As noted above, the fact that many conditions have been found to be associated with OCs, and that OCs may be associated with neuroleptic drug administration years after withdrawal of these drugs (Fitzgerald & Jankovic, 1989) suggest that considering OCs as a pathognomonic sign for EL, particularly acute EL, is questionable. This is particularly the case because almost no association of OCs with acute EL was observed during the epidemic period.

Criterion 4. Sleep (Somnolence and Alterations in the Sleep Cycle/Sleep Inversion)

Although most of the post-1940 EL reports describe sleep alterations in the putative EL cases, it is not clear whether these alterations are the same as those described during the epidemic period. The initial remarkable feature of EL was the tendency of patients to fall asleep in the middle of activities such as walking or eating. The personal self-reports reprinted in Chapter 11 emphasize this overriding desire for sleep in EL patients. This phenomenon is not described in any of the post-1940 cases, although it is consistent with narcolepsy (Bassetti, 2007). Although narcolepsy was known at the time of the EL epidemic, until 1924 only 35 cases of narcolepsy had been reported (Bassetti, 2007); thus, it was not a common diagnosis.

Rail et al.'s (1981) use of the criterion "alterations in sleep cycle" (modern terminology would refer to a "change in sleep architecture") would intuitively seem to be referring to sleep inversion (sleep reversal). However, none of the eight cases they described displayed sleep inversion, and when the authors discussed the two cases listed as having "an alteration of sleep cycle," the descriptions indicate pseudosomnolence (see below). One of Howard and Lees' (1987) patients exhibited sleep inversion and another lethargy.

Pertaining to pseudosomnolence, von Economo (1929) stated that EL's most striking symptom was "a sopor of varying degrees from simple somnolence to the deepest sopor in which the patients may sleep for weeks and months but from which in the majority of cases, it is possible to arouse them" (p. 254). So, in this way, the hypersomnolence of EL typically was similar to normal sleep and therefore different from narcotic-induced sleep and syncope, coma, cerebral concussion, and similar conditions.

Stern (1928) also wrote extensively about the "sleep" of EL. He noted that in relatively "pure" cases, the patient would sleep for long periods of time, continually, day and night. These patients dreamed as healthy people do, suggesting that rapid eye movement (REM) sleep is present. Commenting on pseudosomnolence,

Stern stated that, even if the sleep was deep, the patients could be awakened with strong stimuli and showed complete clarity of consciousness and agility. Stern noted that this was different from soporific comatose conditions. Similarly, van Bogaert and Théodoridès (1979) stated, "Patients in the acute phase of epidemic encephalitis look exactly like a normal person deeply asleep—their eyelids lie down, their pupils are miotic, and the tonus of their limbs is reduced. The depth of sleep is very variable, some patients waking up quickly whereas others need a strong stimulus to do so…" (p. 53).

Sleep inversion was common in EL patients, especially children, but it is also common in mentally retarded children (Rack, 2007) and in idiopathic Parkinson disease (Rodnitzky, 2007). In mentally retarded children, sleep inversion has been associated with encopresis, temper tantrums, mood disturbances, hyperactivity, concentration difficulties, and problems with socialization (Rack, 2007). Thus, sleep inversion cannot be considered pathognomic for EL.

Neither Rail et al. (1981) nor Howard and Lees (1987) listed insomnia as a diagnostic criterion in EL, although it was common in the hyperkinetic type (von Economo, 1929). Von Economo (1929) thought it resulted from a choreiform agitation resembling St. Vitus' dance (Sydenham chorea) or other complex hyper-kinesias associated with lesions in the midbrain and basal ganglia. Depending on the site of the infection and its progression, he suggested that an individual could progress from lethargy to insomnia or the reverse. Insomnia is represented in some of the post-1940 cases (e.g., Drobec & Tschabitscher [1948]; Verschueren & Crols [2001]).

Although lethargy was very common during the epidemic period, Hall (1924) stated that, in some cases, it might have been absent throughout the disease process, even if ocular palsies were present. Similarly, Neal (1942) noted that, in 150 acute cases, 50% showed drowsiness and lethargy, insomnia was present in 16 cases, and reversal of sleep rhythm was apparent in five; 40% of the patients, however, showed no sleep anomaly.

According to van Bogaert and Théodoridès' 1979 biography, von Economo concluded in 1926 that sleep disturbance in EL was a focal sign indicating the selective localization of the infecting agent, rather than a generalized inflamma-tory process in the brain. Von Economo postulated in 1929 that the region of the periaqueductal gray matter connecting the midbrain and the aqueduct, and the posterior wall of the third ventricle as far as the oculomotor nuclei, were prima-rily involved. He recalled that, in one of his cases without somnolence, the cere-bral cortex had been the most affected part of the brain, whereas the di- and mesencephalon were almost entirely normal (von Economo, 1929).

Recent research on narcolepsy may shed more light on the hypersomnolence associated with EL. Narcolepsy has been related to a deficiency in a recently dis-covered neuropeptide hormone, hypocretin (orexin). This deficiency is postulated to result because of autoimmunity and/or an infectious organism with an affinity for hypocretin-secreting cells, which are located in the hypothalamus (Mignot & Zeitzer, 2007).

Hypersomnolence is a very common complaint among contemporary encephalitis patients and may lead to stupor (Hobson et al., 2002; Booss & Esiri, 2003). It is also common among Parkinson disease patients (Hobson et al., 2002). However, the extreme lethargy associated with EL seems to be different from typical hypersomnolence in two ways: pseudosomnolence (see above); and, in EL the desire for sleep is imperative and irresistible. Patients may fall asleep anytime and anywhere.

Recently, Bentivioglio and Kirstensson (2007) found increasing evidence suggesting that the neural mechanisms underlying sleep interact closely with immune-response molecules. They stated that the disease profile of human African trypanosomiasis and the late sequelae of EL resemble the sudden sleep intrusion into wakefulness that is associated with narcolepsy. Bentivioglio and Kirstensson also stated that EL revealed that inflammation in different brain regions can cause functional dysregulation in sleep and wakefulness, and that an infection can cause a narcolepsy-like disorder.

In accordance with von Economo's suggestion that hyperkinesia might cause insomnia in EL, Rodnitzky (2007) stated that the motoric symptoms present in most extrapyramidal disorders have significant potential to interrupt sleep. *Agrypnia excita* is the term applied to an inability to sleep due to overactivity (Provini et al., 2007). Batocchi et al. (2001) related agrypnia to an excess in the activity of central nervous system (CNS) activating systems. In addition, a temporary imbalance between GABAergic and cholinergic systems was suggested to explain a case of agrypnia in a patient who also showed respiratory crises and dysautonomia (Batocchi et al., 2001).

It is interesting that many of the nonsleep signs and symptoms associated with EL have become associated with sleep disorders. Thus, in addition to movement disorders, in recent times, headache, respiratory dysfunction, and autonomic abnormalities have also been associated with sleep disorders (Cortelli & Lombardi, 2007; Culebras, 2007; Rodnitzky, 2007). In this regard, both hypokinetic and hyperkinetic abnormalities can interfere with sleep onset or maintenance. Thus, at least some of the signs and symptoms associated with EL may be secondary to the associated sleep disorders.

Von Economo recognized that attributing both hypersomnolence and insomnia to the same disease was intrinsically inconsistent. He stated (1929) that the fact that they can occur in the same epidemic and in the same individual indicates that they result from the same underlying pathology.

Although the presence of a sleep disorder was not essential for a diagnosis of EL during the epidemic period, this sign would seem to be critical in sporadic cases. Furthermore, the available evidence suggests that, whereas hypersomnolence may be a primary sign of EL, insomnia may be secondary, related to hyperactivity.

Criterion 5. Ocular or Papillary Changes and Ophthalmoplegia

The ocular (extraocular) disturbances associated with EL were, of course, a very early sign (sometimes the first sign) of the disease that von Economo recognized in his original patients, all of whom exhibited some type of ocular abnormality. He stated in his first 1917 article that the ocular muscles were particularly affected by the disease, and that ptosis was typical. He further stated that ptosis can be interpreted as "physiological heaviness of the eyelids due to the somnolence," but that this gradually becomes a paralytic ptosis (von Economo, 1917).

Smith, in his survey of EL in the United States (1921; see Chapter 2), reported that ptosis occurred in 95% of EL patients; he also listed diplopia, strabismus, blurred vision, and nystagmus (see Figure 2.2). Critchley (1928), in an article on the ocular manifestations in the acute and chronic stages of EL, stated that some of the ocular changes were, "so constant as to be most valuable aids to diagnosis both in the early and late stages of the disease" (p. 113). Based on 72 cases, he compiled the ocular abnormalities and their percentage occurrence. Critchley also listed the percentage occurrence of these conditions based on another series of patients (Young, 1927), but it should be noted that Young's cases were all PEP patients (Table 5.3).

Also in 1928, a discussion was held at the Royal College of Medicine on "The ocular complications of encephalitis lethargica," with many of the luminary

Table 5.3 Ocular Abnormalities in Encephalitis Lethargica/Postencephalitic Parkinsonism (EL/PEP)

Condition	Crichley (%)	Young (%)
Blepharoclonus	96	92
Punctate (jerky) eye movements	89	64
Diminished blinking	88	–
Loss of convergence	82	81
"Blinking sign"	65	67
Diplopia	51	41
Lid retraction	26	–
Ptosis	21	–
Unequal pupils	13	–
Limitations of movement	13	–
Pupil reaction poor or lost	11	13
Strabismus	7	10
Sluggish pupils	8	–
Oculogyric crises (found only in PEP)	6	–
Irregular pupils	6	–
Argyll-Robertson pupils	3	–
Nystagmus	3	–

neurologists of the time attending and speaking (e.g., Gordon Holmes and James Collier; Bramwell, 1928a). The speakers differed significantly in what they considered to be important diagnostic ocular signs. Collier stated that there were two kinds of ocular paralysis: a paralysis of the extraocular nerve trunks, usually the abducent, but sometimes the oculomotor nerve; and an irregular ophthalmoplegia that always leaves the optic axes nonparallel. Collier said that there was always recovery from the first, whereas the second may leave some permanent paralysis. He stated that the lesions in the second may involve any part of the nuclear mass of the nerve nuclei, resulting in every variety of change in the size or altered motility both of the palpebral fissures and of the pupils, and every sort of defect in the movements of the eye. He further noted that nystagmus was not common.

In the same session, Williamson-Noble (in Bramwell, 1928a) listed the following ocular conditions as sequelae to EL:

1. Jerky eye movements
2. Lack of blinking
3. Blepharoclonus
4. Partial ptosis
5. Unequal pupils
6. Deficient accommodation
7. Deficient convergence
8. Nystagmoid jerkings
9. Diplopia with squint
10. Lid retraction
11. Oculogyric crises
12. Sluggish reaction to light
13. Argyll-Robertson pupil (rare sign)
14. Squint (rare sign)
15. Tapping on glabella makes the eyelids flicker
16. "Blinking sign" on repeated lateral deviation

Gordon Holmes (in Bramwell, 1928a) observed that, in the acute stage of EL, the ocular palsies may be extraordinarily irregular, but that there were nearly always a predominance of disturbance in convergence, often associated with a complete fixation of the pupil. Accommodation was almost always paralyzed as well. Holmes also agreed that, in the chronic stage, permanent ocular palsies were rare. Finally, Edwin Bramwell, who chaired the session, stated that loss of upward movement of the eyes was not uncommon in EL and that a sign he called "oscillation of the eyeballs" was often found. This latter sign, which he considered pathognomonic, consisted of irregular flickering movements when the eyeballs settled into a new position. Thus, "when the patient was asked to move the eyes.... and the movement was suddenly arrested, the eyes oscillated in different directions for a second or two before coming to rest" (Bramwell, 1928a, p. 996). Bramwell indicated that this phenomenon was sometimes seen in acute cases, but more commonly in association with parkinsonism:"The movements were not like a true nystagmus, but resembled the quivering seen in cases of dislocation of the lens" (p. 996).This sign appears very similar to the "rapid shivering" movement described by Foster Kennedy (see below) and has not been reported for any of the post-1940 cases.

Another well-known early 20th-century neurologist, Robert Foster Kennedy, published an article on the ocular complications of EL in 1929. Foster Kennedy stated that ptosis was a frequent sign and was often accompanied by weakness or paralysis of the lateral rectus muscles. He also cited work by Holden stating that the combination of effects from lesions of the oculomotor and abducent nerves was found only in this disease. Foster Kennedy observed definite spasms of the extrinsic eye muscles during acute EL, resulting in appearance of slow deviations such as those seen in cerebellar disease of the middle peduncle. Foster Kennedy then stated that transient diplopia, usually unaccompanied by strabismus, was per-haps the single most frequent sign of the early stage of EL. He concluded that there was likely to be a special incidence of damage in the region of the tectum, near the oculomotor nuclei. This produced Parinaud syndrome, or a diminution or loss of conjugate associated downward or upward movements of the eyeballs. Furthermore, he noted that nystagmus was "almost the rule" in acute EL. Foster Kennedy further stated that this nystagmus had an extraordinary "electric-like" rapidity ("rapid shivering").

The lack of consistency is striking among these very well-known neurologists pertaining to the ocular disturbances associated with EL. For exam-ple, Critchley (1928) indicated that nystagmus was virtually never found, whereas Foster Kennedy (1929) considered it to be almost always present. Nystagmus was listed as occurring in about 41% of the patients surveyed by Smith (see Chapter 2).

Despite the great variation in ocular signs, agreement does seem apparent among the authors that one or more of these signs is almost requisite for a diag-nosis of EL. Von Economo (1929) noted that, even in the hyperkinetic form, "disturbances of the intra-ocular eye muscles of varying severity are an almost constant feature" (p. 38).

Criterion 6. Involuntary Movements (Torsion Spasm, Myoclonus)

Similar to his concern about hypersomnolence and insomnia being considered signs of the same illness, von Economo (1929) recognized that movement disor-ders would not intuitively be considered part of a "sleeping sickness" disease. "That these disparate kinds of hyperkinesis form actually only one pathological subdivision of encephalitis lethargica... is shown by their simultaneous appear-ance in one and the same epidemic, which they characterize; or by the merging of these different types of motor excitation in an individual patient during his encephalitic affection" (p. 35).

The first cases of the hyperkinetic type of EL were described by Sicard and Kudelsky (1920) at the meeting of the Société des Hópitaux de Paris on January 23, 1920. Four patients were described and diagnosed with a new condition they termed, "encephalite aigue myoclonique." The condition began with lancinating neuralgic pains and fever followed by rhythmic muscular contractions similar to those produced by an electric current. None of the patients showed somnolence, ocular signs, or flu-like symptoms. Rather, all had insomnia, became delirious and comatose, and three of the four died. Sicard and Kudelsky stated that the acute form of this type of encephalitis was characterized by pain, myoclonic jolts, and delirium.

Sicard and Kudelsky (1920) questioned whether these cases were EL. They hypothesized that the virus of EL can localize in nontypical regions, resulting in "excitation." They believed that EL's polymorphism could be compared to that of polio, in which the virus, although typically affecting the anterior horn cells of the spinal cord, could also localize to the mesencephalon, the cerebral "skin," and the meninges.

Ellis, in that same year, described three hyperkinetic cases in England (Ellis, 1920). All three were characterized by vomiting, followed by severe pain in two, delirium, insomnia, and, most strikingly, forceful shock-like contractions of the abdominal muscles. All three showed a marked leucocytosis and widely dilated pupils. All died. Ellis was also not convinced that these cases were the same as EL, particularly because of the leucocytosis and the dilated pupils, which were not common in EL. He speculated that, if these cases were EL, then the virus had fundamentally changed or had found a new localization in the nervous system.

In the United States in 1920, J. Ramsey Hunt, a very well-respected neurologist at the New York Neurological Institute, published a description of hyperkinetic cases (he referred to the condition as "myoclonus multiplex"). He stated that these cases existed both in sporadic and epidemic forms and suggested that the hyperkinetic form was clearly part of the spectrum of EL because it occurred at the same time, and because of the various mixed forms that he had seen (e.g., hyperkinetic forms with cranial nerve palsies). Interestingly, he described two cases of the sporadic form of EL that dated to 1904 and 1914, indicating to him that EL had existed in unrecognized forms prior to von Economo's 1917 description.

Ramsay Hunt (1920) stated that the hyperkinetic form of EL began abruptly with pain that increased rapidly in intensity and became generalized, causing great suffering. Muscle jerks and twitching followed either immediately or after a few days and usually continued after the pain had resolved. All types of muscle contractions could be apparent including fibrillations, muscle waves (myokymia), and contractions of the whole body of a muscle (myoclonus). He also stated, "One of the most striking symptoms was the severity of involvement of the abdomen in all of the cases. This is rather significant, as I have not observed it in anything like the same degree in myoclonus and myokymia multiplex from other causes" (p. 717).

In his 1929 monograph, von Economo stated that, in his first EL publications, he mentioned that athetosis may occasionally accompany the somnolent-ophthalmoplegic form of EL. Accordingly, one of his original cases (case 7) was reported to exhibit "choretic unrest," with stupor, and with bilateral Babinski signs; and, his case 10 showed hyperkinesia of the lower limbs on the day she died.

Von Economo (1929) reported that the hyperkinetic form was very prevalent in Europe in the winter of 1920. Violent pain in the limbs and face was a common initial sign. This was followed by general mental unrest and ceaseless motor activity, with the latter lasting for days and nights without stopping. The patient then typically became delirious, with hallucinations and sleep inversion or insomnia. Von Economo stated that, typically, these patients had unequal and miotic pupils with a sluggish or diminished response. Next, the patients typically showed choretic movements that interfered with normal movements, as in St. Vitus' dance (Sydenham chorea), to such a degree that it was sometimes necessary to put the patients in restraints to prevent self-injury. Myoclonic movements occurred at the same time, accompanied by lancinating pains. Abdominal myoclonus was especially prevalent.

Von Economo related the movement disorders to lesions within the diencephalon, or the striatal or para-striatal systems, although he also thought they might be due to "toxic factors" affecting the whole brain. He observed the patients also showed fascicular twitches, which are due to the inflammatory processes affecting anterior horn cells. He indicated that all the observed cases that had fascicular twitches showed changes in the anterior horn cells upon autopsy. If they didn't die, many of the hyperkinetic patients became somnolent, with ocular signs including ptosis. Sleep became continuous, presumably accompanied by a posterior shift in the center of cerebral inflammation. Other hyperkinetic patients became parkinsonian.

Von Economo indicated that hyperkinetic EL patients may die during any stage, and exhaustion may be responsible. He noted that sequelae are more prevalent in the hyperkinetic form than in the somnolent form. Finally, he stated that the highest incidence of the hyperkinetic form occurred at the same time as the great influenza epidemic and that, in recent years, he had not seen a single case of hyperkinetic EL—rather, they had all been of the somnolent-ophthalmoplegic type.

In Smith's 1921 survey of the symptoms associated with EL in the United States, he reported that tremors occurred in more than 80% of EL patients, whereas choreic movements occurred in less than 20%. Surprisingly, von Economo never mentioned tremor in association with the hyperkinetic form and indicated that it was rare in the amyostatic-akinetic form. However, Ramsay Hunt reported that tremor typically occurred early in the amyostatic-akinetic form of EL. He also stated that choreiform movements may be generalized or localized, and were essential for the neostriatal (choreiform) type of EL (Ramsay Hunt, 1921).

Tilney and Howe's 1920 monograph on EL does not list an EL type that is similar in symptomatology to von Economo's hyperkinetic form. Two cases, however, are described with chorea and myoclonus, but each began with some symptoms associated with the somnolent-ophthalmoplegic form, as well as movement disorders. Hall, in his 1924 monograph, stated that the symptomatology of the hyperkinetic forms, especially during the early 1920s, was in such contrast to the lethargic forms that their relationship to EL was initially obscure. Riley (1930) indicated that hyperkinetic movements typically occur in the chronic form of the disease and result from basal ganglia involvement, which releases lower nervous processes from higher control. Riley also stated that, "As a rule, diagnosis [of EL] depends on the presence of a low-grade infectious process, associated with lethargy, diplopia, headache and most of all, evidence of dissemination of the lesions throughout the length and breadth of the nervous system" (p. 598).

Neal (1942) noted that hyperkinetic cases were often very severe, and the patients were in great pain, with likely intractable insomnia and great psychomotor activity. However, she also stated that she had never seen such severe cases as those described by von Economo. In her series of 150 New York City cases between 1929 and 1940, she noted that about 12% showed some degree of hyperkinesia. Primarily, the hyperkinesia consisted of fascicular twitches of isolated muscle groups, myoclonias, and choreoathoid and dystonic movements.

Two recent textbooks on encephalitis (Johnson, 1998; Booss & Esiri, 2003) do not associate hyperkinetic movements with any form of human encephalitis. Choreoathetosis has infrequently been found in association with herpes simplex encephalitis, with a recent case of an 8-year-old showing good MRI indications of a lesion in the medial thalamus (Kullnat & Morse, 2008).

This lack of association between hyperkinetic movements and any other type of encephalitis reduces the diagnostic value of this sign relative to EL. This is especially the case because, even during the epidemic period, clinicians initially had difficulty accepting this form of the disease. Furthermore, hyperkinetic cases of EL seem primarily to have been prevalent during the peak of the epidemic period, and not later.

Criterion 7. Mental Changes (e.g., Obsessive-Compulsive
Behaviors/Akinetic Mutism)

In his compilation of the signs and symptoms of EL in the United States, Smith did not include any pertaining to mental illness (Fig. 2.4, Chapter 2). However, von Economo (1929) described somnolent-ophthalmoplegic EL patients as often dazed and confused and slightly delirious (hallucinations); they displayed excessive talking, and were apprehensive and restless. Earlier (1917), he referred to EL patients as being "psychically weakened." Nevertheless, they were fully cognizant of their condition and in that way were different from schizophrenics. Stern (1928) similarly stated that delirium did not necessarily accompany the somnolence of EL.

Von Economo in 1929 did describe a relatively rare psychotic type of EL in which only psychiatric signs were initially apparent. Similarly, Kasanin and Petersen (1926) presented four cases in which EL began only with psychiatric signs such as restlessness, agitation, delusions, rambling speech, mutism, and rigidity. Again, however, in this type of EL, cognitive deterioration was not typical. The personal descriptions of EL provided in Chapter 11 suggest that some of the psychiatric signs are associated with a constant feeling of restlessness or hyperactivity rather than being a primary sign.

Wilson (1940) in his review of acute EL said that delirium may alternate with apathy or lethargy, and that mental impairment is seen in reduced attention, orientation, and memory. However, Wilson added a caveat: "[Y]et, even at the height of the illness response to demands is often, surprisingly, rational; the patient can sometimes lift himself to a practically normal level even when conduct and reactions seem 'insane'" (p. 107).

Howard and Lees (1987) described both obsessive-compulsive behavior and akinetic mutism as occurring in acute EL. We can find no indication that obsessive-compulsive behavior was typically exhibited during the EL epidemic period. Howard and Lees also noted that compulsive coprolalia was a sign of acute EL. However, their cited sources refer to chronic EL patients. Akinetic mutism would be consistent with von Economo's amyostatic-akinetic type of EL.

Rail et al. (1981) simply listed "mental changes" as occurring in acute EL and cited an article by Duncan, published in 1924, as a source. However, the Duncan article referred to the *sequelae* of EL, not to signs that occur during the acute phase. Duncan described some of the mental sequelae he observed in his patients, such as defective memory, alteration in disposition, neuroses and psychoneuroses, mental deficiency, manic-depression, and hallucinations. He reported that severe mental sequelae were most common in children under 10 (about 40%) and least common in 21- to 30-year-olds (about 10%).

Psychiatric changes were a very important component of the EL diagnosis within the Soviet Union (Vilensky et al., 2008). Geimanovich (1928) suggested that patients were psychologically "rigid," lacking the ability to inhibit impulses. Margulis (1926) reported that EL patients exhibited changes in personality, agitation, hallucinations, and mental confusion.

This analysis raises the issue of whether the psychiatric components of EL can really be separated from the somatic components. And, as in some of the previously proposed criteria, are these psychiatric factors part of the acute or chronic forms of EL, or part of both? Our suggestion is that psychiatric signs should not be a major component of the differential diagnosis of EL.

Criterion 8. Corticospinal Tract Signs

Rail et al. (1981) listed "corticospinal tract signs" as one criterion for an EL diagnosis. Unfortunately, they did not specifically state what they meant by "corticospinal tract signs." However, all of the patients referred to in their 1981 article as exhibiting such signs showed a Babinski response, so that it is likely that this is the specific corticospinal sign the authors were referring to.

In his original 1917 article, von Economo stated that Babinski responses were often present initially in EL and could persist for a long time, including after the ocular signs had receded. Von Economo reiterated in 1929 that Babinski responses were often present. He accounted for this by noting the close topographical relationship between the inflammatory processes in the pons and medulla, and the pyramidal tract.

In his 1921 survey, Smith found that a high percentage of EL patients in the United States exhibited the Babinski sign (approximately 65%). Wilson (1940) stated that pyramidal signs occurred only early in the progression of the disease.

In contrast, Ramsay Hunt (1920) never observed a Babinski response in his EL patients: "In passing I might say that my experience has been that these pyramidal tract signs are not common, and when they are found they occur late and in the severe cases" (p. 144).

In general, Babinski responses were not commonly recorded in the case descriptions of EL patients. We don't believe the presence or absence of this sign has diagnostic value pertaining to EL.

Criterion 9. Respiratory Symptoms (Respiratory Disturbances/Central Respiratory Irregularities)

Similar to OCs, respiratory disturbances were not present in the initial descriptions of EL. The only respiratory disturbance listed among von Economo's original cases was singultus in one case. Accordingly, Smith (1921) did not list any respiratory signs associated with EL in his chart of EL symptomatology (Chapter 2; Fig. 5.2).

Turner and Critchley (1925) specifically stated that the first example of respiratory abnormalities accompanying EL occurred in 1920, and we could find no evidence contrary to that assertion. Parker (1922) summarized prior reports pertaining to respiratory disturbances, noting that:

1. In the 115 cases analyzed by Dunn in 1920, three patients had hyperpnea that lasted a few days;
2. Sicard and Paraf, in 1921, described a series of patients who suffered from a variety of paroxysmal respiratory disturbances, including hiccups, yawning, stretching, sobbing, and uncontrollable laughing; and,
3. Aronson, in 1921, reported on an 8-year-old boy who, during his recovery from encephalitis, developed hyperpnea that lasted for 7 weeks.

In observing his own patients, Parker (1922) reported that the syndrome consisted of assuming erect posture, breathing noisily, holding the breath with bodily contortions, and releasing the breath in a position best suited for complete expiration. "The epidemic of encephalitis provided many strange and bizarre

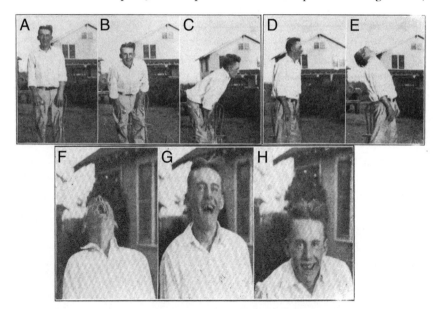

Figure 5.2 Demonstration of respiratory "syndrome" in chronic EL. Positions B–D were repeated from two to seven times before position E was assumed (from Rayburn, 1929).

pictures, but few surpassed the appearance of these little children at the height of their illness" (p. 637).

Bernard (1923) analyzed the cases of respiratory disorders associated with EL/PEP to date, and divided the disorders into eight groups:

1. Disorders of thoracic expansion
2. Tachypnea and bradypnea
3. Respiratory pauses
4. Dyspnea with vasomotor disturbances
5. Inversion of the respiratory formulas or rhythms
6. Sighs
7. Respiratory disorders associated with myoclonus
8. Respiratory tics

For PEP, Bernard (1923) described a much-reduced increase in thoracic "ampliation" (referring to the increase in circumference of the thorax during inspiration) from approximately 6 cm in healthy adults to 1.5 cm. He reported that the intercostal spaces dilated and the thoracic shape became globular, as in emphysema. This resulted because of rigidity, including rigidity of the diaphragm, which was observed fluoroscopically. Bernard noted that, whereas the amplitude of movements of the central part of the diaphragm remained normal, the peripheral part was much reduced, as was apparent from the unchanging costodiaphragmatic recesses. Thus, during inspiration, the abdomen played a much larger role than in normal individuals, in which thoracic expansion predominated. Because of this reduction in thoracic movements, patients showed tachypnea. Tachypnea was also described as occurring in acute EL, with a respiratory rate of up to 80 breaths/minute. It could occur paroxysmally, especially at night, or be permanent, although it was not present during sleep. Rarely, the patients exhibited bradypnea.

Another respiratory phenomenon exhibited by patients was pauses, which differed from the apnea of Cheyne-Stokes. These patients gave the impression that they simply forgot to breathe. Patients often had crises of dyspnea that appeared at night, often associated with anxiety, cyanosis, and a cold feeling in the extremities (Bernard, 1923).

Bernard (1923) reported that, in EL patients, the inhalation phase often was longer than the expiratory phase, which is the reverse of normal except during sleep (so that these patients breathed as if they were asleep). Furthermore, in many patients, the respirations were very inconsistent, suggesting that different fascicles of the diaphragm were contracting with each breath. Sighing was very frequent in EL patients, with long inhales and exhales. This may have "liberated" the patient to resume a normal breathing pattern.

Bernard indicated that respiratory tics and spasmodic coughing were often found in children. During expiration, the air shoots through the nose with a bellowing noise—it appeared as if the patient was trying to blow out a candle using his nose. Their spasmodic coughing was a dry with expectorant. Bernard concluded that the respiratory problems in EL could be based on one of two etiologies: lesions of the respiratory control centers or muscular rigidity, and he noted that, in contrast to PEP, patients, patients with Parkinson disease do not exhibit pauses, sighing, or irregular breathing patterns (Bernard, 1923).

Symonds (in Buzzard, 1923) observed EL cases in which the patient exhibited gasping movements over which he had control. One patient described a sensation of impeded respiration and suffocation that he tried to alleviate by breathing deeply and energetically. Similarly, another patient had a constant sensation of nasal obstruction, causing repetitive blowing of the nose and sniffing.

Hall (1924), in his monograph, reported that disturbances of respiration were frequently noted in the acute stage of EL. In addition to increases in frequency, changes in rhythm of various kinds have been described. Respiratory symptoms may also occur as residua. He cited a 1922 report by Marie et al. dividing these symptoms into three categories: change in rhythm, spasmodic cough, and respiratory tics and abnormal rhinolaryngeal sensations. Respiratory tics were described as taking many forms, including sniffing, blowing, and spitting. In some cases, rhythmic contractions of muscles occurred with each inspiration.

Wimmer (1924), in his monograph on chronic EL, stated, "The peculiar grotesque pictures afforded by these respiratory disorders, their coincidence with psychotic, general nervous, 'hysteriform' or 'neurastheniform' troubles, their being 'punctual to the hour,' their liability to being influenced by psychic factors, and, finally, their frequent monosymptomatic appearance, at any rate for a time, all these features may delude one into conceiving them as purely hysterical. In addition, they often show a considerable resemblance to the respiratory disturbances found in true hysteria" (p. 71). Wimmer also noted that, "A psychogenic blending cannot, of course, be totally disregarded," because of the anxiety displayed by EL patients.

Jelliffe (1927) published an entire monograph on postencephalitic respiratory disturbances, similar to the one he did on OCs (see above), insisting that these abnormalities also occur in the acute phase and referred to a pneumographic study of respiratory alterations occurring in the acute phase of EL. The report found that the respiratory quotient tended to be modified, in that inspiration was longer than expiration and that interruptions in the rhythm were constant (as also described by Bernard, 1923; see above).

Because of his psychosomatic orientation, Jelliffe (1927) suggested that apnea may be viewed as the EL patient trying to strangle himself (self-destruction wish) and agreed that, similar to Wimmer (1924), psychogenic factors may influence the specific phenomenon observed.

In 1929, Von Economo stated that myoclonic twitches of the diaphragm or of isolated parts of the diaphragm were often the cause of hiccup; he was, however, unsure whether epidemic hiccup (see Chapter 2) was EL. Von Economo also stated that other kinds of respiratory abnormalities have occasionally been observed, such as increased rate of respiration, exaggerated respiratory movements of the nostrils, asymmetries of the movements of the halves of the thorax, dissociation of the respiratory rates of the left and right sides, staccato breathing, and other disturbances of inspiration as well as expiration (e.g., myoclonic breathing paroxysms). Chronically, hyperpnea with forced expiration was most frequently seen. Also, he observed that bradypnea, apnea, irregular respirations, nervous cough, spastic cough, sighing, and tics of respiration may occur.

Wilson (1940) indicated that disturbances of breathing may occur early or late in EL. He reported that the disturbances could include (a) altered form and frequency of automatic breathing, (b) respiratory spasms, and (c) respiratory tics.

Respiratory anomalies seem inherent to both the acute and chronic stages of EL, but as with other EL signs, vary greatly in their phenotype. Nothing about them seems particularly diagnostic, although clearly their presence could support an EL diagnosis.

EVALUATION OF POST–1940 REPORTS ON EL

As detailed in Chapter 2 and here, clinicians of the period could not decide on specific criteria by which to conclude that any single patient had EL. Some of them commented that, rather than any single sign/symptom, it was the unusual combination of signs and symptoms that resulted in their diagnosis. Similarly, although the post-1940 criteria compiled by Rail et al. (1981) and Howards and Lees (1987) have merit, both are problematic.

During an epidemic period, diagnosis of ambiguous cases as EL would seem to have some justification. However, diagnoses of ambiguous sporadic cases are much less justified (Pilz & Erhart, 1978). Although EL since 1940 (assuming EL has occurred since then) may have manifested in as many types as were thought to exist during the epidemic period (Table 2.3), comments were made during the period that some of these types were no longer apparent (e.g., hyperkinetic type, see above). Thus, it would be our recommendation that a diagnosis of EL be confined to what was considered the primary (somnolent-ophthalmoplegic) type of EL as originally described by von Economo in 1917; that is, a patient whose signs and symptoms cannot be attributed to any known neurological disease based on clinical examination, serological testing, or imaging studies, and who shows the following signs (see also Chapter 12):

1. *Influenza-like signs*: Relatively recently, but prior to subsequent EL signs/symptoms (days to weeks), patient should have had influenza-like (cold-like) signs/symptoms.
2. *Hypersomnolence*: The patient should sleep (or have slept) for abnormally long periods—days, weeks, months. Sleep should be relatively natural in form (not comatose). Desire for sleep should be overwhelming.
3. *Wakability*: The patient should, at least initially, be relatively easy to rouse and should be aware of time, place, and condition.
4. *Ophthalmoplegia*: One or more (ideally more than one) of the following signs should be present: ptosis, strabismus, diplopia, weakness of convergence, nystagmus, unequal pupils, defective reactions to light, defective reaction on convergence and accommodation, or Argyll-Robertson pupils.
5. *Psychiatric changes*: Children with EL should show profound (negative) changes in emotional behavior; most likely showing aggression, agitation, and/or apathy, but they should also recognize that these behaviors are not socially acceptable. Adults should show mild changes characterized by some emotional rigidity and apathy; mild delirium is possible. Similar to children, they should be aware of their condition.

A criterion that might be included, and that some investigators have considered to be pathognomonic for EL, would be the subsequent development of signs and symptoms consistent with PEP, especially OCs. Based on the analysis presented here and also our discussion of the relationship between EL and PEP presented in Chapter 7, we have not considered PEP signs/symptoms by themselves to be pathognomonic for EL. However, the presence of OCs in an individual who showed some of the other classic somnolent-ophthalmoplegic signs would seem to be consistent with EL. Nevertheless, we want to reemphasize that, during the epidemic period, OCs were virtually never associated with acute EL and have become associated with acute EL only with more recent cases. Therefore, OCs in many recent cases possibly reflect response to medications rather than an inherent part of an acute EL syndrome.

Table 5.4 lists and provides some descriptive information on all of the post-1940 cases of EL reported in the West. In the last column, we provide *our* view as to whether the cases described should be considered as EL, with a brief justification based primarily on the five features listed above. Thus, we are only accepting somnolent-opthamaloplegic cases as most likely being modern cases of EL. Of the 59 reports listed, we consider only 14 to have presented either a case or cases that we would accept as being consistent with a diagnosis of EL.

The post-1940 history of EL in the Soviet Union (Russia) appears to be somewhat different from that of other countries because EL seems to have occurred there at greater frequencies. Accordingly, because of the relatively high number of cases, our inability to separate the cases pre- and post-1940, and the more general nature of the reports, data from the Soviet Union were placed in a separate table (Table 5.5). In 1961, Ulitovsky published an EL review article for the European, Ural Mountain, Mid-Asian, and Dalny Vostok regions of the USSR, and much of the data from Table 5.5 are derived from that review (we are very grateful to Drs. Yuriy and Igor Zhukov for translating this article for us).

Although Table 5.5 indeed suggests a greater post-1940 frequency of EL in the Soviet Union than in the West, some of the case data in Table 5.5 include chronic cases, who likely had their acute episodes during the epidemic period. Thus, the differences in frequency may be more apparent than real. Furthermore, because few specific patient descriptions exist, we did not attempt to determine whether the reports are consistent with a diagnosis of EL. However, as is apparent from Table 5.5, many of the Soviet reports emphasize the hyperkinetic type of EL, which we do not accept for the Western cases.

CONCLUSIONS ON DIAGNOSIS

Encephalitis lethargica cases have been described regularly since 1940, although the reliability of the diagnosis remains limited. In this chapter, we evaluated all of the post-1940 cases based on the original type description of EL—somnolent/ophthalmoplegic—and found that most are not consistent with that typology. Certainly, during the epidemic period, many other types of EL were generally accepted, but some authorities believed that EL was being significantly overdiagnosed (see Chapter 2) and, unfortunately, acceptance of these myriad types outside of an epidemic period permits virtually any neurologic illness to be considered EL. We thus recommend that, until the etiology of EL becomes known, the diagnostic criteria should be limited; it seems that only with such a limitation, unless there is another epidemic, will progress be made on understanding this disease (see Chapter 12).

Table 5.4 Post-1940 Western Cases of Encephalitis Lethargica (EL)

Reference	Patient Data	Treatment/Pathology	Our Evaluation Signs/Symptoms
Lambruschini, 1941 (Argentina)	31 M; somnolence, ptosis, facial paralysis, upper extremity paresis, mental cloudiness; died 6 days after hospitalization	Numerous hemorrhages in white and gray matter of frontal and occipital lobes, hippocampal area, and region of third ventricle; also tumor in temporal-occipital lobe, but author does not attribute EL symptoms to tumor	No initial influenza-like phase, but all other characteristics consistent; seems likely EL
Maciel, 1941 (Brazil)	22 M; sleep inversion only symptom/sign; author considered this new type of EL (monosymptomatic)	Cured with sodium salicylate	Unlikely EL: no cranial nerve or ocular signs
Schulte, 1941 (Germany)	29 M, ?M; two more cases with sex and age not stated; atypical vestibular form: dizziness, ataxia, nystagmus, facial weakness, nausea; all showed virtually complete recovery within a few months		Unlikely EL; "vestibular" form not very apparent during epidemic period
Benedek & Augyal, 1944 (Germany)	18, 30, 34, 36, 39, 43, 48, 53(2), 56 M; 33, 36, 43 F; Babinski, choking fits (one case), headache, insomnia, vertigo, vomiting, diplopia, nystagmus, ataxia, anisocoria, dizziness, diplopia; ataxia; sexual psychopathy		Unlikely EL; primary symptom in patients related to vestibular dysfunction (vertigo, dizziness)
Ernsting, 1946 (Holland)	33M; EL believed to be triggered by fall on head at age 9; emotional lability; currently has PEP signs/symptoms		Trauma to head not likely to cause EL; may have PD: unlikely EL

Leigh, 1946 (England)	38M; 18F; drowsiness and appearance of symptoms associated with nuclear brainstem lesions; diplopia, ptosis, bad-tempered; one patient showed complete recovery and the other much improvement	Sulfathiazole administered; treated with daily injections of "hepolon"; male patient also suffered from Hand-Schüller-Christian disease	Authors diagnose patients with influenza encephalitis, but very consistent with EL
van Deinse, 1946 (Holland)	27F; sinusitis, syncope after injection for typhus, somnolent	Surgery for sinusitis reduced symptoms	Unlikely EL, sinusitis; visual abnormalities
Drobec & Tschabitscher, 1948 (Austria)	38F; 48F; neuritic forms of EL, headache, vertigo, insomnia, nystagmus, weakness, numb hands and feet, tremor, upper extremity weakness, chorea, inability to walk, mentally unstable	Improved with galvanic stimulation of the extremities; sodium salicylate without effect	Unlikely EL (neuritic form?)
Keyserlingk, 1949 (Germany)	28, 48 M; 17, 51 F; all vestibular type; vertigo, ataxia, dysarthria, diplopia, nausea, nystagmus, headache		Primary symptoms vestibular–unlikely EL
Zeiszl, 1949 (Germany)	One case (sex and age not given); neuritic form of EL with sleep disorders and paralysis of axillary and subscapular nerves; extensive remission after 5 weeks		Unlikely EL (neuritic form?)
Geerling, 1950 (South Africa)	100 cases over the last 19 years; called encephalitis africana; various "types" very similar to EL; PEP very common; mild irritability, schizophrenia; confusional states; differentiated from other forms of encephalitis by lack of high temperature; (author does not designate these cases EL but does note that PEP is only common in EL and that this form of encephalitis and EL similarly were not characterized by high temperature	Various sulfonamides; penicillin and streptomycin did not reduce symptoms	Only "ocular" type would be consistent with our definition of EL; does not state how many patients of this type

(Continued)

Table 5.4 continued

Reference	Patient Data	Treatment/Pathology	Our Evaluation Signs/Symptoms
Bickerstaff & Cloake, 1951 (England)	36 M; 24 F(2); drowsiness, oculomotor and facial palsies; ataxia and in two cases total bulbar paralysis and anarthria; catatonia; mania; all three recovered completely; (authors do not believe EL because of severity of symptoms and no sleep inversion, but others have considered these to be EL cases)		No initial influenza-like phase (although slight fever) but all other characteristics consistent; seems likely EL
Nielsen, 1953 (U.S.)	Seven cases EL/PEP but only three appeared to have developed EL after 1940; 33, 34, 38 M; paranoia; fractional Babinski; various parkinsonian signs following earlier acute illness; confusion; trauma precipitated PEP in one case		Patients tended not to have sleep or ocular disturbances; unlikely EL
Wolf, 1953 (Germany)	23 M; headache, pain, drowsiness, followed by development of parkinsonism	Treated with Parpanit (caramiphen hydrochloride)	No ocular signs; unlikely EL
Brewis, 1954 (England)	Describes 93 cases of encephalitis in children; divides into four types, of which type 4 "resembles EL"; 17 cases within type 4 but only five of unknown etiology that could be thus classified as possible EL, with details presented on one case (4 M); masked face; pseudosomnolence; dysphagia; cogwheel rigidity; shallow breathing; mental and emotional instability		Unlikely EL; no ocular signs and no initial influenza-like symptoms

Espir & Spalding, 1956 (England, but two cases from British soldiers stationed in Germany)	16, 19, 28 M; in case 1, PEP developed three years after apparent recovery from EL with hiccups; whereas cases 2 and 3 occurred within a few days of each other in Germany and EL merged into PEP; mutism, pseudosomnolence, Babinski, labile emotional behavior, aggression, ocular signs, fever	Artane (benzhexol hydrochloride)	Likely EL
Machetanz, 1958 (Germany)	13F; PEP with OCs; reported because rare finding in young person		No evidence of influenza-like phase; unlikely EL
Levy, 1959 (U.S.)	100 cases of postencephalitic behavioral disorder in children; 72 males and 26 females; children were hyperactive and destructive; had some earlier illness/trauma that precipitated the behavioral disorder; short attention and concentration spans (details on three cases)	Treated very successfully with Benzedrine sulfate	No evidence of EL
Dobrzynska, 1965 (Poland)	14, 19 F; in case 1 bradykinesia, sleep inversion, catalepsy; development of PEP unilaterally; case 2 had opsoclonus and PEP 5 months after acute illness	Treated with anti-parkinsonian drugs	Both patients initially showed influenza-like signs; very consistent with EL; likely EL
Hunter & Jones, 1966 (England)	?M; 21, 27, 38, 54 F; all six patients were seen in a 3-month period in a psychiatric unit with a combination of cerebral, hypothalamic, and midbrain involvement suggesting EL (confusion, lethargy, sleep disorders, visual disturbances, catatonia, paranoia, irritability, delirium)	Three patients showed dramatic improvement after lumbar puncture	Psychiatric symptoms predominate: unlikely EL

(Continued)

Table 5.4 continued

Reference	Patient Data	Treatment/Pathology	Our Evaluation Signs/Symptoms
Doichinov, 1968 (Bulgaria)	22 F; acute onset followed by parkinsonian signs within 7 days; sleep disturbances; anxiety; completely recovered with signs becoming stationary at 52 days		Definite initial influenza-like signs; unclear whether there were ocular signs; possibly EL
Bojinov, 1971 (Bulgaria)	11, 26 M; 4.5 5.5, 7, 11, 15, 22, 28, 33, 35 F; four died; onset characterized by high fever, headache, vertigo, ocular signs, dyspnea, catalepsy, anxiety, parkinsonian signs; peak between days 7 and 30 and then recede completely or incompletely; residual symptoms static (5-year follow-up); diplopia, ptosis, in one case; possible OCs in one case; disturbed sleep	Postmortem in four cases indicated lesions of brain stem nuclei and severe bilateral destruction of the substantia nigra with perivascular cuffing; treatments included Aturbane, Artane, which alleviated some of the parkinsonian signs	From the details provided on eight cases, very consistent with EL
Misra & Hay, 1971 (England)	18, 19 M; 45 F; all cases presented initially with symptoms of schizophrenia, but later developed signs of encephalitis, hallucinations, Babinski; one case developed PEP	Corticotrophin; one responded very positively to treatment with electroconvulsive therapy	Psychiatric symptoms predominate; unlikely EL
Herishanu & Noah, 1973 (Israel)	2 M; seizures, coma, akinesia, cogwheel rigidity, masked face, shuffling and broad gait, excitation, restlessness, aggression; CSF virus culture grew an enterovirus; complete recovery	Treated with amantadine	Not consistent with EL

Reference	Clinical features	Treatment	Comments
Bonduelle et al., 1975 (France)	16F; hypersomnolence (two successive periods of a few days), pseudosomnolence, headaches, probable strabismus, nausea; increased titre for Coxsackie A2 antibody		No initial influenza-like period; unlikely EL
Pruskauer-Apostol et al., 1977 (Romania)	12, 17, 23F; all three had PEP immediately following presumptive acute EL (headache, fever), Babinski, anxiety	All were successfully treated with L-dopa	Only one showed hypersomnolence; unlikely EL
Pilz & Erhart, 1978 (Austria)	41 M; nausea, somnolence, masked face, emotional lability; 16-fold increase in herpes titre; no PEP	Treated with Vibramycin (doxycycline), dexamethasone and synanthem	No ocular signs; unlikely EL
Gulmann & Pedersen, 1980 (Denmark)	28F; originally diagnosed with Wernicke encephalopathy but later developed PEP; soporific, compulsive weeping	Biperiden (Akineton) markedly reduced PEP symptoms; L-dopa treatment resulted in minimal, if any, improvement	Not consistent with EL
Rail et al., 1981 (England)	29, 32, 43, 44, 50 M; 20, 43, 40 F; all but two developed PEP with initial putative EL episodes 1953–1976; pseudosomnolence, ptosis, OCs in two cases, Babinski, respiratory disturbances, impaired concentration, restlessness, aggression, hallucinations, depression; these authors put forth nine criteria by which EL can be diagnosed (see text)	Treatments included electroconvulsive therapy, imipramine, benzodiazepine, L-dopa, anticholinergics, bromocriptine, dexamethasone, stramonium and benzhexol with variable results (two patients were unresponsive to L-dopa).	EL diagnosis in these cases mainly based on development of PEP; prior hypersomnolent episodes not typically present; not consistent with EL

(Continued)

Table 5.4 continued

Reference	Patient Data	Treatment/Pathology	Our Evaluation Signs/Symptoms
Greenough & Davis, 1983 (England)	11 M (2); 12 F; three presented cases are representative of children who had psychiatric or neurologic symptoms after viral illness (hallucinations, aggression, depression, emotional lability); besides typical EL signs, one had one episode of OCs after a single dose of haloperidol, two had masked face, and one had aggressive feelings toward his family; no serological evidence of viral infection	Haloperidol	Only one showed ocular signs, but other signs very consistent with EL in children: likely EL
Howard & Lees, 1987 (England)	17, 23, 31, 63 F; all had psychiatric disturbances (catatonia, agitation, emotional lability, aggression, mental retardation) sleep inversion, drowsiness, OCs, grasp reflex, rigidity, facial weakness, diplopia, masked face, drowsiness, ptosis, tremor, Babinski, cogwheel rigidity, respiratory abnormalities; three showed cerebrospinal fluid (CSF) oligoclonal IgG banding; one died, and the others did not exhibit notable recovery; authors put forth seven criteria by which EL can be diagnosed (see text)	Autopsy in case 2 showed inflammatory changes throughout cerebral hemispheres, subcortical region and brainstem; in substantia nigra there was mild diffuse neuronal loss	Seems consistent with EL.

Johnson & Lucey, 1987 (England)	17, 23 M; catatonic stupor with compulsive behaviors, akinetic mutism, sleep inversion, flexibilitas cerea, blepharospasm	Treated with sodium pentothal; L-dopa, benserazide; Case 1 markedly improved after 14 electroconvulsive therapy treatments and subsequently improved more with L-dopa; case 2 improved after 12 electroconvulsive treatments	Psychiatric symptoms predominate; unlikely EL
Al-Mateen et al., 1988 (U.S.)	9.5 F; fever, cough, no response to speech, comatose, choreiform movements, sialorrhea, dysphagia, reduced attention span; serologically positive for *Mycoplasma pneumoniae*	CT showed low density lesion in right caudate; MRI suggested inflammatory processes in caudate, putamen, and globus pallidus; improvement with L-dopa treatment although cognitive deficits remain	Not consistent with EL
Kapadia & Grant, 1990 (Scotland)	19 F; hyperactive, obsessive-compulsive, depression, confusion, no focal neurological signs, cranial nerves normal, eyelid twitches, opisthotonus, OCs	CT and MRI normal; treated with midazolam, diazepam, phenytoin, phenobarbitone, clonazepam, thiopentone, propofol	Psychiatric symptoms predominate; unlikely EL
Mellon et al., 1991 (England)	5 M; lethargic, difficult to rouse, headache, masked face, dysphagia, cogwheel rigidity, fecal incontinence; complete recovery	CT normal	No ocular signs but otherwise consistent for child; likely EL
Protheroe & Mellor, 1991 (England)	4 M; 11 F; encephalitis developed within 3 days of respiratory symptoms associated with recent influenza outbreak; seizures, decorticate posturing, akinetic mutism, behavioral problems, Babinski, masked face	Both cases had serological evidence of recent influenza infection; treated with acyclovir, thiamine and dexamethasone; CT showed hypodense regions in thalami; MRI in 1 case showed lesion in pons	Limited ocular signs but generally consistent with EL in children

(Continued)

Table 5.4 continued

Reference	Patient Data	Treatment/Pathology	Our Evaluation Signs/Symptoms
Dolan & Kamil, 1992 (Canada)	23M; sleep inversion, sexually inappropriate behavior, violent behavior, OCs, sialorrhea, masked face, resting tremor, cogwheel rigidity	Treated with thioridazine, chlorpromazine, pipotiazine; CT and MRI normal	No initial influenza-like phase and no initial ocular signs; unlikely EL
Motta et al., 1994 (Poland)	57 F; excessive somnolence (pseudosomnolence), diplopia, ptosis, nystagmus, mental slowness, breathing disturbances	Treated with mannitol, Isoprinosine; CT/MRI showed small-scale cortical and subcortical atrophies	No statement of initial influenza-like stage, but otherwise seems very consistent with EL
Barletta et al., 1995 (Italy)	34 M; fever, confusion, nausea, bradykinesia, bradyphrenia, somnolence, akinetic mutism, ptosis, compulsive behavior, facial paralysis; complete recovery after 5 years	Patients responded well to corticosteroid treatment; side effects of L-dopa negated any effectiveness; CT initially showed diffuse edema; CT/MRI later showed lesions in left pons, right medulla, right thalamus and right parasagittal frontal region	Consistent with EL
Dekleva & Husain, 1995 (U.S.)	34 F; seizures, opisthotonus, catatonia, hallucinations, labile mood, unresponsiveness, flailing of muscles, rigidity, OCs, respiratory crises	Treatment included haloperidol, dantrolene, bromocriptine, pancuronium, diazepam, lorazepam; diphenhydramine; L-dopa did not provide any improvement; 16 electroconvulsive therapy treatments resulted in marked reduction of symptoms	No initial influenza-like stage and no hypersomnolence; unlikely EL

(Continued)

Picard et al., 1996 (France)	42 M; EL at age 5 followed by development of parkinsonian signs; OCs upon awakening from EL coma; upon L-dopa withdrawal at age 40 akinetic, dystonic, and dyskinetic signs appeared	L-dopa treatment suppressed all extrapyramidal signs; CT/MRI showed no major brain lesions, but PET showed bilateral damage to dopaminergic nigrostriatal pathway; suggest virus caused lesion of zona compacta of substantia nigra	seems consistent with EL
Blunt et al., 1997 (England)	23, 26 F; psychosis, akinetic mutism, myoclonus, OCs, catatonia, aggression, agitation, confusion, delusions, chewing movements, lead-pipe rigidity, severe dyskinesia, glaring expression, clawing movements, jerking movements in arms and legs; in both cases CSF oligoclonal banding present	Myoclonus responded to clonazepam; also treated with chlorpromazine, dantrolene, apomorphine, procyclidine; L-dopa improved dyskinesias; methylprednisolone resulted in sustained improvement; CT normal	No hypersomnolence; unlikely EL
Kun et al., 1999 (Singapore)	33 F; ophthalmoplegia, akinetic mutism, extrapyramidal signs, facial bradykinesia, tremor	MRI showed hyperintense lesions bilaterally in substantia nigra; responded to treatment with L-dopa, selegiline, bromocriptine	No hypersomnolence; unlikely EL
McAuley et al., 1999 (England)	16 F; sialorrhea, irregular breathing, catatonia, aggression, rigidity, ophthalmoplegia	MRI normal; needle biopsy frontal cortex revealed non-specific inflammatory changes; apomorphine infusion resulted in improvement; acyclovir used; no response to methylprednisolone; L-dopa also showed continuous benefits with no significant side effects	No hypersomnolence; unlikely EL

Table 5.4 continued

Reference	Patient Data	Treatment/Pathology	Our Evaluation Signs/Symptoms
Shill & Stacey, 2000 (U.S.)	22 F; progressive immobility, mutism, agitation, tremor, catatonia	MRI, brain biopsy negative; FDG-PET showed bilateral cortical hypometabolism and asymmetric thalamic hypometabolism; lorazepam improved motor symptoms; 4 electroconvulsive therapy treatments resulted in dramatic improvement and full recovery	No hypersomnolence, no ocular signs; unlikely EL
Ghaemi et al., 2000 (Germany)	74 F; akinetic–rigid Parkinson syndrome with tremor, hypokinesia, hypomania, cogwheel rigidity, myoclonus, oligoclonal bands; CSF positive for influenza A; patient improved considerably	MRI showed discrete bilateral parieto-occipital leukodystrophic alterations; PET showed pattern of glucose- and dopamine–metabolism different from PD; treated with acyclovir, amantadine and valproic acid	No hypersomnolence, no ocular signs; unlikely EL
Kiley & Esiri, 2001 (England)	26 F; sleep disturbances, nightmares, possible OCs, severe nausea, drowsiness, dysarthria, masked face, bradykinesia; cognitive functions remained intact; oligoclonal bands; authors propose that patient was a "forme cachectisisante" type of PEP in which life is significantly shortened	MRI normal; right frontal lobe biopsy normal; L-dopa was ineffective; methylprednisolone ineffective; postmortem exam revealed active encephalitis mainly concentrated in upper brainstem and diencephalon with extensive Purkinje cell loss and marked plasma cell infiltration and morula cells; perivascular cuffing evident in cerebellar cortex, cerebral cortex and hippocampus	No classic ocular signs and no initial influenza-like stage; probably not EL

Study	Clinical features	Imaging/treatment	Comments
Verschueren & Crols, 2001 (Belgium)	21 M; visual hallucinations, headache, insomnia, gait/limb apraxia, cogwheel rigidity, akinetic mutism	MRI showed hyperintense lesions in substantia nigra and right striatum; acyclovir, ceftriaxone used; L-dopa was of no benefit; methylprednisolone ameliorated symptoms	No hypersomnolence, no ocular signs; unlikely EL
Dale et al., 2004 (England)	20 cases, 11 male; 17/20 less than 18 years old; 19/20 sleep disorders (sleep inversion; pseudosomnolence), emotional lability, mutism, anxiety, depression, apathy, poor social interaction, reduced consciousness, inadequate respiration, inappropriate behavior; all had features of parkinsonism; 10 had rest tremor; 17/20 psychiatric problems; five showed complete recovery; 19/20 were positive for anti–basal ganglia antibodies; authors suggest EL is a PANDA disease (see Chapter 9)	MRI was abnormal in 8 cases with abnormalities present in basal ganglia, midbrain/tegmentum, thalamus, cerebral peduncle and temporal lobe; postmortem in one case showed perivascular cuffing in basal ganglia with lesser cuffing in cerebral cortex and cerebellum	Four cases showed ocular signs and hypersomnolence; no indication of prior influenza-like illness but probable that these four cases are EL; others unlikely
Dewar & Wilson, 2005 (England)	24 F: confusion, paranoid delusion, drowsiness, rigidity; positive for basal ganglia antibodies	CT/MRI normal; treated with steroids and cognitive therapy	Psychiatric symptoms predominate; unlikely EL
McKee & Sussman, 2005 (England)	17 M; lassitude, shuffling gait, dysarthria, rigidity, resting tremor, masked face, akinetic, face, jaw tremor; sialorrhea, bradykinesia; basal ganglia antibodies present	MRI revealed abnormalities in the basal ganglia; treatment with intravenous steroids was very effective (full recovery)	No hypersomnolence, no ocular signs; unlikely EL
Sridam & Phanthumchinda, 2006 (Thailand)	17 M; hypersomnolence, ophthalmoplegia, ptosis, mild facial paresis, head tremor, frequent yawning, masked face, bradykinesia, grasp reflex, inappropriate behavior, orientation intact, PEP	MRI showed lesions in midbrain, basal ganglia and temporal lobes; improved with steroid treatment	Likely EL although no evidence of prior influenza-like illness

(Continued)

Table 5.4 continued

Reference	Patient Data	Treatment/Pathology	Our Evaluation Signs/Symptoms
Dale et al., 2007 (Australia)	3, 8 M; catatonia, coprolalia, agitation, aggression, hallucinations, sleep inversion, dystonic posturing, OCs, respiratory abnormalities, oligoclonal banding	MRI in 1 case normal, in other, subtle changes in right putamen and temporal lobe; treated with haloperidol, midazolam, fentanyl, ketamine, clonidine, thiopentone, chloral, melatonin, lorazepam; L-dopa therapy reduced rigidity and decreased bradykinesia but had adverse effects; dopamine agonists; steroid therapy also used but value unclear	No ocular signs; no initial influenza-like symptoms; unlikely EL
Raghav et al. 2007 (Australia)	21, 23, 36 F; neuropsychiatric symptoms, rigidity, pyrexia, OCs, respiratory disturbances	MRI in one case normal; treated with acyclovir, olanzapine; penicillin, clonazepam; zuclopenthixol. methylprednisolone and IV immunoglobulin infusions; two died and in the third methylprednisolone did not provide any immediate improvement; one postmortem showed mild lymphocytic infiltration; in the leptomeninges and focal infiltration in the brain just ventral to the arcuate nucleus in the tuberal region of the diencephalon, and loss	Psychiatric symptoms predominate; unlikely EL

Study	Clinical features	Findings / Treatment	Comments
Brenneis et al., 2007 (Austria)	16 F; lethargy, dysarthria, oral dyskinesia, respiratory insufficiency, upper limb dystonia, disorientation and behavioral changes; serological testing revealed an increased antibody titre against *Bartonella henselae*; anti–basal ganglia antibodies not found	of pigmented neurons in the locus ceruleus of the pons associated with microglial globules; the other brain was macroscopically normal, with perivascular lymphocyte infiltration in the leptomeninges of the cerebellar vermis and over the hypothalamus, and there was lymphocytic and microglial infiltration in the inferior wall of the third ventricle, and a small number of macrophages in the thalamus	No ocular signs; no initial influenza-like signs; unlikely EL
Ali et al. 2008 (U.S.)	22, 41 F; psychomotor agitation, hallucinations, paranoia, catatonia, bradykinesia, blank expression, chorea, sialorrhea, tremor, ataxic gait	IBZM-SPECT revealed a marked decrease of striatal dopamine D_2 receptor availability; L-dopa, amantadine, erythromycin, methylprednisolone had no effect; complete recovery followed administration of rifampicin and doxycycline, and physical therapy; MRI normal in one case; case 2 revealed left temporal lobe lesion; one case suspicious for herpes simplex encephalitis; treated with olanzapine, lorazepam, haloperidol, gabapentin, benztropine, corticosteroid; both patients showed significant improvement after electroconvulsive therapy	Psychiatric symptoms predominate; unlikely EL

(Continued)

Table 5.4 continued

Reference	Patient Data	Treatment/Pathology	Our Evaluation Signs/Symptoms
Beleza et al., 2008 (Portugal)	16 M; pharyngitis followed by akinetic–rigid parkinsonism; after corticosteroid withdrawal fatal EL-like syndrome	MRI day 5 showed bilateral cortico–subcortical high signal intensity lesions, with insula and putaminal involvement; brain CT on day 32 showed bilateral hypodensity, and brain edema; treated with L–dopa/carbidopa, hydrocortisone, methylprednisolone, acyclovir. Died day 35.	No ocular signs mentioned; unlikely EL
Lopez-Alberola et al., 2008 (U.S.)	2 (2), 6, 24, 28 M; 3, 5, 16 F; authors suggest the eight patients include akinetic, hyperkinetic, and somnolent types of EL; sleep disturbances, emotional lability, mental deterioration, attention deficit hyperactivity, chorea, myoclonus; encephalopathy present in all cases; 3/8 showed OCs; 4/7 showed anti–basal ganglia antibodies	5/8 showed abnormal MRIs including mild atrophy, non-specific white matter changes, perivascular and subcortical white matter abnormalities, basal ganglia abnormalities, and cortical and subcortical abnormalities; treatments included methylprednisolone, tetrabenazine, clonidine, propanolol, morphine, L–dopa/carbidopa, IVIg (immuno modulation); no conclusions made pertaining to treatment	Five patients are considered to be somnolent type, but most comatose; no classic ocular signs (but OCs present); no initial influenza-like phase; most seem unlikely EL although 1–2 cases are nearly consistent assuming OCs are accepted as ocular sign

Study	Clinical features	Investigations/treatment	Comments
van Toorn & Schoeman, 2009 (South Africa)	5, 11, 12 M; 8, 9 F; sleep disturbances (somnolence, insomnia, sleep inversion), dystonia, OCs (3); psychiatric disturbances (hallucinations; obsessive–compulsive symptoms, mutism, apathy, confusion, delirium); streptococcal serology was negative in 3/3 tested; two children recovered completely and three maintained mild learning disorders	CT/MRI were all normal; cerebral SPECT (2) was normal for basal ganglia perfusion; treatments included corticosteroids, L-dopa, melatonin, sodium valproate, biperiden hydrochloride, risperidone, clonazepam, Artane, haloperidol with none showing an immediate effect	Only two showed somnolence and none showed classic ocular signs (one did show OCs, but primarily had visual and auditory hallucinations, which was not an epidemic period finding); unlikely EL
Dale et al., 2009 (Australia)	1-3, 3 (2), 5 (2), 6, 7 (3), 8, 9, 11 F; 5, 8 (2), 10, 13, 14, 152 M; dyskinesias, agitation, seizures, insomnia, somnolence, parkinsonism	All patients had encephalitis based on MRI or CSF analysis; 10 also were serum and/or CSF positive for autoantibodies to the extracellular domain of the NR1/NR2 subunits of the N-methyl-D-aspartate receptor (NMDAR-Ab)	Authors suggest that the dyskinetic form of EL is an NMDAR-Ab encephalitis; suggest that this type of EL much more prevalent in females although this was not the case during EL period; dyskinesia; none of the NMDAR-positive patients were somnolent; findings would suggest that different types of EL had different etiologies; unlikely EL
Chan et al., 2009 (Hong Kong)	12 F; sleep inversion, masked face, limb rigidity, oromotor dyskinesia, OCs, anxiety, emotional lability	L-dopa, carbamazepine, lorazepam; hospitalized for 9 weeks with full motor and cognitive recovery after 2 months	Signs/symptoms generally consistent with EL although OCs not reported during the epidemic period; patient was very responsive to L-dopa

M, male; F, female, CT, computed tomography; MRI, magnetic resonance imaging; OC, oculogyric crises; PEP, postencephalitic parkinsonism.

Table 5.5 Post-1940 Encephalitis Lethargica (EL) Cases in the Soviet Union

Reference	Region/Years	Number of Cases	Comment
Ulitovsky, 1961	Irkutsk, 1932–1956	18 acute, 283 chronic	No epidemics since 1938
Ovechkin★	Sverdlovskaya, 1932–1947	36 acute, 84 chronic	
Amosov★	Azerbaidzhanskaya, 1933–1942	38 acute, 80 chronic	
Michyeyev★	"Northern Region" 1936–1942	50 chronic	
Kanter★	Khabarovskaya, 1939–1947	5 acute, 45 chronic	
Stepanov★	Saratovskaya, 1941–1945	5	
Shukalova★	Kirgizskaya, 1942	"outbreak"	
Limonova★ & Smirnov	Turmenskaya, 1942–1943	61	No cases before 1942
Yershov★	Stalingrad, 1943–1947	8	
Alperovich★	Vinnitskaya, 1944–1948	4 acute, 64 chronic	
Dyakonova & Papova★	Voronezh region, 1945–1946	33	Small epidemic
Klyuchikov★	Region north of Moscow, ?–1949	45	Second most prevalent neurological infection (polio first)
Lovtskaya & Kostrova, 1957	Leningrad, 1936–1950	31 acute, 19 chronic	New forms of disease (pseudoasthenic, diencephalic); some of the older types no longer found (choreic, myoclonic, pseudotabetic)
Davidenkova-Kulkova & Kostrova, 1957	Leningrad, 1957	Describes one case of spinal EL	Characterized by tetraparesis, ptosis, oculogyric crises (OCs), drowsiness, sphincter disturbances
Alperovich, Bilyk, & Rudaya, 1964	Vinnitsa 1943–1962	Description of hyperkinetic form (21 patients)	Modern hyperkinetic form characterized by polymorphism, e.g., choreiform, myoclonic, athetotic, and torsion-dystonic movements; also spastic torticollis

Table 5.5 continued

Reference	Region / Years	Number of Cases	Comment
Konovalova, 1971	Moscow	21, all children, acute and chronic	Usually diagnosed as acute respiratory infection; neurological signs indicate lesion in diencephalon
Legkonogov & Bezrukova, 1973	Vladivostok, 1968–1971	18 cases	Observed all classic forms; in addition reported that acute form may resemble appendicitis
Strokina, Guliaeva, & Strokin, 1976	Vladivostok, 1967–1974	48 acute, 56 chronic; all forms showed sleep disorders; oculomotor disturbances (diplopia, anisocoria, and ocular spasm); OCs in acute stage	High frequency of vestibular type of EL in acute stage, and hyperkinetic form in chronic stage
Zinchenko, Komlik, Perepelitsa, & Klepikov, 1980	Kharkov, 1972–1980	147 acute and chronic	Concludes that clinical picture of EL has changed with hyperkinetic types becoming more frequent; also, acute stages now milder
Alperovich, Bylik, & Rudaya, 1982	Vinnica, 1944–1981	46 acute, 272 chronic	Current cases less severe than during epidemic period; most patients recover; transmitted by virus carriers and patients with subclinical forms

* From Ulitovsky (1961)

POST-1940 TREATMENT OF ENCEPHALITIS LETHARGICA

As shown in Table 5.4, treatments used in the putative post-1940 EL cases differed widely, with varying results. Probably the most unexpectedly successful reported treatment for EL was the use of electroconvulsive shock therapy (ECT). Electroconvulsive shock therapy is not commonly associated with the treatment of encephalitis and its application to EL would seem to be related more to the neuropsychiatric aspects of the disease than to other features. Furthermore, the number of actual patients treated with ECT is very small (six). Misra and

Hay (1971) described a 19-year-old man who was believed to have developed schizophrenia following encephalitis. He showed significant improvement after ECT. Case 2 in Rail et al. (1981) was initially treated with ECT in a psychiatric hospital, with no improvement noted. All of the remaining four cases (Dekleva & Husain, 1995; Shill & Stacey, 2000; Ali et al., 2008) were characterized by catatonia and showed improvement. Accordingly, ECT is considered to be an effective therapy in malignant catatonia (Ali et al., 2008). One of the cases presented in the Chapter 11 (case 4) also reported positive results from ECT therapy.

Table 5.6 provides a compilation of the reported drugs by type used to treat EL since 1940. The efficacy of most of these drugs for EL is not clear, either because it was not clarified in the respective reports, insufficient data exist, or contrary findings are reported in different studies. Recent reports have emphasized the

Table 5.6 Drugs Used to Treat Encephalitis Lethargica Since 1940

Drug Class	Specific Drugs
Neuroleptics	Chlorpromazine
	Haloperidol
	Olanzapine
	Pipotiazine
	Zuclopenthixol
Antidepressants	Imipramine
Anticholinergic	Amantadine (Viregyt)
	Aturbane (phenglutarimide)
	Benzhexol (Artane)
	Benztropine
	Biperiden
	Parpanit (caramiphen)
	Procyclidine
Corticosteroids	Corticotrophin
	Dexamethasone
	Methylprednisolone
	Synacthen
Alkaloid	Stramonium
Dopamine agonist	Apomorphine
	Bromocriptine
	Benserazide
	Levodopa

Table 5.6 continued

Drug Class	Specific Drugs
Antiviral	Acyclovir
	Isoprinosine
Antibiotic	Ceftriaxone
	Doxycycline
	Erythromycin
	Penicillin
	Rifampicin
	Sulfonamide
Anti-hypertensive	Clonidine
	Propanolol
	(also antiessential tremor)
Opiate	Morphine
Anti-inflammatory	Intravenous immunoglobulin
	Fentanyl
	Gabapentin
	Ketamine
	Sodium salicylate (aspirin)
Amphetamine	Benzedrine sulfate
Tranquilizer and antiepileptic	Benzodiazepines (clonazepam, midazolam, diazepam)
	Chloral hydrate
	Diphenhydramine
	Lorazepam
	Risperidone
	Phenobarbitone
	Phenytoin
	Propofol
	Sodium pentothal (thiopentone)
	Tetrabenazine
	Valproic acid
Diuretic	Mannitol
Dietary supplement	Melatonin
	Nootropil
Muscle relaxant	Dantrolene
	Pancuronium

use of L-dopa, corticosteroids, and intravenous immunoglobin therapies, but there is no consistent evidence of effectiveness.

The variable success of these pharmaceutical agents does not permit any conclusions to be made on the best treatment options for new cases of EL.

REFERENCES CITED

Abrahamson, I. (1920).The epidemic of lethargic encephalitis. *Medical Record, 98,* 969–973.
Ali, S., Welch, C. A., Park, L. T., Pliakas, A. M., Wilson, A., Nicolson, S., Huffman, J., & Fricchione, G. L. (2008). Encephalitis and catatonia treated with ECT. *Cognitive and Behavioral Neurology, 21,* 46–51.
Al-Mateen, M., Gibbs, M., Dietrich, R., Mitchell, W. G., & Menkes, J. H. (1988). Encephalitis lethargica-like illness in a girl with mycoplasma infection. *Neurology, 38,* 1155–1158.
Alperowicz, P. M., Bilyk, V. D., & Roudaia, B. I. (1964). Clinical presentation of hyperkinetic form of modern EL [in Russian]. *Zhurnal nevropatologii i psikhiatrii, 64,* 340–345.
Alperowicz, P. M., Bilyk, V. D., & Roudaia, B. I. (1982). Clinico-epidermiological characteristics of epidemic encephalitis. *Klinicheskaia meditsina, 60,* 50–54.
Aramideh, M., Bour, L. J., Koelman, J. H. T. M., Speelman, J. D., & Ongerborer de Visser, B. W. (1994). Abnormal eye movements in blepharospasm and involuntary levator palpebrae inhibition: Clinical and pathophysiological considerations. *Brain, 117,* 1457–1474.
Aronson, L. S. (1921). Epidemic encephalitis with unusual sequelae. *Neurological Bulletin, 3,* 113–116.
Barkas, M. (1926).Tonic spasms of the eyes in conjugate deviation. *Lancet, 2,* 330.
Barletta, L., Simonetti, F., Karau, J., Manni, R., Uggetti, C., Poloni, T. E., Pergami, P., Savoldi, F., & Ceroni, M. (1995). Encephalitis lethargica. *Nervenarzt, 66,* 781–784.
Bassetti, C. L. (2007). Narcolepsy. In A. Culebras (Ed.), *Sleep Disorders and Neurologic Diseases* (pp. 83–116). New York: Informa Healthcare.
Batocchi, A. P., Della Marca, G., Mirabella, M., Caggiula, M., Frisullo, G., Mennuni, G., & Tonali, P. (2001). Relapsing-remitting autoimmune agrypnia. *Annals of Neurology, 50,* 668–671.
Beleza, P., Soares-Fernandes, J., Jordão, M. J., & Almeida, F. (2008). From juvenile parkinsonism to encephalitis lethargica, a new phenotype of post-streptococcal disorders: Case report. *European Journal of Paediatric Neurology, 12,* 505–507.
Benedek, L., & Angyal, L. (1944). Gehäuftes Vorkommen von vestibulotropen Encephalitis-Fällen. *Archiv für Psychiatrie und Nervenkrankheiten, 117,* 52–67.
Bennett, A. E., & Patton, J. M. (1930). Oculogyric crises in postencephalitic states. *Archives of Ophthalmology, 4,* 361–367.
Ben-Pazi, H., Livne, A., Shapra, Y., & Dale, R. (2003). Parkinsonian features after streptococcal pharyngitis. *The Journal of Pediatrics, 143,* 267–269.
Bentivoglio, M., & Kristensson, K. (2007). Neural-immune interactions in disorders of sleep-wakefulness organization. *Trends in Neuroscience, 30,* 645–652.
Bernard, E. (1923).Troubles respiratoires dans l'encephalite lethargique. *Gazette des hopitaux ciuils et militaries, 96,* 85–90.
Bickerstaff, E. R., & Cloake, P. C. P. (1951). Mesencephalitis and rhombencephalitis. *British Medical Journal, 2,* 77–81.
Blunt, S. B., Lane, R. J. M., Turjanski, N., & Perkin, G. D. (1997). Clinical features and management of two cases of encephalitis lethargica. *Movement Disorders, 12,* 354–359.

Bojinov, S. (1971). Encephalitis with acute parkinsonian syndrome and bilateral inflammatory necrosis of the substantia nigra. *Journal of the Neurological Sciences, 12*, 383–415.

Bonduelle, M., Bouygues, P., Lormeau, G., & Degos, C. (1975). Note au sujet d'une observation d'hypersomnie de type léthargique [Case of lethargic-type hypersomnia]. *Revue Neurologique, 131*, 737–739.

Booss, J., & Esiri, M. M. (2003). *Viral Encephalitis in Humans.* Washington DC: ASM Press.

Bramwell, E. (1928a). The ocular complications of lethargic encephalitis. Joint discussion No. 4: Sections of Ophthalmology and Neurology. *Proceedings of the Royal Society of Medicine (London), 21*, 985–996.

Bramwell, E. (1928b). The upward movement of the eyes. *Brain, 51*, 1–17.

Breggin, P. R. (1993). Parallels between neuroleptic effects and lethargic encephalitis: The production of dyskinesias and cognitive disorders. *Brain and Cognition, 23*, 8–27.

Brenneis, C., Scherfler, C., Engelhardt, K., Helbok, R., Brössner, G., Beer, R., Lackner, P., Walder G., Pfausler, P., & Schmutzhard, E. (2007). Encephalitis lethargica following Bartonella henselae infection. *Journal of Neurology, 254*, 546–547.

Brewis, E. G. (1954). Recent experience of encephalitis in childhood. *British Medical Journal, 1*, 1298–1302.

Buzzard, E. F. (1923). Discussion on the sequelae of lethargic encephalitis. Proceedings of Sections at the Annual Meeting: Sections of Neurology and Psychological Medicine. *British Medical Journal, 2*, 1083–1090.

Cardoso, F. (2006). Infectious and transmissible movement disorders. In J. J. Jankovic & E. Tolosa (Eds.), *Parkinson's Disease and Movement Disorders* (pp. 584–595). Philadelphia: Lippincott Williams & Wilkins.

Chan, B., Chan, K. Y., & Yau, K. C. (2009). Encephalitis lethargic in a twelve-year-old girl; the response to Levodopa therapy. *Hong Kong Journal of Pediatrics, 14*, 122–125.

Chinnery, P. F., Crompton, D. E., Birchall, D., Jackson, M. J., Coulthard, A., Lombes, A., et al. (2007). Clinical features and natural history of neuroferritinopathy caused by the *FTL1* 460InsA mutation. *Brain, 130*, 110–119.

Cords, R. (1921). Die augensymptome bei der encephalitis epidemica. *Zentralblatt für die gesamte Ophthalmologie und ihre Grenzgebiete, 5*, 225–258.

Cortelli, P., & Lombardi, C. (2007). Autonomic dysfunctions in sleep disorders. In A. Culebras (Ed.), *Sleep Disorders and Neurologic Diseases* (pp. 337–348). New York: Informa Healthcare.

Critchley, A. M. (1928). Ocular manifestations following encephalitis lethargica. *Bristol Medico-Chirurgical Journal, 45*, 113–124.

Cruchet, R. (1925). The relation of paralysis agitans to the parkinsonian syndrome of epidemic encephalitis. *Lancet, 2*, 263–268.

Culebras, A. (2007). Headache disorders and sleep. In A. Culebras (Ed.), *Sleep Disorders and Neurologic Diseases* (pp. 349–359). New York: Informa Healthcare.

Dale, R. C., Church, A. J., Surtees, R. A. H., Lees, A. J., Adcock, J. E., Harding, B., et al. (2004). Encephalitis lethargica syndrome: 20 new cases and evidence of basal ganglia autoimmunity. *Brain, 127*, 21–33.

Dale, R. C., Irani, S. R., Brilot, F., Pillai, S., Webster, W., Gill, D., et al. (2009). N-methyl-D-aspartate receptor antibodies in pediatric dyskinetic encephalitis lethargica. *Annuals of Neurology, 66*, 705–709.

Dale, R., Webster, R., & Gill, D. (2007). Contemporary encephalitis lethargica presenting with agitated catatonia, stereotypy, and dystonia-parkinsonism. *Movement Disorders, 22*, 2281–2284.

Davidenkova-Kulkova, E. F., & Kostrova, E. S. (1957). Diagnosis of separate variants of epidemic encephalitis [in Russian]. In S. N. Davidenkov (Ed.), *Questions of Neurology:*

Collection of Works Dedicated to the Memory of Professor L. V. Blumenau (pp. 243–251). Leningrad: Institute for the Advancement of Physicians.

Dekleva, K., & Husain, M. M. (1995). Sporadic encephalitis lethargica: A case treated successfully with ECT. *The Journal of Neuropsychiatry and Clinical Neurosciences, 7,* 237–239.

Dewar, B. K., & Wilson, B. A. (2005). Cognitive recovery from encephalitis lethargica. *Brain Injury, 19,* 1285–1291.

Dobryzynska, L. (1965). Two cases of lethargic encephalitis. *Polski Tygodnik Lekarski, 20,* 1945–1946.

Doichinov, D. (1968). To the question of the modern acute postencephalitic Parkinson syndrome [in Russian]. *Nevrologiia, Psikhiatriia i Nevrokhirugiia, 7,* 459–464.

Dolan, J. D., & Kamil, R. (1992). Atypical affective disorder with episodic dyscontrol: A case of von Economo's disease (encephalitis lethargica). *Canadian Journal of Psychiatry, 37,* 140–142.

Drobec, E., & Tschabitscher, H. (1948). Zur neuritischen Form der Encephalitis lethargica. *Klinische Medizin; östereichische Zeitschrift für wissenschaftliche und praktische Medizin, 3,* 877–880.

Duncan, A. G. (1924). The sequelae of encephalitis lethargica. *Brain, 47,* 76–95.

Dunn, A. D., & Heagey, F. W. (1920). Epidemic encephalitis: Including a review of 115 American cases. *American Journal of the Medical Science, 160,* 568–582.

Ellis, A. (1920). The myoclonic form of acute epidemic encephalitis. *Lancet, 2,* 114–116.

Ernsting, W. (1946). Encephalitis lethargica after cranial injury followed by diabetes insipidus and disturbances of sleep. *Nederlands Tijdschrift voor Geneeskunde, 90,* 884–887.

Espir, M. L. E., & Spalding, J. M. K. (1956). Three recent cases of encephalitis lethargica. *British Medical Journal, 1,* 1141–1144.

Ewald, G. (1924). Schauanfälle als postenzephalitische Störung (Zugleich ein Beitrag zur Frage psychischer Störungen bei postenzephalitischen Zuständen). *Monatsschrift für Psychiatrie und Neurologie, 57,* 222–253.

Fischer, B. (1924). Uber vestibulare Beeinflussung der Augenmuskelstarre bei der Encephalitis epidemica. *Deutsche Zeitschrift für Nervenheilkunde, 81,* 164–169.

Fitzgerald, P. M., & Jankovic, J. (1989). Tardive oculogyric crisis. *Neurology, 39,* 1434–1437.

Ford, Frank R. (1937). *Diseases of the Nervous System in Infancy, Childhood and Adolescence.* Springfield, IL: Charles C. Thomas.

Geerling, R. (1950). Encephalitis africana: A preliminary report. *South African Medical Journal, 24,* 339–343.

Geimanowitsch, A. I. (1928). Epidemic encephalitides and their investigation in the USSR [in Russian]. *Central Medical Journal, 5,* 837–847.

Geimanowitsch, A., Beilin, B., & Leschtschenko, G. (1924). Augenmuskelsymptome bie epidemischer Encephalitis. *Zentralblatt für die Gesamte Neurologie und Psychiatrie, 38,* 146. [Abstract]

Ghaemi, M., Rudolf, J., Schmülling, S., Bamborschke, S., & Heiss, W. D. (2000). FDG- and Dopa-PET in postencephalitic parkinsonism. *Journal of Neural Transmission, 107,* 1289–1295.

Greenough, A., & Davis, J. A. (1983). Encephalitis lethargica: Mystery of the past or undiagnosed disease of the present? *Lancet, 1,* 922–923.

Gulmann, N. C., & Pedersen, H. E. (1980). Parkinsonism after acute encephalopathy. *Ugeskrift for Laeger, 142,* 960–961.

Hall, Arthur J. (1924). *Epidemic Encephalitis (Encephalitis Lethargica).* Bristol: John Wright & Sons.

Hanagasi, H. A., Lees, A., Johnson, J. O., Singleton, A., & Emre, M. (2007). Smoking-responsive juvenile-onset parkinsonism. *Movement Disorders, 22,* 115–118.

Herishanu, Y., & Noah, Z. (1973). On acute encephalitic parkinsonian syndrome: Case report and review of the recent literature. *European Neurology, 10*, 117–124.

Hobson, D. E., Lang, A. E., Martin, W. R. W., Razmy, A., Rivest, J., & Fleming, J. (2002). Excessive daytime sleepiness and sudden-onset sleep in Parkinson Disease. *Journal of the American Medical Association, 287*, 455–463.

Hohman, L. B. (1925). Forced conjugate upward movements of the eyes. *Journal of the American Medical Association, 84*, 1489–1490.

Holmes, G. (1928). Encephalitis: Ocular complications. *Proceedings of the Royal Society of Medicine, 21*, 994–996.

Houin, D-H. (1922). *Les troubles des mouvements oculaires associés au cours de l'encéphalite léthargique épidémique.* Thesis, Universite de Nancy, Faculté de Médeciné, 2 Serie, No. 177.

Howard, R. S., & Lees, A. J. (1987). Encephalitis lethargica: A report of four recent cases. *Brain, 110*, 19–33.

Hunter, R., & Jones, M. (1966). Acute lethargica-type encephalitis. *Lancet, 2*, 1023–1024.

Jelliffe, S. E. (1927). *Postencephalitic Respiratory Disorders: Review of Syndromy, Case Reports, Physiopathology, Psychopathology and Therapy.* New York & Washington: Nervous and Mental Disease Publishing Company, Monograph Series No. 45.

Jelliffe, S. E. (1932). *Psychopathology of Forced Movements and the Oculogyric Crises of Lethargic Encephalitis.* New York & Washington: Nervous and Mental Disease Publishing Company, Monograph Series No. 55.

Johnson, R.T. (1998). *Viral Infections of the Nervous System.* Philadelphia: Lippincott-Raven.

Johnson, J., & Lucey, P.A. (1987). Encephalitis lethargica, a contemporary cause of catatonic stupor: A report of two cases. *British Journal of Psychiatry, 151*, 550–552.

Kakigi, R., Shibasaki, H., Katafuchi, Y., Iyatomi, I., & Kuroda, Y. (1986). The syndrome of bilateral paramedian thalamic infarction associated with oculogyric crisis. *Rinsho Shinkeigaku (Clinical Neurology), 26*, 1100–1105.

Kapadia, F., & Grant, I. S. (1990). Encephalitis lethargica. *Intensive Care Medicine, 16*, 338–339.

Kasanin, J., & Petersen, J. N. (1926). Psychosis as an early sign of epidemic encephalitis. *Journal of Nervous and Mental Disorders, 64*, 352–358.

Foster Kennedy, R. (1929). Ocular disturbances in epidemic encephalitis. *Archives of Ophthalmology, 1*, 346–350.

Keyserlingk, H. (1949). Akute Encephalitis mit vorwiegend vestibulärer Symptomatik. *Medizinishe Klinik, 36*, 1155–1157.

Kiley, M., & Esiri, M. M. (2001). A contemporary case of encephalitis lethargica. *Clinical Neuropathology, 20*, 2–7.

Kim, J. S., Kim, H. K., Im, J. H., & Lee, M. C. (1996). Oculogyric crisis and abnormal magnetic resonance imaging signals in bilateral lentiform nuclei. *Movement Disorders, 11*, 756–758.

Konovalova, G. I. (1971). Clinical picture and duration of epidemic encephalitis in children. *Journal of Neurology and Psychiatry in Korsakova, 71*, 1486–1490.

Kullnat, M. W., & Morse, R. P. (2008). Choreoathetosis after herpes simplex encephalitis with basal ganglia involvement on MRI. *Pediatrics, 121*, e1003–e1007.

Kun, L. N., Yian, S. Y., Haur, L. S., & Tjia, H. (1999). Bilateral substantia nigra changes on MRI in a patient with encephalitis lethargica. *Neurology, 53*, 1860–1862.

Lambruschini, C. (1941). Contribución al estudio de la encephalitis letárgica aguda [Contribution to the study of acute encephalitis lethargica]. *Revista Argentina de Neurologia, Psiquiatria y Neurocirugia, 6*, 164–181.

Legkonogov, V. A., & Bezrukova, L. V. (1973). Clinical forms of acute period of epidemic encephalities. *Journal of Neurology and Psychiatry in Korsakova, 73*, 185–188.

Leigh, A. D. (1946). Infections of the nervous system occurring during an epidemic of Influenza B. *British Medical Journal, 2,* 936–938.

Leigh J., Foley, J. M., Remler, B. F, & Civil, R. H. (1987). Oculogyric crisis: A syndrome of thought disorder and ocular deviation. *Annals of Neurology, 22,* 13–17.

Lemos, M. (1924). Claudication intermittente, crampe des écrivains, deviation conjuguée de la tête et des yeux, spasme des muscles masticateurs glosso-palato-laryngés et des membres supérieurs, apparus au cours du syndrome parkinsonien: Encéphalite prolongée–Localisation striée probable. *Revue Neurologique, 2,* 425–449.

Levy, S. (1959). Post-encephalitic behavior disorder: A forgotten entity–A report of 100 cases. *American Journal of Psychiatry, 115,* 1062–1067.

Liu, G. T., Carrazana, E. J., Macklis, J. D., & Mikati, M. A. (1991). Delayed oculogyric crises associated with striatocapsular infarction. *Journal of Clinical Neuro-Ophthalmology, 11,* 198–201.

Lopez-Alberola, R., Georgiou, M., Sfakianakis, G. N., Singer, C., & Papapetropoulos, S. (2009). Contemporary encephalitis lethargica: Phenotype, laboratory findings and treatment outcomes. *Journal of Neurology, 256,* 396–404.

Lovtskaya, A. Y., & Kostrova, E. S. (1957). Clinical picture of modern encephalitis [in Russian]. In S. N. Davidenkov (Ed.), *Questions of Neurology: Collection of Works Dedicated to the Memory of Professor L. V. Blumenau* (pp. 233–242). Leningrad: Institute for the Advancement of Physicians.

Maciel, Z. (1941). Epidemic encephalitis of pure lethargic form with regression after intravenous sodium salicylate. *Brazil-Medico, 55,* 804–806.

Machetanz, E. (1958). Postencephalitischer Parkinsonismus mit Blickkrämpfen im Kindesalter. *Zeitschrift für Kinderheilkunde, 81,* 555–566.

Margulis, M. S. (1926). Apercu general de l'epidemi d'encephalie en 1923-24 a Moscou. *Archives De Neurologie, 4,* 1–13.

McAuley, J., Shahmanesh, M., & Swash, M. (1999). Dopaminergic therapy in acute encephalitis lethargica. *Journal of the European Federation of Neurological Societies, 6,* 235–237.

McCowan, P. K., & Cook, L. C. (1928). Oculogyric crises in chronic epidemic encephalitis. *Brain, 51,* 285–309.

McKee, D. H., & Sussman, J. D. (2005). Case report: Severe acute parkinsonism associated with streptococcal infection and antibasal ganglia antibodies. *Movement Disorders, 20,* 1661–1663.

Mellon, A. F., Appleton, R. E., Gardner-Medwin, D., & Aynsley-Green, A. (1991). Encephalitis lethargica-like illness in a five-year-old. *Developmental Medicine and Child Neurology, 33,* 158–161.

Meyer, A. (1924). Beitrage zur Encephalitis epidemica. *Archiv für Psychiatrie und Nervenkrankheiten, 70,* 466–528.

Mignot, E., & Zeitzer, J. M. (2007). Neurobiology of narcolepsy and hypersomnia. In S. Gilman (Ed.), *Neurobiology of Disease* (pp. 715–722). Amsterdam: Elsevier Academic Press.

Misra, P. C., & Hay, G. G. (1971). Encephalitis presenting as acute schizophrenia. *British Medical Journal, 1,* 532–533.

Misra, U. K, & Kalita, J. (2002). Prognosis of Japanese encephalitis patients with dystonia compared to those with parkinsonian features only. *Postgraduate Medical Journal, 78,* 238–241.

Motta, E., Rosciszewska, D., & Piela, Z. (1994). Diagnostic difficulties in the case of a 57-year-old. *Przeglad Epidemiologiczny, 48,* 495–497.

Mulder, D. W., Parrott, M., & Tahler, M. (1951). Sequelae of Western equine encephalitis. *Neurology, 1,* 318–327.

Nangaku, M., Motoyoshi, Y., Kwak, S., Yoshikawa, H., & Iwata, M. (1990). MRI pathology of the globus pallidus in a patient with oculogyric crisis and tremor. *Rinsho Shinkeigaku (Clinical Neurology), 30,* 760–764.

Neal, J. B. (1942). *Encephalitis: A Clinical Study.* New York: Grune & Stratton.

Nielsen, J. M. (1953). Complications of encephalitis of the von Economo type. *Bulletin of the Los Angeles Neurological Association, 18,* 84–90.

Oeckinghaus, W. (1921). Encephalitis epidemica and Wilsonsches Krankheitsbild. *Deutsche Zeitschrift für Nervenheikunde, 72,* 294–309.

Onuaguluchi, G. (1961). Crises in post-encephalitic parkinsonism. *Brain, 84,* 395–414.

Parker, H. L. (1922). Disturbances of the respiratory rhythm in children: A sequela to epidemic encephalitis. *Archives of Neurology and Psychiatry, 8,* 630–638.

Paviour, D. C., Surtees, R., & Lees, A. (2004). Diagnostic considerations in juvenile parkinsonism. *Movement Disorders, 19,* 123–135.

Picard, F., Hirsch, E., Salmon, E., Marescaux, C., & Collard, M. (1996). Syndrome Parkinsonien et mouvements involontaires stéréotypés post-encéphalitiques, sensibles a la L-dopa. *Revue Neurologique (Paris), 152,* 267–271.

Pilz, P., & Erhart, P. (1978). Gibt es noch eine Encephalitis lethargic Economo? Zur Problematik virologisch-serologischer Diagnostik neurologischer Krankheitsbilder. [Is there still an encephalitis lethargica Economo? On the problems of virological-serological diagnosis of neurologic diseases.] *Wiener Medizinische Wochenschrift, 128,* 762–763.

Poser, C. M., Huntley, C. J., & Poland, J. D. (1969). Para-encephalitic parkinsonism. *Acta Neurologica Scandinavica, 45,* 199–215.

Protheroe, S. M., & Mellor, D. H. (1991). Imaging in influenza A encephalitis. *Archives of Disease in Childhood, 66,* 702–705.

Provini, F., Lombardi, C., & Lugaresi, E. (2007). Insomnia in neurology. In A. Culebras (Ed.), *Sleep Disorders and Neurologic Diseases* (pp. 39–52). New York: Informa Healthcare.

Pruskauer-Apostol, B., Popescu-Pretor, R., Plăiaşu, D., Tăturu, E., Ciobanu, I., & Voiculescu, V. (1977). The present status of encephalitis lethargica. *Neurologie et Psychiatrie, 15,* 125–128.

Rack, M. J. (2007). Sleep disorders associated with mental retardation. In A. Culebras (Ed.), *Sleep Disorders and Neurologic Diseases* (pp. 27–37). New York: Informa Healthcare.

Raghav, S., Seneviratne, J., McKelvie, P. A., Chapman, C., Talman, P. S., & Kemster, P. A. (2007). Sporadic encephalitic lethargica. *Journal of Clinical Neuroscience, 14,* 696–700.

Rail, D., Scholtz, C., & Swash, M. (1981). Post-encephalitic parkinsonism: Current experience. *Journal of Neurology, Neurosurgery, & Psychiatry, 44,* 670–676.

Ramsay Hunt, J. (1920). Acute infectious myoclonus multiplex and epidemic myoclonus multiplex. *Journal of the American Medical Association, 75,* 713–718.

Ramsay Hunt, J. (1921). A consideration of the symptoms and syndromes referable to the basal ganglia in epidemic encephalitis. *American Journal of the Medical Sciences, 162,* 481–498.

Rayburn, C. R. (1929). Epidemic encephalitis. *Fiske Fund Prize Essay, 63,* 7–49.

Riley, H. A. (1930). Epidemic encephalitis. *Archives of Neurology, 24,* 574–604.

Rodnitzky, R. L. (2007). Sleep in Parkinson's disease. In A. Culebras (Ed.), *Sleep Disorders and Neurologic Diseases* (pp. 205–228). New York: Informa Healthcare.

Roselli, F., Russo, H., Fraddosio, A., Aniello, M., DeMari, M., Lamberti, P., et al. (2006). Reversible parkinsonian syndrome associated with anti-neuronal antibodies in acute EBV encephalitis: A case report. *Parkinsonism and Related Disorders, 12,* 257–260.

Rossi, C. (1922). Note clinche sull encefalite epidemica con speciale riguardo ai sintomi del periodo tardivo. *Rivista di Patologia Nervosa, 27,* 135–137.

Schrag, A., & Scott, J. M. (2006). Epidemiological, clinical and genetic characteristics of early-onset parkinsonism. *Lancet Neurology, 5(4)*, 355–363.

Schulte, W. (1941). ber atypische vestibulotrope Encephalitiserkrankungen. *Deutsche Zeitschrift für Nervenheilkunde, 153*, 50–63.

Shapiro, S. L. (1935). Otologic findings in oculogyric crises. *Archives of Neurology and Psychiatry, 34*, 714–733.

Shevell, M. (2009). The tripartite origins of the tonic neck reflex: Gesell, Gerstmann, and Magnus. *Neurology, 72*, 850–853.

Shill, H. A. & Stacy, M. (2000). Malignant catatonia secondary to sporadic encephalitis lethargica. *Journal of Neurology, Neurosurgery & Psychiatry, 69*, 402–403.

Shimpo, T., Fuse, S. & Yoshizawa, A. (1993). Retrocollis and oculogyric crisis in association with bilateral putaminal hemorrhages. *Rinsho Shinkeigaku (Clinical Neurology), 33*, 40–44.

Sicard, J. A., & Kudelski, C. (1920). Mésocéphalite léthargique à rechute et type alterne. *Bulletins et Mémoires de la Societe Médicale des Hôpitaux de Paris, 44*, 93–98.

Smith, H. F. (1921). Epidemic encephalitis (encephalitis lethargica, Nona): Report of studies conducted in the United States. *Public Health Reports, 36*, 207–242.

Sridam, N., & Phanthumchinda, K. (2006). Encephalitis lethargica-like illness: Case report and literature review. *Journal of the Medical Association of Thailand, 89*, 1521–1527.

Stern, F. (1928). *Die Epidemische Encephalitis.* Berlin: Julius Springer.

Strokina, T. I., Guliaeva, S. E., & Strokin, V. A. (1976). Clinical variants of epidemic encephalitis in Primor'e [in Russian]. *Zhurnal Nevropatologii i Psikhiatrii Imeni S. S. Korsakova, 76*, 194–197.

Taylor, E. W., & McDonald, C. A. (1928). Forced conjugate upward movement of the eyes following epidemic encephalitis. *Archives of Neurology and Psychiatry, 19*, 95–103.

Tilney, F., & Howe, H. S. (1920). *Epidemic Encephalitis (Encephalitis Lethargica).* New York: Paul B. Hoeber.

Turner, W. A., & Critchley, M. (1925). Respiratory disorders in epidemic encephalitis. *Brain, 48*, 72–104.

Ulitovsky, D. A. (1961). Epidemic (lethargic) encephalitis. In K. G. Khodos (Ed.) *Infectious and Toxic Diseases of the Nervous System* [in Russian]. Irkutsk: Irkutsk Book Publishers.

Van Bogaert, L., & Théodoridès, J. (1979). *Constantin von Economo (1876–1931): The Man and the Scientist.* Wien: Ernst Becvar.

Van Deinse, J. B. (1946). Een bijzonder geval van encephalitis lethargica [A strange case of encephalitis lethargica]. *Nederlands Tijdschrift voor Geneeskunde, 90*, 653–656.

van Toorn, R., & Schoeman, J. F. (2009). Encephalitis lethargica in 5 South African children. *European Journal of Paediatric Neurology, 13*, 41–46.

Verschueren, H., & Crols, R. (2001). Bilateral substantia nigra lesions on magnetic resonance imaging in a patient with encephalitis lethargica. *Journal of Neurology, Neurosurgery and Psychiatry, 71*, 275.

Vilensky, J. A., & Gilman, S. (2006). Encephalitis lethargica: Could this disease be recognised if the epidemic recurred? *Practical Neurology, 6*, 360–367.

Vilensky, J., Mukhamedzyanov, R., & Gilman, S. (2008). Encephalitis lethargica in the Soviet Union. *European Neurology, 60*, 113–121.

von Economo, C. (1917). Encephalitis lethargica. *Wiener klinische Wochenschrift, 30*, 581–585.

von Economo, C. (1929). *Die Encephalitis lethargica, ihre Nachkrankheiten und ihre Behardlung.* Berlin: Urban & Schwarzenberg. (Published in English in 1931; translated by K. O. Newman, London: Oxford University Press.)

Wilson, S. A. K. (1940). *Neurology.* Baltimore: Williams & Wilkins.

Wimmer, A. (1924). *Chronic Epidemic Encephalitis.* London: William Heinemann.

Wimmer, A. (1926). Tonic eye fits ("oculogyric crises") in chronic epidemic encephalitis. *Acta Psychiatrica et Neurologica, 1*, 173–187.

Wolf, G. (1953). Sporadic incidence of encephalitis lethargica. *Deutsche medizinische Wochenschrift, 78*, 968–970.

Young, A. W. (1927). A clinical analysis of an extrapyramidal syndrome: Paralysis agitans and postencephalitic parkinsonism. *Journal of Neurology & Psychopathology, 8*, 9–18.

Zeiszl, E. (1949). Neuritische Formeneiner sporadische Encephalitis lethargica. *Wiener klinische Wochenschrift*, pp. *352*.

Zinchenko, A. P., Komlik, R. K., Perepelitsa, A. L., & Klepikov, E. N. (1980). The evolution of epidemic encephalitis. *Journal of Neurology and Psychiatry in Korsakova, 80*, 180–184.

6

TRANSMISSIBILITY (CONTAGIOUSNESS) OF ENCEPHALITIS LETHARGICA

Joel A. Vilensky

In the vast majority of encephalitis lethargica (EL) outbreaks, the rarity of familial and case-to-case infections is notable. Cruchet, with reference to his original 1916 cases within the French military hospitals, noted the absence of any evidence of contagion (Cruchet, 1928). He believed that those soldiers with EL whom he diagnosed did not come from the same regiment or even neighboring regiments. Nevertheless, Mauss (1931) referred to a German soldier who was granted military compensation for chronic EL because he was placed in a French prisoner of war camp in which "the flu" was known to be present, and thus it was assumed that he developed EL because of his exposure to the virus within that camp.

Evidence of transmission of EL through direct contact could not be ascertained for 1,156 cases in Vienna or for 520 patients in Germany seen in clinics during the early epidemic period (Matheson Commission, 1929; Gerstenbrand et al., 1958). Similarly, a French Institute of Hygiene paper (Bernard & Renault, 1920) reported that, among 464 notified EL cases from January to May 1920, there were no obvious cases of contagion. In Smith's 1921 report on 181 cases in the United States (see Chapter 2), he did not find secondary infections in any family member of the patients, and he specifically noted that he searched for abortive and/or mild cases among family members. Von Economo (1929) observed that in not more than 4.5% of the total number of cases was a mode of transmission apparent. He also stated that, if direct transmission does occur, it probably occurs only in the prodromal state of the disease, through saliva. (Von Economo believed that the virus was primarily spread through the air. He noted the remarkable "coincidence" that, at the time of the spread of the disease from Italy to the Alps and Austria, there were warm northwardly winds that could have carried the disease.)

In 1921, C. Dopter published *La contagiosité de l'encéphalite épidémique* (Contagion in Epidemic Encephalitis) in *Paris Médical*, which was a very thorough review of the evidence for and against direct transmission of EL. Dopter noted that epidemic diseases are generally contagious but, based on its manifestations, EL does not appear to be. Whereas in a typical epidemic there is also usually an initial concentrated series of patients, often in a single home, in EL there was usually a first case in a locality, followed by a second and a third, but the three were generally not in close proximity (i.e., the victims were scattered in the community, with no apparent affiliation). Dopter also stated that if EL is spread via saliva, lethargic patients would not likely be very effective spreaders. But Dopter also argued that EL is contagious and that the ambulatory or *frustes formes* play a central role in transmission. In other words, patients with virtually asymptomatic forms (and/or completely healthy "carriers") of EL play an important role in spreading the disease. Dopter noted that the spread of epidemic hiccups undoubtedly demonstrates the contagiousness of EL. He cited a case in which a student at school developed epidemic hiccups along with other students. He was visited by his brother who, 4 days later, developed classic EL. Dopter also thought that "convalescents" (i.e., those recovering from acute infections) also transmit the disease. He concluded that EL was definitely contagious.

Tilney and Howe, in their 1920 monograph on EL, *Epidemic Encephalitis (Encephalitis Lethargica)*, also suggested that EL was probably communicable, based on the fact that it was a notifiable disease in England and Wales. The first Matheson report (1929), although acknowledging that person-to-person transmission was rare, listed approximately 50 references that presented evidence for person-to-person transmission. Roques, in a 1928 monograph that carefully reviewed all of the available data on EL during pregnancy and in newborns (Fig. 6.1), concluded that the EL virus is capable of crossing the placenta and infecting a fetus in utero, but doubted that an infant could be infected via mother's milk or from other maternal sources (e.g., saliva).

Thus, although the general perception today is that EL is not particularly contagious (if at all), as suggested by Dopter and the Matheson report, some studies provide striking evidence that person-to-person transmission occurred, implying that some particular forms (viral strains?) of EL were more contagious than others, or that some combinations of factors at a specific time and place made the disease directly transmissible. In this chapter, I first describe the most well-known report suggesting a high rate of contagion, the Derby girls' school case in England, and I next provide summaries/abridgements of some other similarly strong reports that generally support direct transmission (although I also provide a few examples

EPIDEMIC ENCEPHALITIS

IN

Association with Pregnancy, Labour, and the Puerperium

BY

FREDERICK ROQUES,

M.A., M.D., M.Chir., (Cantab.), F.R.C.S., (Eng.),

Obstetric and Gynaecological Registrar, the Middlesex Hospital ;
Obstetric Tutor, the Middlesex Hospital.

Published for the MIDDLESEX HOSPITAL PRESS, LONDON,

BY

SHERRATT & HUGHES

MANCHESTER

1928

Figure 6.1 Title page of book on encephalitis lethargica and pregnancy by Roques (1928).

of noncontagion, in which contagion might be expected). I selected these reports to provide examples of contagion in a variety of contexts (e.g., schools, hospitals, families) and also from a variety of countries, especially non–English speaking countries, because I felt that some of these reports have been ignored because they were published in French, German, or Russian. Although most of the descriptions here present examples of transmission of EL during the acute phase, I also present some examples in which EL was thought to have been transmitted by patients in the chronic phase.

Following the presentations of specific case descriptions pertaining to the transmission of EL, I discuss "epidemic hiccups" and describe a pamphlet published by the Illinois Department of Public Health, which assumed EL was contagious pertaining to the control of the disease in 1928.

REPORTS OF CONTAGION

Derby and Derbyshire Rescue and Training Home

The director of the investigation into this case, as well as the author of the Ministry of Health article describing it, was Dr. A. Salusbury MacNalty who, previous to his work on EL, had been especially interested in tuberculosis. He had a distinguished medical career and later (in 1935) became Chief Medical Officer for England. He is also mentioned in Chapter 2 for his initial (1918) categorization of EL.

The documented outbreak occurred in the Derby and Derbyshire Rescue and Training Home (for Girls, in the United Kingdom (Fig. 6.2). By the end of the outbreak, 12 of 21 girls and women in the house were affected, and six died within 10 days of onset. The patients were all initially affected between August 14 and August 27, 1919, and ranged in age from 16 to 40 (three of the victims were staff who were older than 30; all the others ranged in age from 15 to 22). Nine of the victims had very classic somnolent-ophthalmoplegic EL including pseudo-somnolence, masked facies, and ocular signs. The other three had what MacNalty referred to as the "abortive" type of the disease, without localizing signs. As a specialist in epidemiology, MacNalty considered noncontagious causes of the outbreak including diet, environmental factors, or toxic effects of drugs, and excluded them. Autopsies on the fatal cases were done, and only one victim's brain showed marked congestion; the other brains were almost normal in appearance. MacNalty was concerned about the relative lack of confirmatory pathological findings but, because the clinical picture was so consistent with previous cases of EL that he had treated, he concluded that the cases at Derby had died before the characteristic brain lesions had developed. MacNalty also noted no contemporaneous cases of EL or any similar illness in this remote village, and that there was no indication of illness in the remaining residents of the school.

The clinical descriptions in this report are very good and highly consistent with EL, and the investigation was done by an experienced EL clinician who examined the outbreak epidemiologically and concluded that person-to-person transmission had occurred. Stallybrass discussed this case in 1923 and concluded that these patients had been exposed to an aberrant EL virus with enhanced virulence. He also stated that, based on this report and others, "case-to-case infection is not infrequent."

In 1923, L.L Fyfe, in *The Lancet*, described a very similar type of EL outbreak in a school in the remote village of Eden Hill in England. Four of 18 girls were affected, none fatally. Fyfe suggested that this epidemic was similar to that in

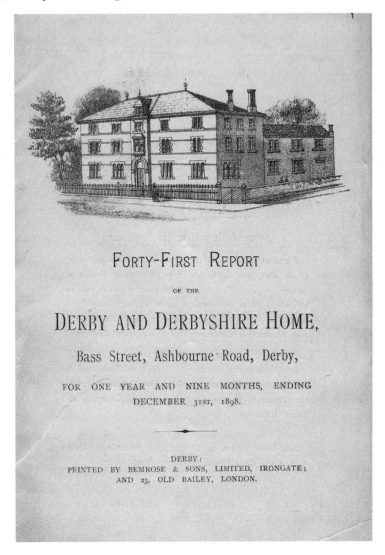

FORTY-FIRST REPORT

OF THE

DERBY AND DERBYSHIRE HOME,

Bass Street, Ashbourne Road, Derby,

FOR ONE YEAR AND NINE MONTHS, ENDING
DECEMBER 31ST, 1898.

DERBY:
PRINTED BY BEMROSE & SONS, LIMITED, IRONGATE;
AND 23, OLD BAILEY, LONDON.

Figure 6.2 Image of Derby and Derbyshire Rescue and Training Home (for girls).

Derby and that EL had an incubation period of about 9 days. A note added to the article by the county medical officer, Dr. Hamilton Wood, discussed the importance of the report and also noted that Dr. Fyfe's investigation was conducted in cooperation with the Ministry of Health.

Netter's Report on the Transmissibility of Encephalitis Lethargica

Arnold Netter was a renowned French Professor of Medicine who first characterized EL in France (see Chapter 2). In 1921, he authored, *Sur l'étiologie et la prophylaxie de l'encéphalite léthargique; sa declaration obligatoire* (On the Etiology and Prophylaxis of Encephalitis Lethargica; Its Obligatory Declaration). This report (abridged below) described the results of a commission composed of selected members of the French Academy of Medicine who were asked by the Ministry of Hygiene to investigate the transmissibility of EL:

There are two conflicting theorems about EL that are nevertheless compatible: (1) The EL epidemic is typically limited pertaining to locality and time; and (2) EL is transmissible by contagion. Furthermore, EL's transmissibility, which may be so limited that it can be doubted to exist, in some cases reaches a proportion as high as in the most contagious diseases. Examples of both extremes are presented below, with examples of noncontagion presented first.

In a family with five children living in a single apartment, a 4-year-old infant remained sick with EL for many weeks without any of her siblings showing signs of the disease. Similarly, because of the absence of separate rooms at the children's hospital, contagious diseases spread easily. Nevertheless, we have been required to hold in our wards more than 50 infants with EL. None of our other children showed signs of encephalitis, not even of the abortive type; and, none of the staff showed signs of EL.

We were asked to see a girl suffering from encephalitis in an institution with more than 500 patients and with numerous personnel. There were no other patients with EL.

We note the case of a female postal employee who was affected with EL between September 1919 and January 1921, but who continued to work during this period. The post office at which she was assigned had a workforce of 350 people. She was in charge of the electric stamping of letters, which in turn were sent to 23 other employees assigned to the sorting of them. None of these employees or any other employee in the post office developed EL.

Pertaining to the troops at land or at sea, the cases of encephalitis remained isolated.

Judging by these findings, as well as by the absence of reports on contagion from the earlier observers), the disease is not contagious.

To the contrary, one of the most demonstrative cases in support of contagion is one that we reported on April 20, 1920 to the Academy of Medicine and that appeared in a family from the 15th District of Paris in which three children caught EL one after the other. The first came down with the disease in Puy-de-Dôme, in which the treating physician, Dr. Laroche, observed at that time other contagious cases of EL. The child was brought to Paris, where she remained ill for many weeks. She was released from the hospital on November 16, placed in a small, poorly ventilated room on the ground floor with her eldest sister and younger, breastfeeding brother. The sister showed the first symptoms of fatal encephalitis on December 12, and the infant showed signs in January.

In the next example, EL made its appearance almost simultaneously in siblings who were together at rather rare times in a family. They had been bridesmaids at the same wedding. The younger, aged 4 years, developed the disease on April 26 in the middle of the ceremony. The older had been hospitalized the same day for encephalitis that had "erupted" on the 24th. The younger girl had been at a boarding school prior to the wedding in which another young girl had been affected 3 weeks previously. This observation provides proof of the transmissibility of EL from a subject during the incubation period of the disease.

Monsieur René Mathieu communicated to us the history of two sisters treated for EL at a clinic of nervous diseases at the Salpêtrière (a Paris hospital). One became ill in January, and the other in December of 1919. They lived with their respective families, but worked in the same establishment. This would tend to establish that the sister first taken ill could still spread the disease 11 months after its debut.

Similar to the cases of familial contagion, are examples of contagion occurring in hospitals, barracks, and schools. Twice, we have had two children affected, at an interval of 3–4 weeks, in a boarding school. These children were in direct contact. The population of one of these establishments was greater than 500 children whereas the other had more than 100 residents.

Monsieur Henri Claude observed at Saint-Antoine (hospital) two cases of encephalitis: one, 5 months, and the other 4 weeks of age, after their entry into rooms in which patients affected with EL were being treated. Messieurs Henri Roger and André Blanchard had treated at Marseille, at 15-day intervals, two soldiers affected with encephalitis. They had been recruited at the beginning of October, 1920, apparently to the same position of student corporal, shared almost adjacent beds in the barracks, and worked at length in the same office days before they first showed the initial symptoms.

In all of the observations described so far, the starting point of transmission was a patient, a convalescent, or a subject in the course of incubation. In the following observations, the contagion was unquestionably due to a healthy subject (one or both the parents or a servant in this case) who was not showing signs of encephalitis, but had visited a patient. We have seen a little boy, the last victim in a family of which M. Pierre-Paul Lévy reported his observations to the Society of Hospitals on July 9, 1920, and of which this is summarily the history. The eldest girl became ill January 10, 1920, and died 8 days later. The two remaining children left the apartment January 12 without contact with the patient. The house was disinfected with formalin on January 20 and abandoned by all the family on this date. On February 6, the parents, the two children, and the servant left for Hendaye, where they stayed for 4 months, until June 1920. At the beginning of May 1920, the son became ill at Hendaye with paralysis of the soft palate and some constriction of the pharynx, presumably an attack on the nuclei of the ninth and tenth cranial nerves and for which one could confirm the absence of any relationship with diphtheria. The youngest child, upon returning to Paris, became ill on June 13. In addition to headache, the child showed irregular heartbeats and respirations. On June 18, the second child developed choreoathetoid movements, and walked stiffly with a head tremor. Somnolence developed on June 19, followed by myoclonic spasms in the face and limbs. For 20 hours, the child had retention of urine. A lumbar puncture revealed clear liquid with normal albumin, and 41 lymphocytes. The heart beat irregularities persisted for 2 weeks. The child was treated with an injection of turpentine, which resulted in rapid improvement. The interval between the first two cases was 4 months, and 1 month passed between the second and third. The interval is longer between the two following familial cases.

A girl of 14 years developed EL on June 25, 1920. The sister of this young girl, 22 years old, had died on January 8, 1919 from EL, which debuted on December 25, 1918. The patient is assumed to have been exposed to the virus while in the presence of her sister, although not developing symptoms until 1.5 years after her sister's death. A man, 36 years of age, developed encephalitis in Paris on the 4th of September. His father had died on February 5, the ninth day of myoclonic encephalitis in a village in the center of France. The son had not returned to this city before August 5. From August 5 through the 20, he lived in the house where his father died, put into order his diverse affairs, arranged his cabinets, wore the interior part of his father's suit coat, and made use of his linens, in particular, his handkerchiefs. However, the widow and the brother, who had looked after the father, and who also lived in the house from August −20, did not develop any form of EL. The suspicion here is that the objects contained and transmitted the virus of EL.

We suggest that, although contagion is seldom highlighted in EL, it still plays an indisputable role in its propagation and that is sometimes very prominent. This paradoxical observation of contagiousness rarely manifesting but indisputable is not special to encephalitis. It is seen in poliomyelitis, of which the contagious character had been for a long time overlooked, and in cerebral-spinal meningitis, where it is often exaggerated. In encephalitis, as in poliomyelitis and meningitis, the portal of entry is most commonly within the nasal passages [author's note: this was later shown to be incorrect; polio is spread via ingestion of contaminated liquid]. M. Duret pointed out to us that the cerebral peduncles, the primary area of the lesions of encephalitis, are situated precisely above the sphenoidal sinus.

We have, with M. Durand, reported the importance of the alterations in the salivary glands in EL, and expressed the idea that, as in rabies, it is there that the virus of encephalitis attaches to nervous elements. If this hypothesis is confirmed, it will explain the intermittent presence, irregularity of the virus and, by consequence, the variable transmissibility, as well as the long duration of contagiousness. The relative rarity of contagion may be due to the necessity for a nervous predisposition in certain subjects and the emotional disturbances in these years of war, which, without a doubt also contribute to the vulnerability of the brain.

These considerations dictate appropriate conduct when one recognizes the existence of a case of EL. One should try very hard to isolate the patients. It should not be forgotten that the diagnosis is not always easy because of the extreme polymorphism of the disease so that, in certain cases, EL can manifest simply as neuralgia pain, chorea, or even a simple hiccup. Isolation should be continued for the convalescent, and may have to be continued for many months and even many years.

Although Netter seemed to be convinced that these cases demonstrate contagiousness, they seem much less convincing than the Derby school case——and for all these cases, it would be relatively easy to postulate coincidence rather than contagion.

Kling and Liljenquist's Report on the Spread of Encephalitis Lethargica in Lapland, Sweden

In 1921, C. Kling and F. Liljenquist published *Epidemiologie de l'encephalitie lethargique* (Epidemiology of Encephalitis Lethargica), which detailed the spread of EL in rural Sweden. It is abridged here:

In autumn, 1919, EL made its appearance in Sweden. We conducted our studies there in February, 1921, specifically in the parish of Vilhelmina in Lapland—the most northern province in Sweden—where the disease was very severe. The town of Vilhelmina, consisting of an area of 8,700 square kilometers and a very sparse population of 9,000 individuals, presented favorable conditions for the study of the stages of the epidemic. This large town is composed of the administrative center, with 1,000 inhabitants, and a large number of outlying regions with 25–300 habitants. We have chosen for our research four of the smaller of these regions, of which we have examined all the inhabitants. Our results are as follows:

1. We noticed that, apart from the typical cases of the disease, there were a large number of mild cases. The morbidity of those varied between 7.1% and 45%. In certain families, many members were affected with the disease simultaneously, and in two households, all of the inhabitants were affected.
2. Near some of the most serious cases, we found other subjects affected with less pronounced nervous system manifestations. These individuals were suddenly taken ill and stayed in bed for hours or even 1 or 2 days. The symptoms were: catarrhal complaints in the upper respiratory tract (cold, bronchitis), insomnia, fever, headache, strong sensitivity to the scalp, pain in the neck and chest, dilated pupils and slow reaction to

light, dissociation of ocular movements, and sometimes facial paresis. Some patients had relentless hiccups that lasted from 1 to 4 days.

3. Our epidemiological research did not suggest that EL could be transmitted by water, milk, bedbugs, fleas, or lice (body or head). In winter, there are not any insects in this region. The dogs and cats, which we have examined, were found to be unaffected.

4. Accordingly, the disease thus presumably was spread here by human contact, and the number of minor cases, most of who continued with their daily business, contributed to the multiple occasions for the diffusion of the virus. The catarrhal symptoms of the respiratory tract indicated that the virus is contained in the nasopharyngeal and tracheal secretions. The diarrhea, which is often apparent, explains the elimination of the virus by way of intestinal tract.

The incubation period was evaluated in three cases. It appeared to be around 10 days. In the large territory of Vilhelmina, the disease was spread in the short space of 2 months; a diffusion so rapid that it virtually cannot be explained by anything other than human contact.

Kling and Liljenquist seemed to have performed a very thorough epidemiological investigation and reached conclusions very similar to MacNalty, and also similar to Netter, in terms of the role of nasopharyngeal secretions (saliva) in propagating the disease. Their conclusion that human contact was involved in the propagation of the disease is hard to dispute.

Duzár and Balo's Report of the Spread of Encephalitis Lethargica in a Newborn Ward in Hungary

In 1922, J. Duzár and J. Balois published *Eine interessante "Encephalitis-Epidemica"-Endemie an einer Säuglingsabteilung* (An Interesting Encephalitis Epidemic in a Newborn Ward). This is an important report because, although there were many descriptions of hospital wards in which contagion was not apparent, in this case, EL appeared to be highly contagious.

On October 17, 1921, a 2.5-month-old child was admitted to the children's Hospital of Elizabeth University in Budapest with EL. On the fourth day after admittance, the 2-month-old infant in the neighboring bed, who had been admitted 1 day before with minimal bronchitis, fell ill as the first link in a chain of fatal epidemic affecting the whole ward. The illness spreads like a raging fire without our being able to stop it. One infant after another was attacked with the same symptoms. It should be noted that our ward is divided into box-systems assuring a high degree of isolation; and, our staff is recruited from intelligent, well-practiced welfare workers who graduate from our nursing course. Thus, the infectious disease among the infants, if it was not transferred through an illness of the staff, was most likely to have been spread during bathing when the infants were in close proximity. Of our 11 ill children, one recovered (it later died with pertussis in a hospital specializing in infections). Another child with initial symptoms was taken home by its parents and we do not know its final fate. All the other infants died, on average, 6–8 days after onset (in one case after 2, in another, after 14 days).

Although there seems little doubt that some infectious agent spread through the newborns, diagnosis of EL in such young children would seem especially tenuous, and I am reticent to accept this report as definitive pertaining to EL contagiousness. On the other hand, we could assume that these were experienced physicians who were familiar with EL, so the diagnosis may have been valid.

Chasanow's Description of Encephalitis Lethargica in White Russia

In 1930, M. Chasanow wrote *Beobachtungen über die epidemische Encephalitis in Weissrussland* (Some Numbers and Observations About Epidemic Encephalitis in White Russia). The term "White Russia" is an English translation from the Slavonic "Byelaya Ruś," and refers to an eastern region of the former Soviet Union that borders the Baltic States and Poland, currently Belarus.

We observed two cases of encephalitis in White Russia in 1918. More cases of EL appeared in White Russia in 1919, and increased steadily after 1920. Our material includes 919 cases from the years 1918 to 1928.

The first case in 1918 seems to have spread from Germany. Two cases observed by us developed shortly after occupation of White Russian territory by the German army; both were in families where German soldiers had been quartered. In one village, after German soldiers were quartered there, about 10 persons fell ill "with sleeping sickness, fever, and disturbances of the eyes" lasting 12–14 days. Of these, we later observed several with typical postencephalitic symptoms.

In 1918–1919, the encephalitis epidemic flared up in Poland, and seemed to spread across White Russia with Polish troops who occupied White Russia in 1919–1920. In 1919, we personally observed several cases of sleeping sickness, fever, and diplopia both in Polish soldiers (from Poznan) and among the local population with whom they had contact. The number of cases tripled from 1919 to 1920. Irrespective of the great typhus epidemic that peaked in White Russia in 1920–1921, the encephalitis cases steadily increased. In 1921, we had the opportunity to follow the continued development and course of the epidemic in one town.

The spread of this epidemic, which could be followed from house to house in the sparsely populated little towns and which took place within 4 to 5 months, confirms to some extent the investigations of Kling and Liljenquist (cf. above), and others: (1) on the contagiousness of EL through direct contact as well as indirectly via virus carriers; (2) on the appearance, in the vicinity of encephalitis patients, of flu-like illnesses that can be considered rudimentary, abortive cases of encephalitis; and, (3) that the incubation period is 2 to 30 days.

As did Maier, Orlow, Rapoport, Tschetwerikow, and others, we were also able to confirm a significant number of cases of EL among railroad employees and their families, and also in professions connected to ongoing social/ business contact with many people.

As noted by the author, there are many similarities in these examples to the report by Kling and Liljenquist; Chasanow seemed to be very well-versed in EL, and his data are hard to dispute as evidence of anything other than person-to-person transmission.

Geimanowitsch's Report on Encephalitis Lethargica in the USSR

A.I. Geimanowitsch (sometimes spelled Heimanovitsch) published extensively on EL in the Soviet Union (see Vilensky et al. 2008). In a 1928 review article, he indicated that Astvatzaturov (from Saint Petersburg) discussed one family with hiccups and a 4-year-old son who then developed a fatal case of EL. Geimanowitsch also stated that Andres reported an EL epidemic at a military unit in Karkov, and Korganov at the orphanage in Vladikavkaz. Geimanowitsch found records for one family in Stavropole in which four members developed EL. Finally, Geimanowitsch stated that Rapoport reported three contagious cases from among 95, Krontovsky identified two cases among 507 in Kiev, and he found five cases among 1,500.

Geimanowitsch's data are not very convincing of contagion; they are included here because data from the USSR are not typically found in the EL monographs.

Stiefler Report on Contagiousness of Encephalitis Lethargica in Austria

In 1922, G. Stiefler published *Zur Frage der Kontagiostät der Encephalitis Lethargica Epidemica* (About the Contagiousness of Encephalitis Lethargica), which discussed the contagiousness of EL in Austria. He concluded that EL was contagious based on the following observations:

1. The 33-year-old wife of a merchant with definitive EL died during an abortion (done because she had EL). Her mother, 72 years old, lived in an apartment in a part of the city far away from the daughter. However, 11 days after visiting her daughter (kissing her repeatedly), the mother became ill with flickering before her eyes, rapid fatigue of eyes while reading, and diplopia. After 8 days, she recovered.

2. In the hospital of the Merciful Sisters, there were four new cases of EL in the same ward, all of whom became ill between Jan. 14 and Feb. 16, 1920. They were typical EL cases, who had a strong/considerable sleeping sickness apart from the well-known other symptoms: pupillary disturbances; eye muscle and facial paresis; unclear, monotonous speech; weakness and differences between the tendon reflexes of the legs; nervous irritations; and sometimes myoclonus, which occasionally had a choreic character. There were no cold symptoms of the nasal and throat passages or of the bronchial airways.

   On March 1, 1920, a 34-year-old nun, who had been taking care of the EL patients, became ill with headaches, sleeplessness, fatigue, and fever. She continued her duties at first, and then developed light chorea in both arms that lasted a few days. Somnolence then appeared, but from which she was easily awakened and oriented. Other symptoms followed, with full recovery by July 4.

3. A 44-year-old male teacher became ill on Jan. 2 without warning, with shivers, nausea, light fever, pains in the back of the head, double vision, and light stiffness of the neck. He was very restless, rushed out of bed, and spoke nonsensically, mostly about his professional duties. Upon examination, he had a strong headache in the back of the head; feelings of dizziness when sitting up; slight ptosis on both sides; a left pupil that was somewhat wider than the right; slight and slow reaction to light and convergence on both sides; and dysarthria. After a variable course in the beginning, gradual improvement occurred. Upon examination on March 14, there were no more local symptoms of illness. He offered a picture of a postinfection nervous and weak condition with heightened excitability, sleeplessness with increased need of sleep, rapid fatigue, and lightly depressed mood. After 5 more weeks, the patient was fully recovered and was able to work.

   On January 23, 3 weeks after the beginning of the illness, his 17-year-old daughter, who lived with him and his wife, and who was a sales clerk in a business, developed shivers, general feeling of illness, and fatigue. During the next few days, she developed intense head and body aches, nausea, and sweating. She fully recovered within 3 weeks. In this observation, assumption of a transfer of the illness from father to daughter is very probable, although neither his wife nor his two other children developed the disease. This transmission suggests a 3-week incubation time.

4. A 47-year-old unskilled worker at a shipyard was admitted to the hospital on March 3, 1921 with ophthalmoplegia. The patient said that he became ill suddenly on the 1st of March with chills, headache, fatigue, and diplopia. He recovered by the end of June but had been bedridden for 5 weeks.

   A 19-year-old female clerk lived in a room directly next to the worker's apartment and interacted with him often. On February 24, she entered his apartment and told him that she had had strong headaches since yesterday, sniffles, and a sore throat. She became bedridden the same day. She next became delirious, which was followed by a deep lethargy of several weeks. She completely recovered after about 8 weeks.

5. The 51-year-old wife of a government clerk became ill on November 14, 1919, with general ill feelings, light shivers, sweating suddenly overnight, with a strong right-sided facial paralysis. The paralysis regressed very slowly but is still currently slightly recognizable: shallower furrowing of the brow to the right than to the left, almost complete but powerless closing of the right eyelid. On the day before the appearance of symptoms, she had undertaken a train trip, and a broken window exposed the right side of the face to a cold draft. Her 69-year-old governmental clerk husband became ill on November 27, 1919, with a paralysis of the left half of the face with flickering before his eyes and strong pains in the area behind the ear.

   Because of the medical history given by the woman, I considered it a cold paralysis and tended to see the same etiology for her husband although there was no analogous medical history. However, I was not entirely satisfied with this assumption because there was observed in Linz at that time an outbreak of peripheral facial paralysis that suggested that the cause was an infectious agent associated with EL. Both patients lived in one house and saw each other almost every day, so that the assumption of a contagious transfer seems rather obvious.

6. A 46-year-old carpenter became suddenly ill on Jan. 25, 1920, with light fever and shivers, general fatigue, and diplopia. Mentally, there was a mild delirium that alternated with somnolence. The latter became stronger after a 1-week delirious phase. A peripheral facial paralysis was present bilaterally. On February 25, the patient was subjectively free of complaints and was able to return to work. Nose, throat, and bronchia remained free of catarrh-like symptoms during the entire course of the illness.

   A 12-year-old neighboring female became ill with fever, headache, nausea, sleeplessness, and delirious confusion in mid-February 1920. Following the delirious state, there was a deep lethargy of several weeks. In the middle of May, the patient began recovering. These two individuals lived in two neighboring streets. Their apartments didn't touch each other but were about 400 steps from each other. However, the carpenter's daughter sat next to this girl in school. A few days later, I examined the carpenter's daughter, who remained well. Epidemiologically, this case thus shows a contagious connection through a healthy virus carrier.

7. A 23-year-old farmer became ill in the middle of March 1920 with light fever, headache, double vision, and sleep sickness that lasted several weeks. Later, one noticed unsteadiness of the hands when grasping objects and of the legs when standing and walking. His condition became better gradually, but then worsened.

   A farmer's 11-year-old son developed in June 1919 a feverish flu for several days with full recovery. He became ill again on the 10th of February, 1921, with similar symptoms to the first farmer. His family lived in an isolated farm that was located about a 30-minute walk from the first farmer's residence. The interaction between the families was not espe-cially active, but his 13-year-old sister visited the ill farmer at the end of January 1921 and 10–12 days later, he became ill with EL. Both patients gave the symptomatic picture of an acute cerebral ataxia with a chronic course. The relationship to EL can hardly be called into doubt despite the generally rarer cerebellar localization in this illness. The contagiousness can be assumed to be likely because of the described interaction, whereby the mode of infection can be considered to be a healthy virus carrier—the older sister of the boy who visited the farmer. The incubation time could be seen as 10–12 days.

8. The 9-year-old boy became ill at the beginning of March 1920 with chills and fever, strong headache, double vision, hallucinations, and somno-lence. He was bedridden for several months and developed a stiff pos-ture, slowness of movement, and quiet, misunderstood speech. Upon examination on April 16, 1921, we found double-sided ptosis, slowness of pupillary light reaction, paresis of the right side of the mouth, mask-like facial expression, drooling, monotonous speech, forward bending of the trunk of the body, flexion position of the arms and legs, poverty of move-ment, slowness and difficulty of active movements—the Parkinson syn-drome. The mother of the patient shared with me upon questioning that in a farm 2 hours away from her property an 11-year-old girl had fallen ill with the same symptoms and currently had the same symptoms as her son. Further research showed that the parents of the 9-year-old had visited on Easter 1920 (April 4) the family of the 11-year-old, who 8 days later developed EL.

For many of his observations, Steifler seemed to rely on the transmission of EL with very similar symptomatology from one person to another. On the other hand, the symptomatology of EL was very variable both among patients and within patients (transitory). Thus, these cases seem less convincing, although the transmission of EL to the nun in case 2 is the most credible as an example of EL contagion.

Freeman's Report on Contagion in Chronic Encephalitis Lethargica in the United States

In 1926, Walter Freeman, who was a senior medical officer at St. Elizabeth's Hospital in Washington, D.C., and who later became famous (infamous) for his development of transorbital lobotomy as a treatment of psychiatric disorders, published *Chronic Epidemic Encephalitis,* which includes a description of eight cases of acute EL, which he believed were derived from contact with individuals who had chronic EL. He reported that:

1. A young girl developed and recovered from acute EL in March of 1918, but EL returned with diplopia and fever in September 1920. In November of 1920, her father developed acute EL.
2. A tuberculosis patient in a hospital was in the same ward as a postencephalitic parkinsonism (PEP) patient in August 1920. In December of that year, the tuberculosis patient developed fever, diplopia, and somnolence.
3. A boy had acute EL from May to July 1920; he recovered, but residual signs remained. His cousin, who visited him every day, developed EL on December 23, 1920.
4. A young woman initially developed EL in October 1919, which progressed to PEP. In the spring of 1922, she had a recurrence of acute symptoms; at this time, her father also developed acute EL.
5. In July 1919, a woman developed EL with lassitude and vertigo. In January 1920, EL recurred, but this time with insomnia and muscular rigidity. A year later, her husband showed signs of EL and was diagnosed with PEP by October of that year.
6. A 46-year-old-man was hospitalized with chronic EL in December 1922, with death occurring in January 1923. A few days after his death, an 18-year-old boy who occupied the same ward contracted acute EL.
7. A 22-year-old male polio victim was located between two PEP patients in a hospital. Although there were no cases of acute EL in the hospital, the man developed EL.

Freeman believed these cases implied the persistence of the causative agent of EL long after the subsidence of the acute disease. He suggested that patients with the chronic form of EL are suffering from a continuance of the infection, just as patients with dementia paralytica (tertiary syphilis; general paresis of the insane) are suffering from the persistence of the spirochete. Although Freeman may be correct about the persistence of the EL virus in chronic cases, the cases he described are generally not very convincing relative to simple conincidence.

MacGregor and Craig's Report on Transmission from Postencephalitic Parkinsonism Patients to Young Children in Scotland

In 1934, A. R. MacGregor and W. S. Craig published, *An Epidemic of Acute Encephalitis in Young Children.*

Two hospital PEP patients with excessive salivation, on a hot day, held, kissed, and played with four children during their outings in the garden for "long periods" of time. Cases 1–3 were in the same ward and, cases 1 and 2 were in adjacent cots. Case 4 was in a different ward. The four children were attended to by the same nurses.

All four children fell ill within a period of 36 to 48 hours. Each of the four cases was very similar in nature, i.e., each child experienced severe, writhing pain upon examination and having their head touched. Cases 1 and 2 resulted in a "rapidly fatal course." Cases 3 and 4 recovered.

The four cases occurred so close together, and followed such similar courses, that the term "epidemic" can be used. The afebrile course, the results of blood examination, and the failure to discover any source of toxemia either clinically, or at autopsy confirmed the diagnosis of EL. The almost simultaneous occurrence of the four cases seemed to indicate a common source of infection rather than case-to-case transmission. No member of the staff in attendance on the four children reported sick at any time during the month. There were no other recognized cases of EL in the wards. Apart from the possible presence of an unrecognized carrier, there is little likelihood that infection was derived from any member of the staff or patient in the wards.

The infection in the case of our two adult patients with chronic encephalitis dated from acute attacks 9 and 11 years earlier. There was no history of any exacerbation in either case, but it may be mentioned that one of the patients had suffered from an attack of unexplained vomiting shortly before the outbreak among the children. The intimate contact occurring between these patients and the affected children has already been emphasized. On the assumption that the PEP patients were still infective, the risk of the children contracting infection could hardly have been greater.

Although I am reticent to criticize physicians of the time, the description of EL in these children is very unusual and limited. Thus, EL is, at best, at very tentative diagnosis and the notion of contagion of EL in these cases can similarly be questioned.

EPIDEMIC HICCUPS

Many "epidemics" of hiccups occurred during the EL epidemic period. Von Economo (1929) considered these epidemics to represent the most common form of the monosymptomatic type of EL. He noted that, in Vienna, in 1920, a small epidemic appeared of singultus without any other symptom, which affected many people and disappeared in hours to days. Von Economo noted that similar epidemics were seen in Paris, and that MacNalty described a hiccup epidemic in London as late as 1929.

Von Economo expressed some doubt as to whether these epidemics of hiccups actually represented EL because none of those affected (except for one case) had been noted to develop chronic EL. But his general view appears to be that they did represent some form of EL. Similarly, Dopter (1921) suggested that they represented a fragmented, myoclonic form of EL (see above).

The most well-known hiccup epidemics occurred in Winnipeg, Canada. Winnipeg experienced hiccup epidemics in 1919, 1922, and 1924. More than 100 cases were recorded during both the 1919 and 1924 epidemics. The epidemics began in November of each year, generally while more serious EL epidemics were also occurring. But there was not a single case of EL in a patient who had had a prior episode of hiccups, thus suggesting some sort of common immunity. Similar to EL, evidence of direct transmissibility of the hiccups could not be found in the Winnipeg epidemics (in contrast to the French hiccup epidemics mentioned by Dopter; see above). Finally, whereas EL generally affected both sexes approximately equally, 90% of those affected with hiccups in the Winnipeg epidemic were male (Cadham, 1925).

These hiccup epidemics were and still are perplexing. It seems likely that they did represent some form of EL, but similar to other forms of EL, the hiccups were contagious in some epidemics but not most.

ILLINOIS DEPARTMENT OF PUBLIC HEALTH (ISAAC
D. RAWLINGS, DIRECTOR). RULES AND REGULATIONS
FOR THE CONTROL OF EPIDEMIC (LETHARGIC)
ENCEPHALITIS

This nine-page pamphlet (Fig. 6.3) noted that the described regulations were in force throughout the state beginning August 1, 1928. The first sentence reads, "The Illinois Department of Public Health hereby declares epidemic (lethargic) encephalitis to be a contagious, infectious, and communicable disease and dangerous to the public health." It further states, pertaining to the specific rules, "It shall be the duty of all local boards of health, health authorities and officers, police officers, sheriffs, constables, and all other officers and employees of the State or any county, village, city, or township thereof, to enforce the rules and regulations that may be adopted by the State Board of Health."

The pamphlet differentiates between cases and carriers of the disease (the latter can disseminate the disease although do not show symptoms). It then declares that any case of suspected EL must immediately be reported to the local

ILLINOIS DEPARTMENT OF PUBLIC HEALTH
Isaac D. Rawlings, M. D., Director,
Springfield, Ill.

Rules and Regulations

FOR THE

Control of

Epidemic (Lethargic) Encephalitis

IN FORCE THROUGHOUT ILLINOIS

Revised August 1, 1928

[Printed by authority of the State of Illinois.]

Figure 6.3 Cover of Illinois pamphlet on regulations for the containment of EL.

health authority. Subsequently, the physician in charge of the case should either isolate the patient or instruct the family to do so. Such a patient should be isolated for 2 weeks, and no one other than attending medical personnel may be in contact with the patient. The pamphlet requires that all discharges from the respiratory tract, mouth, nose, and throat of the patient be contained in paper napkins and either burned immediately or immersed in a vessel containing an approved disinfecting solution. Similar instructions were given for soiled bedclothes. Once the case "terminated," the premises were to be thoroughly cleaned, aired, and "sunned."

If a patient died from EL, the body had to be disposed of within 48 hours unless properly embalmed. These rules went into effect on August 1, 1928. Penalty for violation of the rules consisted of a fine not exceeding $200 for each offense and/or imprisonment in the county jail for a period not exceeding 6 months. Although these rules are no longer technically in force, any current EL case would still be reportable in Illinois.

CONCLUSION

In this chapter, I have highlighted some of the reports suggesting that EL, at specific times and places, could be highly contagious. I must emphasize, however, that the vast majority of reports suggested that it typically was not. Of course, it is also possible that the lack of evidence for contagion in most reports may simply reflect that EL was ubiquitous, but phenotypic expression was not common (i.e., most people were carriers, as surmised by some of the above reports), perhaps being dependent on genetic predisposition. Nevertheless, the fact that EL was a reportable disease in many countries suggests that at least the respective Ministries of Health were concerned about contagion. Similarly, the publication of the Illinois Department of Public Health pamphlet indicates that, at least among some medical professionals as late as 1928, there was a firm belief that EL was highly infectious. Currently, I cannot explain the rather rare but convincing cases of EL contagion (e.g., Derby School, Lapland, White Russia) relative to the many examples of non-transmission. Perhaps, as suggested by others, these cases were based on rare strains. Or, as we suggest in other chapters as well, EL may not have been a unitary condition, and thus some forms could have been highly contagious whereas others were not. Pertaining to the epidemics of hiccups, they remain very enigmatic, but seemingly again may be explained by some rare strain of the virus that presumably caused EL. Regardless, the presented data do suggest that if EL recurs, measures to control its spread via person-to-person contact may need to be instituted.

REFERENCES CITED

Bernard, L. & Renault, J. (1920). L'enquête épidémiologique du ministère de l'Hygiéne sur l'encéphalite léthargique en France. *Bulletin de l'Académie Nationale de Médecine, 3,* 470–474.

Cadham, F. T. (1925). Hiccup: The Winnipeg epidemic. *Journal of the American Medical Association, 84,* 580–582.

Cruchet, R. Encéphalite Épidémique. (1928). Paris: Gaston Doin & C.

Chasanow, M. (1930). Einige zahlen und beobachtungen über die epidemische encephalitis in Weissrussland. *Archiv für Psychiatrie und Nervenkrankheiten, 93,* 116–129.

Dopter, C. (1921). Contagiosite de l'encephalite epidemique. *Paris Medical, 39,* 458–466.

Duzár, J. & Baló, J. (1922). Eine interessante "Encephalitis-Epidemica"-Endimie an einer Säuglingsabteilung. In v. Bokay, J., Czerny, A., Feer, E., Heubner, O. & Moro, E. (Eds.), *Jahrbuch Für Kinderheilkunde Und Physische Erziehung* (pp. 209–228). Berlin: Verlag Von S. Karger.

Freeman, W. (1926). Chronic epidemic encephalitis. *The Journal of the American Medical Association*, *87*, 1601–1603.

Fyfe, L. L. (1923). Encephalitis lethargica: an intensive outbreak in a small school. *Lancet*, *1*, 379–381.

Geimanowitsch, A. I. (1928). Epidemic encephalitides and their investigation in the USSR [in Russian]. *Central Medical Journal*, *5*, 837–847.

Gerstenbrand, F., Hoff, H., & Weingarten, K. (1958). Klinischer bericht über enzephalitis nach grippe. *Weiner Medizinische Wochenschrift*, *108*, 1–3.

Illinois Department of Public Health. (1928). *Rules and Regulations for the Control of Epidemic (Lethargic) Encephalitis; In Force Throughout Illinois, August 1928* (No. 401442A). Springfield, Illinois: Isaac D. Rawlings, M.D., Director.

Kling, C., & Liljenquist, F. (1921). Epidemiologie de l'encephalitie lethargique. *Comptes Rendus des Séances de la Societi de Biologie*, *74*, 521–524.

Matheson Commission. (1929). *Epidemic Encephalitis: Etiology, Epidemiology, Treatment*. New York: Columbia University Press.

MacGregor, A. R., & Craig, W. S. (1934). An epidemic of acute encephalitis in young children. *Archives of Disease in Childhood*, *9*, 153–170.

MacNalty, A. S. (1919). Report on outbreak of encephalitis lethargica in a girls' home. *Great Britain Ministry of Health: On the State of the Public Health* (Appendix VII), 357–368.

Netter, A. (1918). L'encéphalite léthargique épidémique. *Bulletin de l'Académie Nationale de Médecine*, *79*, 337–347.

Netter, A. (1921). Sur l'étiologie et la prophylaxie de l'encéphalite léthargique; sa declaration obligatoire. *Bulletin de l'Académie de Médecine*, *85*, 278–298.

Roques, F. (1928). Epidemic encephalitis in association with pregnancy, labour and the puerperium–A review and report of twenty-one cases. *The Journal of Obstetrics and Gynecology of the British Empire*, *35*, 48–113.

Smith, H. F. (1921). Epidemic encephalitis (encephalitis lethargica, nona): report of studies conducted in the United States. *Public Health Reports*, *36*, 207–242.

Stallybrass, C. O. (1923). Encephalitis lethargica: some observations on a recent outbreak. *Lancet*, *2*, 922–925.

Stiefler, G. (1922). Zur frage der kontagiosität der encephalitis lethargica epidemica. *Zeitschrift für die gesamte Neurologie und Psychiatrie*, *74*, 396–414.

Tilney, F., & Howe, H. S. (1920). *Epidemic Encephalitis (Encephalitis Lethargica)*. New York: Paul B. Hoeber.

Vilensky, J., Mukhamedzyanov, R., & Gilman, S. (2008). Encephalitis lethargica in the Soviet Union. *European Neurology*, *60*, 113–121.

von Economo, C. (1929). *Die Encephalitis Lethargica, ihre Nachkrankheiten und ihre Behardlung*. Berlin: Urban & Schwarzenberg. (Published in English in 1931: Translated by K. O. Newman; London: Oxford University Press).

7

SECONDARY (CHRONIC) ENCEPHALTIS LETHARGICA

Joel A. Vilensky and Sid Gilman

Part of the mystery and apprehension pertaining to encephalitis lethargica (EL) was its secondary (chronic) symptomatology, which could variably be called residuae, complications, or sequelae. The secondary stage of EL could arise directly from the acute stage, might appear and disappear as relapses with the same or a different set of symptoms than those exhibited during the acute stage, or might appear at some time (weeks to months to years) after apparent recovery or near-recovery. And, the symptomatology of these secondary stages could be as variable as that exhibited during the acute stage.

The most well-known chronic manifestation of EL in adults is postencephalitic parkinsonism (PEP). In children, the behavioral disturbances described in Chapter 2 are the most common sequel (von Economo, 1929), and the reader is referred to that chapter or to the article on these manifestations by Vilensky et al. (2008).

Von Economo (1929) listed some of the more common non-PEP sequelae as palsies, tremors, chorea, torticollis, ocular pareses, and various psychological conditions such as aphasia, agnosia, and bradyphrenia. He also indicated the presence of autonomic signs, such as sialorrhea and seborrhea, various neuralgias, especially limb pain, and vertigo. Wilson (1940) noted that hemiplegia, monoplegia, and hemianopia were common sequelae. And both noted how variable the signs could be, in accord with the variable signs of the acute phase.

In the EL/PEP literature, a great deal of confusion and ambiguity pertains to whether the non-PEP types of chronic EL persisted or whether PEP was the final outcome in virtually all cases of secondary EL. Among 925 EL patients, Wilson (1940) found that 334 (36.1%) became PEP cases. However, Neal (1942) stated that 80% of chronic cases were PEP. Certainly, as time passed from the epidemic period, the knowledge of non-PEP chronic sequelae diminished. Nielson (1953) indicated that all cases eventually developed parkinsonism. Duvoisin and Yahr, in 1965, stated that the majority of EL patients who survived eventually developed PEP. They suggested that even those who were not classified as having PEP may have been misclassified because minimal signs of parkinsonism may have been overshadowed by other encephalitic sequelae. Earlier, in 1931, Borthwick classified 265 cases of chronic EL (Table 7.1); he too considered all chronic conditions other than behavioral disorders, which are typically found in children, as manifestation of a parkinsonian syndrome, although the signs and symptoms would not all be consistent with parkinsonism (e.g., respiratory disorders, ocular palsy, hemiplegia). And even earlier, in 1922, House reported that parkinsonism only accounted for about 10% of chronic EL cases.

To some extent, the question as to whether all the chronic cases are PEP is a semantic one, in that virtually any one of the common chronic signs and symptoms could be consistent with a parkinsonian syndrome although probably not considered "Parkinson disease." The dichotomy is the classic "splitters" versus "lumpers" issue (i.e., those who view a syndrome as multiple, separate disease states versus those who assume that a variety of signs/symptoms arises from a single disease state).

One forgotten aspect of secondary EL is that it was not reported to develop uniformly during the epidemic period. Von Economo (1929) indicated that the number of chronic cases varied in different epidemics, so that the likelihood for a

Table 7.1 Chronic Encephalitis Lethargica Symptomatology (Modified from Borthwick, 1931) Based on 265 Cases

Behavioral Disorders
    Nocturnal excitement, etc. (4 cases)
    Mild, moderate, and severe behavioral disorders (48, 26, 33)
    Behavioral disorder of mentally deficient class (9)

Parkinsonian Syndromes
    Generalized: mild, moderate, severe (24, 36, 42)
    Hemi-parkinsonism (21)
    Hyperkinesias (6)
    Respiratory disorders (7)
    Dyspituitarism (4)
    Epilepsy (3)
    Ocular palsies (1)
    Pyramidal hemiplegia (1)

chronic phase to develop was dependent on the local and chronological peculiarities of the separate epidemics: "I saw, for instance, particularly in the wake of the epidemics of 1920–1921, a very striking number of such cases [chronic EL] and the number of mental and physical invalids who owe their disability to that epidemic is legion. In the epidemic of 1916–1917, I know of only two cases which took a chronic course" (p. 111). He went on to note that varying "types" of sequelae were also not uniformly distributed. For example, he observed that PEP was particularly prevalent in the London epidemic of 1918, and the one in Hamburg in 1919.

Because almost no data exist on non-PEP cases since the epidemic period, the remainder of this chapter pertains almost entirely to PEP.

POSTENCEPHALITIC PARKINSONISM

Von Economo referred to PEP patients as being frozen in position (catatonia), although they tended to be less rigid in the evenings. This "frozen in space and time" element is the prominent feature in the 1973 book by Oliver Sacks, *Awakenings*, and the 1990 movie of the same name. Von Economo also stated that, although PEP patients may show a rest tremor, it is rarely of the "pill-rolling" type sometimes seen in idiopathic Parkinson disease (PD). Because PEP and the use of L-dopa is so connected to Oliver Sacks and *Awakenings*, a separate chapter (Chapter 8) is devoted to this subject, and it will only be briefly mentioned further in this chapter.

Neal (1942) suggested that a single symptom typically appeared first in PEP: localized tremor, slight loss of facial expression, loss of fine movements, drowsiness, diplopia, bradykinesia, weakness in the arm or leg, or rigidity. Tremor was the earliest sign in about 50% of the cases, which is very consistent with the more recent Hoehn and Yahr data (1967; see below). The patient often complained of a feeling of mental fatigue, as well as loss of quickness in thinking and ability to concentrate (see self-reports in Chapter 11). With time, symptoms intensified, and new symptoms developed: oculogyric crises (OCs), blepharospasm, sialorrhea, and slowness or other difficulty in speech. Next, loss of or diminution in associated movements, masked facies, and infrequency in blinking almost always occurred. Rigidity could increase to the point that it became impossible for the patient to rise from a chair, and there were disturbances in gait. Other signs were obesity, disturbances of sexual function, cachexia, and constipation. The rate of progression varied, and there might be periods of apparent improvement or exacerbations. Only a few patients reached a stationary phase.

The rigidity and bradykinesia in PEP are similar to that in PD, but PEP may typically be distinguished from PD clinically (Table 7.2; Figs. 7.1–7.3) with age at onset being the best differentiator. Twenty years after Neal published her findings, Hoehn and Yahr (1967) also examined the differences between PEP and PD and

Table 7.2 Features that Distinguish Parkinson Disease from Postencephalitic Parkinsonism (from Neal, 1942)

Sign	PD	PEP
Age at onset	Typically 50–60	Any age; typically under 40
Onset	Gradual	Gradual
Course	Regular progression	Progresses rather quickly; but may then become stationary
Extent	Usually generalized	Body parts affected may be limited but may also be generalized
Tremor	Both rigidity and tremor almost always present	Tremor not common; rigidity almost always present
Complications		Encephalitis residua: tics, spasms, respiratory disorders; behavioral changes
Special features	Sialorrhea not common; diplopia not common; papillary reactions normal	Sialorrhea common; wet tongue; greasy skin; pupillary reactions impaired; diplopia

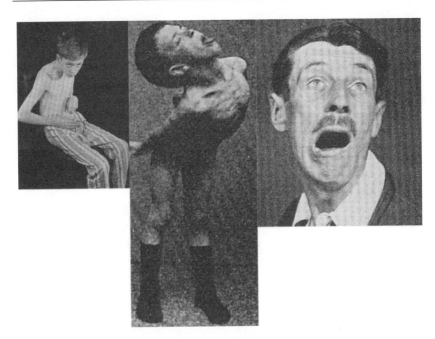

Figure 7.1 *Left*: Illustration of postencephalitic parkinsonism (PEP) attitude in male adolescent. *Middle*: Postencephalitic torsions spasm. *Right*: PEP patient with mandibular tic. (From Wilson, 1940.)

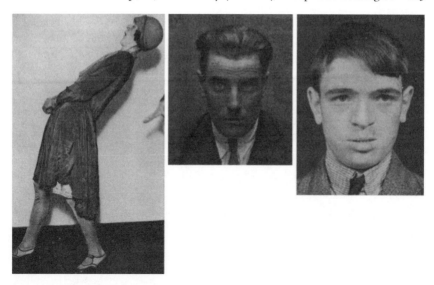

Figure 7.2 *Left*: An unusual case of postencephalitic parkinsonism (PEP) in extension. *Middle* and *right*: PEP cases with narcolepsy; note expressionless face. (From Wilson, 1940.)

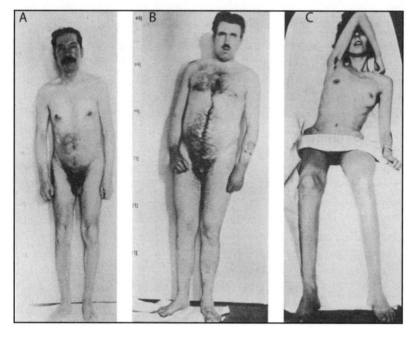

Figure 7.3 **A**: Parkinsonian syndrome, following epidemic encephalitis. **B**: Parkinsonian syndrome in man 23 years old, following epidemic encephalitis 10 years earlier; right arm and leg are rigid. **C**: The peculiar position of the right upper extremity in this PEP patient frequently assumed and long maintained. (From Barker, 1930.)

Table 7.3 Age at Onset of Parkinson Disease versus Postencephalitic Parkinsonism (from Hoehn and Yahr, 1967)

	Age at onset	Standard deviation	Range
PD (n = 672)	55.3	11.3	17–89
PEP (n = 96)	28.2	8.8	12–53

reported that age again was the best differentiator (Table 7.3; Fig. 7.1–7.3). Note that, in Table 7.3, the mean age of onset of PD (55.3) is almost double that of PEP (28.2). Parkinson disease also had much greater age range (17–89) than did PEP (12–53). In 1998, Litvan et al. reported that contemporary neurologists could separate PEP from PD using medical records with almost 100% accuracy, based mostly on age at onset (younger in PEP), duration (longer in PEP), and the presence of OCs in PEP.

Hoehn and Yahr (1967) found, similar to Neal (1942; see above), that tremor was typically the initial sign in both PEP and PD, although it constituted the initial sign in 70% of their PD patients and 52% of their PEP patients. Sleep, psychiatric, and speech disorders were more frequent initial signs in PEP than in PD. Neither group had a pure intention tremor. The mean age of death in the PD group was 65.9 years and that of the PEP group was 54 years, but age at death did not differ between PEP and the PD patients who began their parkinsonism at comparable (young) ages. Thus, age of death seems to be a consequence of age at onset rather than type of parkinsonism.

In 1963, Poskanzer and Schwab suggested that PEP and PD were dissimilar only quantitatively, presumably based on the longer disease span and younger age at onset in the PEP patients. They postulated that the vast majority of parkinsonian patients living at the time had contracted EL during the epidemic period (in many cases, subclinically) and the effects became evident as parkinsonism up to 40 years later. However, based on their analysis, a sharp drop in the number of cases of parkinsonism should have occurred after 1980, and this did not happen. Poskanzer and Schwab's theory was featured in a *New York Times* article, "*New Theory Links Palsy to a Virus*," which appeared October 19, 1962. Duvoisin et al. (1963) sharply criticized this work, asserting that PD has multiple causes and that the disease would remain a prominent neurologic entity (cf. below).

Although sialorrhea is found in both PD and PEP patients, there may be a difference in the etiology between them. Whereas in PD patients it is typically attributed to difficulty in swallowing, in PEP patients it was believed to be due to increased secretion of the parotid gland (Neal, 1942; three of the physician self-reports in Chapter 12 specifically refer to excessive salivation). This is not generally known, and it suggests some differences in the underlying pathophysiology between the two disorders (although the physicians and patients of the time may not have detected a decrease in reflex swallowing).

Neal (1942) noted that the development of the chronic stage of EL seemed to be correlated with certain events, such as physical and emotional trauma, illness, mental or physical overexertion, and pregnancy. She believed this apparent relationship was probably coincidental, but exogenous factors were typically mentioned in Russian articles on EL as contributing to the development of the acute or chronic phases (Vilensky et al. 2008). Similarly, Crafts (1927) stated that trauma can be "important in activating the virus of EL" (p. 196). He described five cases in which he believed trauma (e.g., head injury) may have triggered the initiation of the disease process.

Neal reported that the beginning of the chronic stage of EL was often associated with pregnancy and recommended abortion in those cases because pregnancy tended to exacerbate EL's symptoms (see case 8 in Chapter 11). Although rarely reported, the hyperhydrosis in PEP patients could be of a crisis type; it would occur paroxysmally and be unrelated to the environment. Typically, these crises occurred late in the night or early in the day and could be so intense as to require a change in clothing. In these crises, there was marked skin hyperemia, and axillary temperature could exceed 100°F [37.8°C] (Onuaguluchi, 1964).

Finally, the phenomenon of paradoxical kinesis was very prominent in PEP patients. Von Economo (1929) noted that it was interesting that akinesia and hypertonia can be overcome in PEP patients because sometimes patients who could only walk with difficulty could dance quite well to musical accompaniment or might, in a state of excitement, run after a moving vehicle (this is also true of some PD patients).

Except for OCs, which are described in Chapter 5 and were a rather uncommon characteristic of PEP, none of the features listed in Table 7.2 is unique to PEP and may occasionally be found in other parkinsonian disorders. Thus, diagnosis of PEP is somewhat indefinite, usually depending on the presence of some combination of the features listed in the table plus the prior occurrence of an encephalitic illness, presumably EL. However, as will be discussed later in this chapter, many cases of parkinsonism were considered PEP despite the complete lack of any evidence that the patient had an acute EL episode. Thus, PEP, similar to EL, cannot typically be diagnosed with certainty.

In order to further understand the presumed relationship among EL, PEP, and PD, it is important to examine whether PEP existed prior to the EL epidemic period.

EVIDENCE FOR PRE-ENCEPHALITIS LETHARGICA EXISTENCE OFF POSTENCEPHALITIC PARKINSONISM

In 1917, Dr. James Parkinson published *Essay on the Shaking Palsy*, which portrayed parkinsonism in far greater cohesiveness than had ever been done previously.

He described its cardinal features, "involuntary tremulous motion with lessened muscular power, in parts not in action and even when supported; with a propensity to bend the trunk forwards and to pass from a walking to a running pace; the senses and intellect being uninjured" (p. 223, Parkinson, 2002 [reprinted]). After Parkinson, Charcot, who became Chair of Diseases of the Nervous System at the Salpêtriére hospital in Paris, in 1882 "filled in the outline which Parkinson had drawn" (Sacks, 1990; p. 4). Charcot recognized the major symptoms of the condition: tremor, rigidity, postural problems, and bradykinesia.

There is no indication that either Parkinson or Charcot identified individuals with an unusual parkinsonian disorder similar to PEP, based on its relatively distinctive symptomatology. However, in 1921, Catola noted that PEP was observed in the 17th century, although he does not provide details.

In 2000, Brusa and Pramstaller published the results of their examination of more than 1,000 articles from the neurologic literature published between 1850 and 1916, and identified three cases that they considered "atypical parkinsonian cases" from 1895, 1905, and 1909. All three lacked a tremor and the authors concluded that, "…clinical syndromes characterized by the presence of extrapyramidal, pseudobulbar, and ocular symptoms, and the absence of tremor, were also present in the pre-encephalitic era" (p. 408). Thus, these reports are at least suggestive of the presence of PEP prior to the definitive existence of EL, although the described symptomatology would also be consistent with progressive supranuclear palsy (PSP).

Another approach to investigating whether PEP existed prior to the EL epidemic is to examine the early 20th-century descriptions of juvenile and early-onset parkinsonism because early onset (compared to PD) was characteristic of PEP. In 1911, Willige provided a detailed analysis of all previously described cases of early-onset PD (47 cases). He considered many of his cases to be nonstandard parkinsonism. He also found that parkinsonism often occurred in young people (18–20 years of age was his earliest-aged case) following an infection, typically typhus (it is unclear exactly what he meant by "typhus" in today's terminology), and it is also possible that many of these patients had Wilson disease rather than parkinsonism. He found that many of the young patients had a history of parkinsonism in their families, which is consistent with the currently understood genetic contribution to juvenile PD (see Chapter 5). Willige suggested that juvenile PD might be different from adult PD, and he also believed that some of his cases might have been complicated by multiple sclerosis. Ramsay Hunt (1917) described four cases of juvenile parkinsonism in detail, and these cases appeared very similar to classical PD. However, one (case 2), had the slow "rhythmical oscillation of eyeballs," which we described in Chapter 5 and which Bramwell (1928) believed was pathognomonic for EL/PEP. This patient first developed parkinsonian signs in 1896, so this possibly was a pre-EL case of PEP. Ramsay Hunt (1918), similar to Willige, also reported a strong familial component to juvenile PD, suggesting that most forms were probably of the genetic type (see Chapter 5).

Based on these reports, evidence seems suggestive that PEP existed prior to EL, but this conclusion is based on incomplete information and must be considered speculative.

IDENTIFICATION OF POSTENCEPHALITIC PARKINSONISM AND/ OR A PARKINSONIAN TYPE OF ENCEPHALITIS LETHARGICA DURING THE EPIDEMIC PERIOD

By the time of the EL epidemic, PD was a well-known and well-recognized neurologic disorder. One can then readily imagine the great confusion that was undoubtedly present during the epidemic period, first by the large increase in parkinsonism in the general population and then by its unknown relationship to the idiopathic form of the disease. Certainly, clinicians of the time wondered whether PD was really different from amyostatic EL and PEP, or if perhaps all forms of parkinsonism were caused by encephalitis. (Interestingly, a recent and well-cited theory on the etiology of PD also suggests that it is due to a neurotrophic virus; Hawkes et al., 2007; see Chapter 9) Many clinicians of the time thought that PEP simply resulted from parkinsonism striking younger-aged individuals. This confusion was further confounded by some EL patients showing parkinsonism during acute EL and/or immediately following EL, whereas others showed virtually complete recoveries only to develop PEP many years later.

All of the EL cases von Economo described in his original two 1917 articles were acute cases and, at the time, he clearly had no idea that EL had long-term sequelae. Furthermore, he did not describe in either of his original EL articles any constellation of symptoms that could be viewed as parkinsonian. He did note, however, that three of the initial patients showed a "peculiar rigidity" of the extremities, which disappeared. However, any relationship with parkinsonism seems tenuous because these same patients and two others also showed ataxic features that suggested cerebellar involvement. But, by the time he published his 1929 monograph on EL, sequelae were well-known and PEP was relatively well-defined.

Netter's 1918 description of EL in France also did not mention any sequelae, although the first major British report on EL, also appearing in 1918 (Newsholme et al.), did mention sequelae but only paresis and contractures. It is significant that this British report did not include any type of EL that appeared related to the basal ganglia, although these structures were by this time believed to be associated with PD. In fact, nowhere in the entire 74-page monograph is parkinsonian or "amyostatic" ever mentioned. The authors considered the lesions of EL to be very similar to those of African sleeping sickness rather than any basal ganglia disease.

In 1918, British clinician E. Buzzard published an article on EL, noting that he made a mental diagnosis of paralysis agitans when a 59-year-old patient entered the examination room, based solely on the patient's gait and mask-like face.

Buzzard also reported that the patient had greatly recovered 2 months after his initial consultation, thus implying that these features were part of a transitory phase of EL. This article is the earliest to mention parkinsonism in relation to EL. Later in this same article, Buzzard reported that, in some cases of severe EL, the patients appeared to recover, but were, "overtaken by more or less disabling seque-lae at varying intervals of time" (p. 60). These sequelae consisted of involuntary movements affecting the limbs, jaw, or tongue. There is no mention of any seque-lae with parkinsonian features, and this seems important considering that Buzzard had mentioned a parkinsonian type of acute EL.

Also in 1918, another British clinician, A. J. Hall (1918a) remarked that the facial expression of an encephalitic patient was, "so suggestive of Parkinson's mask that I thought at first she must have paralysis agitans" (p. 569). Hall also noted that the symptoms disappeared in a few days and that the patient's tremor was very different from that in paralysis agitans.

A third British physician in that same year, Kinnier Wilson, described seven EL cases, each representing a different type of EL, including a paralysis agitans type. This patient showed bradykinesia, tremor, and a masked face; after 5 weeks, his symptoms markedly declined in severity (Wilson, 1918).

In the United States, the first mention of parkinsonism being related to EL appeared in the 1920 monograph by Tilney and Howe. They described five cases of EL as the "paralysis agitans" type: suppression of automatic movements, brady-kinesia, flexed attitude, masked facies, and the "agitans" tremor; only two showed any degree of somnolence, and three showed marked restlessness; three suffered from an episode of influenza just prior to the onset of EL.

Von Economo, in his 1929 monograph, noted that the French physicians Sicard and Paraf in 1920 were the first to call attention to the frequency of par-kinsonian signs in chronic EL. Sicard and Paraf initially described five patients suffering from PEP, noting that the patients showed rigidity, bradykinesia, and a shuffling gait. These patients did not show the pill-rolling tremor often associated with idiopathic PD. All of these patients initially suffered from the somnolent-ophthalmoplegic form of EL, and the authors stated that they have never seen PEP develop from the myoclonic type of EL (Sicard & Paraf, 1920). In comment-ing on this work, Souques (1921) maintained that so-called idiopathic PD can in fact also develop from EL. He referred to PEP as "pseudo-parkinsonism."

In 1921, additional American and European reports describing a "parkinso-nian" type of EL and PEP sequelae appeared. A world conference on EL met in Paris, in 1921, chaired by M. A. Souques and A. Netter, in which PEP was a major topic of discussion. Both the U.S. and European observers at the conference were struck by the "absolute resemblance" of PEP to parkinsonism. Souques referred to the case seen by Kinnier Wilson and noted that, in France, some differences in opinion existed as to the relationship between PEP and PD, but that he believed that encephalitic parkinsonism could lead to the disease of Parkinson, and that EL is one of the causes of paralysis agitans. Souques indicated that the lesions are the same in both conditions and that, if EL causes minor and repairable lesions, a "parkinsonian syndrome" will result, whereas if the lesions are serious and irreparable, the patient will develop true parkinsonism. Souques related the earlier age of onset of PEP compared to PD to the fact that data indicated that EL typically did not affect the middle-aged or elderly. Souque also stated that, in most cases, PEP followed the somnolence-ophthalmoplegic form of EL, and that the parkinsonian signs appeared shortly after the lethargic symptoms disappeared. He believed that, when a PEP syndrome lasted for more than 2 years, it should be assimilated under the disease of Parkinson. Souques did admit that some of the signs and symptoms of parkinsonism appear in different frequencies and intensities in PEP compared to PD, but he did not believe that the two differed pathologically.

In 1922, the British Ministry of Health published a 344-page volume on EL that was authored by Parsons et al. Table 47 in that volume detailed EL sequelae; it is reproduced here as Table 7.4. Parkinsonism is not listed as a separate category in any of the 271 cases of EL that had sequelae 2–18 months after the acute episode. Tremors were reported for 45 patients, but rigidity for only nine. Mental impairment was found to be the most frequent sequel (57 cases). The authors did state, however, "Express references to *symptomatic paralysis agitans* do not occur, but mention is made of the mask-like face, stiffness, festinant gait, and other features of the parkinsonian picture" (p. 113). In modern English, this means that there were no prior references relating EL to PD, although some articles do mention masked face, rigidity, festination, and other features associated with PD. Hence, these authors, clearly aware that EL had been related to parkinsonism, did not consider any of the EL sequelae to be similar to PD and were thus apparently unaware of some of the publications described earlier.

Drysdale, in 1922, published an article in which he assumed that paralysis agitans and the parkinsonian syndrome that "apparently" results as a direct sequel to EL are the same disease. He also questioned whether some of his American patients might have developed PD, regardless of whether they had EL. He raised this issue because he was uncertain that these patients had definitely developed a previous phase of EL (see below).

Wimmer, in the preface to his 1924 book on chronic EL, indicated that, by this date, PEP had become well known to "medical men." Thus, if we assume his statement to be accurate, by 1924, PEP had become well-established as a common and direct sequel of EL. This perspective has persisted since that time.

THE RELATIONSHIP BETWEEN ENCEPHALITIS LETHARGICA AND POSTENCEPHALITIC PARKINSONISM

In contrast to the perspective that PEP consistently developed as a direct sequel to EL, in recent publications, we suggest that the relationship between EL and

Table 7.4 Sequelae of Encephalitis Lethargica

Sequelae	# Cases
Mental impairment	57
Psychiatric changes	47
Tremors	45
General weakness, asthenia	35
Ocular defects (65):	
Indefinite palsies	17
Impaired vision	16
Squint	16
Nystagmus	6
Diplopia	4
Blindness	3
Ptosis	3
Paralysis or paresis face	17
Paralysis or paresis upper limbs	17
Paralysis or paresis lower limbs	15
Drowsiness	15
Speech changes	14
Insomnia	12
Headache	11
Athetosis	10
Rigidity	9
Neurasthenia	7
Loss of memory	6
Abnormal gait	4
Fits	4
Melancholia	4
"Chorea" (chronic movements)	3
Exaggerated tendon reflexes	3
Incontinence of urine	3
Pain	3
Paralysis or paresis upper and lower limbs	3
Adiposity	2
Constipation	1
Enlarged thyroid	1
Exophthalmos	1
Incoordination upper and lower limbs	1
Muscular wasting	1
Vertigo	1
Vomiting	1

From Parsons, MacNalty, and Perdrau, 1922; 271 cases.

PEP may not be as simple or direct as is commonly believed (Vilensky et al., 2010a,b). In our review of the EL/PEP literature, we repeatedly found reports describing patients with PEP who had no prior history of an acute phase of EL. Furthermore, we noted that PEP and OCs were not considered as sequelae to EL until well after it was clear that EL resulted in other chronic sequelae (see above), and that the amyostatic-akinetic (parkinsonian) form of acute EL, which is one of the reasons EL and PEP were linked, was not universally recognized initially and even later may have had a rather limited distribution. We concluded by suggesting that, whereas EL was probably a factor in the etiology of PEP, it may not have been the only factor. The complete argument relative to our thesis is described in these articles (Vilensky et al. 2010a,b). Here, we provide some of our supporting data relative to patients who seemed to have developed PEP without a prior episode of EL.

In his 1924 monograph, *Chronic Epidemic Encephalitis*, Wimmer stated:

> Among my own patients, it was only in a minority of cases that I was able to obtain information which indicated a fairly typical "encephalitis lethargica." Far more frequently there was an indication of a short, common febrile phase, without the encephalitis triad [fever, lethargy, eye symptoms], and which was designated by the physician in charge of the patient, or by the patient himself, sometimes as "influenza," sometimes as "the Spanish disease" (commonly called "the flu"). (p. 3)

Wimmer attributed cases that showed no acute symptoms at all to "ambulatory encephalitis." Many other clinicians of this period, including von Economo, also indicated that a varying percentage (in some cases a majority) of their PEP patients had no prior history of an acute phase of EL. Krabbe, in 1932, in addition to noting that many cases of EL were originally diagnosed as influenza, indicated the difficulty in distinguishing EL from multiple sclerosis. Similarly, Corral-Corral and Quereda Rodriguez-Navarro, in a 2007 review of chronic EL in Spain, reported that in Galicia, many PEP cases occurred, although there had not been a previous EL epidemic in that city. Similarly, von Economo (1929) noted that there were cities such as Buenos Aires that had a substantial number of PEP cases but no serious prior EL epidemics.

The development of PEP in patients without prior EL symptomatology was repeatedly explained by suggesting that these patients had had asymptomatic EL. This argument could be considered circular; it assumes EL caused PEP, and therefore assumes that if a patient had PEP without any evidence of EL, we must be missing the evidence of EL. It is noteworthy that seven of the 20 PEP patients described by Oliver Sacks in *Awakenings* had no prior illness that could be diagnosed as EL except influenza in two (see Table 8.1). Furthermore, another of his patients, Margaret A., did not develop parkinsonian signs until 30 years after EL (Table 8.1).

The issue of the presumed relationship between EL and PEP had particular significance for the military because compensation was paid if it could be demonstrated that a patient developed a condition during his time spent in a military unit. Many such cases relating to PEP were decided by panels within the German military system that were detailed in a 1931 monograph by Dr. W. Mauss, *Die Encephalitis epidemica in ihren Beziehungen zum Militardienst* (The Relations Between Encephalitis Lethargica and the Military). At the time, Dr. Mauss was "staff doctor in the sixth Prussian Medical Department, assigned to the hospital."

Mauss, pertaining to these appeals for compensation, noted how not just laymen confused EL and influenza, but also physicians. He indicated that a single feverish incident during the war could not be definitively used to affirm a relationship with the later development of chronic EL; the applicant would have to at least show some "bridging" symptoms between the initial and PEP symptoms, and/or needed to show specific initial signs associated with encephalitis (e.g., diplopia). Mauss suggested that the bridging symptoms may have been interpreted as pseudoneurasthenia or signs that show the beginning of parkinsonism. Thus, German military panels were reticent to directly ascribe flu-like symptoms alone as being EL.

In 1965, Duvoisin and Yahr argued that only a small percentage of PEP cases developed in patients who did not have symptomatic EL, citing reports by Ziegler (1928) and Hall (1934). Ziegler's 1928 study of Mayo Clinic patients reported that only about 15% of chronic cases did not have a history of acute EL. Ziegler's study, however, was not limited to PEP patients but included all of the types of EL sequelae; PEP cases constituted 78% of this cohort. Furthermore, Ziegler noted that, in 22%, the acute attack had been diagnosed as influenza but that careful clinical analysis revealed it to be EL. In addition to influenza, the acute attacks had also been initially diagnosed as "...smallpox, measles, mumps, acute rheumatic fever, pleurisy, sore eyes, diarrhea, injury to the head or back, brain tumor, acute appendicitis, typhoid, meningitis, skin rash, pelvic abscess, neuritis, tonsillitis, and so forth" (p. 139).

In his report of 1934, Hall stated, "Out of 480 cases of parkinsonism of which I have full records, about 5% are of this kind, in which there has never been a day's illness which could not be *construed* [our italics] as the acute infection" (p. 27). Thus, in both of the reports cited by Duvoisin and Yahr, the authors made post hoc diagnoses of EL based on the current manifestations of a disease (see above).

In 1967, Hoehn and Yahr presented data on 586 cases of parkinsonism of all types who were seen at the Vanderbilt Clinic of the Columbia-Presbyterian Medical Center from 1949 to 1964. They found that :

> In reviewing charts, it was found that many patients, when first seen in the 1930s and 1940s, had been diagnosed as postencephalitic parkinsonism only because the onset of disease occurred at an early age. They had no history of encephalitis lethargica or any other infectious illness which might be confused with it; they have neither the pathognomonic sequelae (oculogyria and palilalia) nor the other common neurologic sequelae of encephalitis lethargica. Clinically they are

in no way different from patients seen more recently with an early age of onset who are now classified as primary parkinsonism and in this study are classified in that group. (p. 431)

Hoehn and Yahr (1967) also noted a category of parkinsonian patients, whom they termed *indeterminate parkinsonism patients*, for which it was impossible to determine whether the disease was primary or secondary, as in PEP, noting in particular that the retrospective diagnosis of EL may have been in error. Thus, these authors also expressed doubts about the post hoc diagnoses of EL during the epidemic period. This ambiguity is quite evident in case 6 in Chapter 11, in which the patient appears to have had EL, but symptomatically he seems to have developed idiopathic PD.

Interestingly, relative to the post-diagnoses of influenza as EL, Martilla and Rinne in their 1976 review of PD in Finland specifically stated that, in differentiating PD from PEP, a history of Spanish influenza was not considered equivalent to encephalitis. Alford (1971) also suggested that the flu had been incorrectly diagnosed as EL in cases of presumed PEP.

Further interpretation of these data relative to the relationship between EL and PEP is presented in the concluding section after we present data on PEP and PD in the post-epidemic period. This relationship is important for understanding the current perspective on PEP.

POSTENCEPHALITIC PARKINSONISM AND PARKINSON DISEASE IN THE POST–EPIDEMIC PERIOD

In 1940, Rudolf Klaue published "Parkinsonsche krankheit und postencephalitischer parkinsonismus" (Parkinson's Disease [paralysis agitans] and Postencephalitic Parkinsonism). In contrast to many earlier and later studies, he indicated that the clinical symptomatic picture of PD and PEP fundamentally agree with each other. He suggested that the characteristic differences listed in the literature were only of a quantitative nature, or that they only applied to a percentage of the cases. Klaue insisted that not one *pathognomonic* sign could distinguish between them. He also stated that PEP and PD do not differ fundamentally in their neuropathology and therefore suggested that a closer etiologic relationship existed between them than was previously assumed.

In 1946, Dimsdale published a very well-cited article on the relationship between PEP and PD. Her data were based on British patient records of 320 cases of parkinsonism from 1900 to 1942. She found that during the epidemic period the interval between the acute (EL) phase and the development of PEP seldom exceeded 6 months, and that frequently the two phases blended together. Furthermore, young adults were almost exclusively affected, with the modal age of onset being the second decade of life; symptoms developed rapidly, with "shakiness" often the presenting sign; mental symptoms (especially emotional instability) were very prominent; and tremor, when present, was coarse and nonrhythmic. In contrast, from 1931 to 1942, the latency between EL and PEP varied from immediate onset to 19 years, with a latency of some years being typical; the age of onset shifted to the third decade of life, with almost no cases occurring between 11 and 20 years of age; hemiplegic forms became much more common; onset was insidious and the course prolonged; and tremor was present in 90% of the cases and was frequently described as "fine" or "pill-rolling." Dimsdale, similarly to Hoehn and Yahr (1967), also identified a group of patients whom she classified with "indeterminate parkinsonism." These were patients who resembled PEP patients in clinical symptomatology, but who did not have a history of EL.

In 1963, Poskanzer and Schwab examined 1,576 parkinsonian cases treated at Massachusetts General Hospital (MGH) from 1875 to 1961 (193 were eliminated from consideration for various reasons). The authors reported that, from 1875 to 1915, only 17 cases of parkinsonism were diagnosed, whereas 1,366 cases were diagnosed in the following 45 years. There was also a progressive increase in the mean age of onset beginning in 1924. Based on these data, Poskanzer and Schwab concluded that the vast majority of current parkinsonian patients were of encephalitic origin, even though only 11.2% reported a history of EL: "One must therefore conclude that the greatest number of our patients who would be classified as idiopathic PD on the basis of medical history are in fact many of the cohort at which EL occurred" (p. 970). Furthermore, the authors concluded that, as the cohort affected by EL aged and died, the number of cases of the disease should diminish markedly. Poskanzer and Schwab further predicted that, by 1980, only the disease described by James Parkinson in 1817 would still be apparent, and it would be occurring in a much reduced frequency and be a less important neurologic problem.

The Poskanzer article was covered by the popular media. *The New York Times,* on October 19, 1962, published the article "New Theory Links Palsy to Virus." In a second article, which appeared on December 11, 1963, *The Times* noted that some scientists disputed the claims by these authors that parkinsonism would almost disappear. This was based primarily on a report by Duvoisin et al. that was published in the *Archives of Neurology* in 1963.

In that article, Duvoisin et al. argued that PD was a well-recognized entity and a major neurologic disease prior to EL. They presented additional data, concluding that parkinsonism had its usual onset in midlife from the time it was first recognized by Parkinson until the EL epidemic, 100 years later. Encephalitis lethargica occurred in younger ages and depressed the mean age for parkinsonism. The authors believed that all recent cases represent classic PD and not PEP. According to *The New York Times,* these arguments did not change Poskanzer and Schwab's views, although time has clearly shown their conclusions to have been wrong.

In their 1963 article countering Poskanzar and Schwab, Duvoisin et al. did not mention that they had discovered an error in Poskanzar's data collection. Poskanzar had looked at the annual statistical reports of the MGH and noted a sharp increase in the number of parkinsonian patients seen there in 1920 and thereafter, as compared to the earlier years. However, they did not realize that MGH published the statistics for outpatients and inpatients in separate volumes through 1919, and that, in 1920, MGH consolidated the reports into one volume. Poskanzar had only used the inpatient data, and prior to 1920, very few parkinsonian patients had been inpatients (Duvoisin, personal communication).

In 1965, Duvoisin and Yahr published an article that was designed to document the then-current status of PEP. Of 49 PEP patients, 27 were considered definite based on a clear history of EL or the presence of OCs; seven were considered probable PEP patients because of symptomatology despite the absence of a clear history of EL; three patients with less definitive PEP symptomatology were considered possible PEP cases; and, seven patients were symptomatically similar to PD patients but gave a history suggestive of EL. The age of onset of PEP was less than 40 years in 33/38 cases comprising the first two groups, whereas there was no onset under 40 in the last group. The patients in the first two groups had been rather stable, with progression in less than 50%. The authors concluded that the PEP patients had been exposed to EL during the 1920s and were long-term survivors of that epidemic.

In 1967, Hoehn and Yahr published, "Parkinsonism: Onset, Progression and Mortality." Their patient group included 82 cases who had had a definite history of EL or its "pathognomonic" stigmata, oculogyria and palilalia. They had a second group of 14 patients whom they classified as probable PEP patients, "with a less definite history of sleeping sickness and without oculogyria who, nevertheless, exhibit some nonpathognomonic but frequent sequelae of encephalitis lethargica: these include oculomotor and other cranial nerve palsies, pyramidal tract signs, dystonic phenomenon, sleep disturbances, personality changes, and autonomic dysfunction" (p. 130). Hoehn and Yahr reported that there were few differences in initial symptomatology among the various types of parkinsonism, except that speech, psychiatric, and sleep disturbances were more frequent in PEP patients. Interestingly, however, some recent studies in PD have emphasized the early onset of neurovegetative signs (Lees, 2009). As noted above, PEP patients also died at younger ages and had longer disease durations than the did PD patients.

Also in 1967, James Purdon Martin published *The Basal Ganglia and Posture*, which was a study of the role of the basal ganglia in movement and posture based on experimental studies of the PEP patients at Highlands Hospital in England (this hospital, similar to Mount Carmel Hospital in New York [Beth Abraham Hospital; see Chapter 8] housed chronic EL patients). The first part of the book's dedication reads: "To the postencephalitic patients in the Highlands Hospital who have helped eagerly, in the hope that their broken lives might help others"(p. vi).

Although the book presents much data on the postural and movement disorders characterizing PEP patients, it contains virtually no information about the patients themselves and in that way it is very different from Oliver Sack's *Awakenings* (see below). But, similar to *Awakenings*, L-dopa was used to treat these patients, and the results were published (see Chapter 8).

After the 1967 reports, the next notable study pertaining to PEP did not occur until 14 years later, in 1981. This study, by Rail et al., is discussed in detail in Chapter 5. The authors presented eight patients whom they proposed had had recent episodes of EL that progressed to PEP. They thus concluded that PEP could still be diagnosed in 1981 based on a history of a prior EL-like illness.

In 1997, Wenning et al. published a paper that called attention to the potential relationship between PEP and progressive supranuclear palsy (PSP), which is also discussed in Chapter 10, They described six patients with clinically confirmed PEP; four of these patients also had supranuclear gaze palsy and two had eyelid apraxia, both of which are associated with PSP. The authors suggested that these patients blur the differences between PEP and PSP, and that disorders of ocular and eyelid movement cannot alone be used to distinguish the two. However, although all the patients seemed to have had EL, very large time spans typically passed between their acute EL phase and the development of PEP (in one case, 44 years); thus, the diagnosis of PEP is open to question.

The following year, in 1998, Casals et al. wrote a major review on PEP. They noted that, although PEP is generally thought to be caused by the same virus that caused EL, primary encephalitides as well as encephalopathies caused by established viruses seldom if ever lead to parkinsonism. They reviewed recent putative cases of PEP due to EL, noting that, although the clinical and pathologic data are convincing, the lack of a pathognomonic indicator casts some doubt on the authenticity of the diagnosis.

Also in 1998, Litvan et al. investigated whether the great decrease in the incidence of PEP since earlier periods could be due to misdiagnosis (e.g., diagnosing current PEP patients as PSP patients) or to cases of multiple-system atrophy. The study population consisted of 105 autopsy-confirmed cases of parkinsonism or dementia, of which seven were PEP (24 PSP, 16 multiple-system atrophy, 15 PD, 14 dementia with Lewy bodies, ten corticobasal degeneration, seven Picks disease, four Alzheimer disease, four Creutzfeldt-Jakob disease, three vascular parkinsonism, and one Whipple disease). The PEP patients were diagnosed based on a "clinical history compatible with PEP." Cases were presented to six neurologists, who were asked to diagnose the cases based on their written histories. The authors found that the neurologists could very accurately diagnose PEP relative to the other disorders. Key distinguishers were prolonged duration (>16 years), the presence of OCs, and onset before middle age. The neurologists made no false-positive diagnoses (wrongly classifying other diseases as PEP), but occasionally did mistake PEP cases for other parkinsonian disorders. The authors concluded that the decreasing incidence of PEP is not due to mistaken diagnosis.

CONCLUSION

Neal et al. (1925) suggested that the percentage of EL patients who developed sequelae may have been highly exaggerated because mostly those who did not recover from acute EL were identified. This seems a very reasonable argument, especially from a world expert on EL, and thus it is probable that a far smaller percentage of EL patients actually developed secondary signs than is currently believed (see Chapter 13).

Did virtually all of the types of secondary EL (except perhaps the neurobehavioral disturbances found in children) eventually progress to PEP? As noted, to some extent, this is a semantic issue depending on how broadly one accepts a clinical definition of parkinsonism. Furthermore, just as PD may actually represent an umbrella term for a number of distinct clinical syndromes (Lees, 2009), we believe that PEP may not be a unitary entity but rather represents a number of distinct disorders, some of which may stem directly from EL, but not all. This argument is based on the clinical variability, the lack of a definite EL phase in many of if not most PEP patients, the fact that the chronic form of EL did not follow uniformly among the EL epidemics, the differences in PEP noted by Dimsdale (1946) between the epidemic and later periods, and the variation in neuropathology, which is discussed in detail in Chapter 10. We are not the first to suggest this. Jakob (1923; cited in Neustaaedtler & Lieber, 1937), and Forno and Alvord (1971) suggested this view based on pathological grounds. We also believe that EL itself may not have been a uniform entity (see Chapter 12).

Perhaps the most valuable aspect of the review presented here is its depiction of the confusion during the epidemic period pertaining to the amyostatic form of EL, PEP, and PD. From this confusion, the prominent view that developed was that EL progressed in certain cases either directly or after a period of "recovery"—which could be very long—to PEP. This conclusion was severely limited by the lack of knowledge of disease processes and the poor understanding of pathophysiologic mechanisms at the time. Even during the epidemic period, prominent clinicians of the time could not agree on whether specific patients had EL—for example, in Chapter 2, we noted that Cruchet believed he had identified 40 EL cases, whereas von Economo disputed all but one of these cases (considering two more to be possible EL). Furthermore, the course of EL and the presumptive later development of PEP may have been strongly influenced by an apparent similarity between EL/PEP and the stages of syphilis (Hall, 1924; von Economo, 1929).

Finally, some features of chronic EL seem to have been forgotten in recent times: for example, paradoxical kinesis, that sialorrhea might have been primarily due to excess salivary gland secretions rather than a reduced swallowing reflex, the paroxysmal nature of some of the signs, perhaps the role of trauma and pregnancy in initiating some cases, and the reasonable possibility that PEP existed before the EL epidemic. Furthermore, a notable proportion of clinicians through the 1920s did not believe that PEP and PD were fundamentally distinct disorders.

Finally, there is the surprising finding that PEP patients responded to lower dosages of L-dopa than did PD patients, despite the presumed longer disease duration (see Chapter 8). These factors should be considered in any attempt to understand the underlying pathophysiology of chronic EL (PEP).

REFERENCES CITED

Alvord, E. C. Jr. (1971). The pathology of parkinsonism. Part II. An interpretation with special reference to other changes in the aging brain. *Contemporary Neurology Series, 8,* 131–161.

Borthwick, G. A. (1931). The sequelae of epidemic encephalitis. *Clinical Journal, 60,* 510–514, 521–524.

Bramwell, E. (1928). The ocular complications of lethargic encephalitis. Joint discussions no. 4 (Sections of Ophthalmology and Neurology). *Proceedings Royal Society of Medicine (London), 21,* 985–996.

Brusa, A., & Pramstaller, P. P. (2000). Ante litteram description of atypical parkinsonian cases. *Journal of the Neurological Sciences, 21,* 407–409.

Buzzard, E. F. (1918b). Encephalitis lethargica. *Proceedings Royal Society Medicine* (Section on Neurology), *12,* 56–64.

Casals, J., Elizan, T.S., & Yahr, M.D. (1998). Postencephalitic parkinsonism - a review. *Journal of Neural Transmission, 105,* 645–676.

Catola, G. (1921). A propos de l'evolution et du pronostic du Parkinsonisme postencephalitique. *Revue Neurologique, 28,* 694–715.

Corral-Corral, I., Quereda Rodriguez-Navarro, C. (2007). Sindromes postencefaliticos en la literatura medica espanola. *Revue Neurologique, 44,* 499–506.

Crafts, L. M. (1927). *Epidemic Encephalitis (Encephalo-Myelitis).* Boston: Richard G. Badger.

Dimsdale, H. (1946). Changes in the parkinsonian syndrome in the twentieth century. *Quarterly Journal of Medicine, 15,* 155–170.

Drysdale, H. H. (1922). Parkinson's disease as sequelae to lethargic encephalitis. *Ohio State Medical Journal. 18,* 842–849.

Duvoisin, R. C., & Yahr, M. D. (1965). Encephalitis and Parkinsonism. *Archives of Neurology, 12,* 227–239.

Duvoisin, R. C., Yahr, M. D., Schweitzer, M. D., & Merritt H. H. (1963). Parkinsonism before and since the epidemic of encephalitis lethargica. *Archives of Neurology, 9,* 232–236.

Von Economo, C. (1929). *Die Encephalitis lethargica, ihre Nachkrankheiten und ihre Behardlung.* Berlin: Urban & Schwarzenberg. (Published in English in 1931; translated by K. O. Newman, London: Oxford University Press.)

Forno, L.S., & Avord, E. C. Jr. (1971). The pathology of Parkinsonism. Part I. Some new observations and correlations. *Contemporary Neurology Series, 8,* 119–130.

Hall, A. J. (1918). Epidemic encephalitis. *British Medical Journal, 2,* 461–463.

Hall, A. J. (1924). *Epidemic Encephalitis (Encephalitis Lethargica).* Bristol: John Wright & Sons.

Hall, A. J. (1934). Prognosis and treatment of chronic epidemic encephalitis. *Practitioner, 133,* 26–36.

Hawkes, C. H., Del Tredici, K., & Braak, H. (2007). Review: Parkinson's disease: A dual-hit hypothesis. *Neuropathology and Applied Neurobiology, 33,* 599–614.

Hoehn, M. M. & Yahr, M. D. (1967). Parkinsonian onset, progression and mortality. *Neurology, 17,* 427–442.

House, W. (1919). Epidemic (lethargic) encephalitis. Clinical review of cases in the Pacific Northwest. *Journal of American Medical Association, 74*, 372–375.

Klaue, R. (1940). Parkinsonsche Krankheit (Paralysis agitans) und postencephalitischer Parkinsonismus. *Archiv für Psychiatrie und Nervenkrankheiten, 111*, 252–321.

Krabbe, K. H. (1932). The Initial Stages of the Parkinsonian Forms in Chronic Epidemic Encephalitis. *Acta Psychiatrica et Neurologica Scandinavica 7*, 317–337.

Lees, A. J. (2009). The Parkinson chimera. *Neurology, 72*, S2–S11.

Litvan, I., Jankovic, J., Goetz, C. G., Wenning, G. K., Sastry, N., Jellinger, K., et al. (1998). Accuracy of the clinical diagnosis of postencephalitic parkinsonism: a clinicopathologic study. *European Journal of Neurology, 5*, 451–457.

Marttila, R. J., & Rinne, U. K. (1976). Epidemiology of Parkinson's disease in Finland. *Acta Neurologica Scandinavica, 53*, 81–102.

Martin, J. P. (1967). *The Basal Ganglia and Posture.* London: Pitman Medical Publishing Co.

Mauss, W. (1931). *The Encephalitis Epidemica in Its Relations to the Military Service.* Berlin: E.S. Mittler & Sohn.

Neal, J. B. (1942). *Encephalitis: A Clinical Study.* New York: Grune & Stratton.

Neal, J. B., Jackson, H. W., & Appelbaum, E. (1925). A study of four hundred and fifty cases of epidemic encephalitis. *American Journal of Medical Science, 170*, 708–722.

Nielsen, J. M. (1953). Complications of encephalitis of the Von Economo type. *Bulletin of the Los Angeles Neurological Association, 18*, 84–90.

Netter, A. (1918). Encephalite lethargique epidemique. *Bulletin de l'Academie Nationale de Medecine, 79*, 337–347.

Neustaedter, M., & Liber, A. F. (1937). Concerning the pathology of parkinsonism (idiopathic, arteriosclerotic, and post-encephalitic). *Journal of Nervous and Mental Disease, 86*, 264–283.

Newsholme, A., James, S. P., MacNalty, A. S., Marinesco, G., McIntosh, J., & Draper, G. (1918). *Report of an Enquiry into an Obscure Disease, Encephalitis Lethargica.* Reports to the Local Government Board on public health and medical subjects, new ser., no. 121. London: Printed under the authority of His Majesty's Stationery Office by Jas. Truscott and Son.

Onuaguluchi, G. (1964). *Parkinsonism.* London: Butterworths.

Parkinson, J. (2002). An essay on the shaking palsy. *Journal of Neuropsychiatry Clinical Neuroscience, 14*, 223–236.

Parsons, A. C., MacNalty, A. S., & Perdrau, J. R. (1922). *Report on EL: Being an Account of Further Enquiries into the Epidemiology and Clinical Features of the Disease; Including the Analysis of over 1,250 Reports on Cases Notified in England and Wales during 1919 and 1920, Together with Comprehensive Bibliography of the Subject.* London: H.M.S.O.

Poskanzer, D. C., & Schwab, R. S. (1963). Cohort analysis of Parkinson's syndrome. *Journal of Chronic Diseases, 16*, 961–973.

Rail, D., Scholtz, C., & Swash, M. (1981). Post-encephalitic Parkinsonism: current experience. *Journal of Neurology, Neurosurgery, & Psychiatry, 8*, 670–676.

Ramsay Hunt, J. (1917). Atrophy of the large motor cells (giant cells) of the corpus striatum in the presenile type of paralysis agitans. *Transactions Association of American Physicians, 32*, 567–570.

Ramsay Hunt, J. (1918). A case of juvenile paralysis agitans primary atrophy of the pallidal system of the corpus striatum. *Neurological Bulletin, 1*, 237–242.

Sacks, O. (1990). *Awakenings.* New York: HarperCollins Publishers.

Sicard, J. A., & Paraf, J. (1920). Parkinsonnisme et Parkinson, reliquats d'Encephalite epidemique. *Revue Neurologique, 28*, 465–470.

Souques, M. A. (1921). Rapport sur les syndromes Parkinsoniens. *Revue Neurologique, 37*, 534–573.

Tilney, F. & Howe, H. S. (1920). *Epidemic Encephalitis (Encephalitis Lethargica)*. New York: Paul B. Hoeber.

Vilensky, J. A., Foley P., & Gilman S. (2007). Children and encephalitis lethargica: A historical review. *Pediatric Neurology*, *37*, 79–84.

Vilensky, J. A., Gilman, S., & McCall, S. (2010a). Does the historical literature on Encephalitis Lethargica support a simple (direct) relationship with Postencephalitic Parkinsonism? *Movement Disorders, 25*, 1124–1130.

Vilensky, J. A., Gilman, S., & McCall, S. (2010b). A historical analysis of the relationship between Encephalitis Lethargica and Postencephalitic Parkinsonism: a complex rather than a direct relationship. *Movement Disorders, 25*, 1116–1123.

Vilensky, J., Mukhamedzyanov, R., & Gilman, S. (2008). Encephalitis lethargica in the Soviet Union. *European Neurology, 60*, 113–121.

Wenning, G. K., Jellinger, K., & Litvan, I. (1997). Supranuclear gaze palsy and eyelid apraxia in postencephalitic parkinsonism. *Journal of Neural Transmission, 104*, 845–865.

Willige, H. (1911). Uber paralysis agitans in jugendichen Alter. *Z Neurol Psychiat Zeitschrift für die gesamte Neurologie und Psychiatrie, 4*, 520–587.

Wilson, S. A. K. (1940). *Neurology*. Baltimore: The Williams & Wilkins Company.

Wimmer, A. (1924). *Chronic Epidemic Encephalitis*. London: William Heinemann.

Ziegler, L. H. (1928). Follow-up studies on persons who have had epidemic encephalitis. *Journal of the American Medical Association, 3*, 138–141.

8

OLIVER SACKS, *AWAKENINGS*, AND POSTENCEPHALITIC PARKINSONISM

Joel A. Vilensky, Roger C. Duvoisin, and Sid Gilman

The publication of *Awakenings* by Oliver Sacks in 1973 and the release of the movie of the same name in 1990 resulted in an increase in public awareness of postencephalitic parkinsonism (PEP) and the treatment of Parkinson disease (PD) with dopamine precursors (L-dopa). Because of the importance of this phenomenon relative to PEP, the treatment of PEP patients with L-dopa will be described here in some detail. Some of the information presented here is summarized from *Beans, Roots and Leaves* by Paul B. Foley, which is a marvelous book about the history of the chemical treatment of parkinsonism.

In 1960, Oleh Hornykiewicz published a landmark article in which he showed a marked depletion of dopamine in the caudate nucleus and putamen of patients with PD and PEP. Six years later, he published a major review suggesting that striatal dopamine deficiency is correlated with most of the motor symptoms of parkinsonism. In 1961, a colleague of Hornykiewicz', Walter Birkmayer, administered 50 mg of L-dopa to a female PEP patient, who showed dramatic improvement, especially a great reduction in akinesia. The benefits of this treatment were recorded on film, and the film is vividly described in *Beans, Roots and Leaves* (p. 414).

Following that work, many reports appeared on the treatment of parkinsonism with L-dopa, with varying results, probably due to the form and dosage of L-dopa used and perhaps also to the patients themselves, because PEP patients tended to have more dramatic responses than did PD patients. However, in 1969,

Cotzias and colleagues published a definitive report in the *New England Journal of Medicine* on the use of L-dopa in parkinsonism. Their results had been publicly released earlier, and an article about them with the headline, *Parkinson Victims Reported Relieved by Drugs in Tests*, was published in the *New York Times* on May 8, 1968. An editorial in the *British Medical Journal* in 1969 described the trials as follows:

> They treated 28 patients over periods of up to 2 years, and of these 20 were substantially improved. They began by giving 100 mg three times a day, and every 2 to 4 days the dose was increased by 200–300 mg, though some patients could tolerate increments of only 50 mg per day. The maximum therapeutic effect and the maximum tolerated dose varied from individual to individual, but normally fell within the range of 3 g–16 g daily. Perhaps the most exciting outcome of this and similar carefully conducted clinical trials has been the demonstration that the most disabling clinical manifestations, such as akinesia, may be dramatically relieved by the use of this drug. Improvement was also seen in speech, in swallowing, and in reduction of salivation, and there was general improvement in posture, gait, and facial expression. (p. 202)

Cotzias et al.'s patients included both postencephalitic and idiopathic patients, although they do not present the numbers of each. The authors noted that because all responded similarly, the cause of the dopamine deficiency is irrelevant to the beneficial effects of L-dopa.

The value of L-dopa for PEP patients was confirmed in England with the 1969 publication of a study by Calne et al. in *The Lancet* using patients at the Highlands Hospital (see Chapter 7). Calne et al. administered oral L-dopa over 6 weeks, with maximum dosages ranging from 0.5 to 2.5 g/day. They noted that this dosage was not as high as that used by Cotzias et al. (1969) or in a study by Duvoisin et al. (1968), probably because PEP patients had longer disease durations and more severe brain damage. Seven of the 20 treated patients improved substantially, and three moderately; five showed no notable response and treatment had to be withdrawn because of side effects. Calne et al. stated:

> The beneficial effects of L-dopa were exemplified in three patients who had required considerable assistance in walking for up to 4 years; on L-dopa they were able to walk unaided. Drooling saliva improved in five patients… Three showed an increase in chairbound activity, which reduced their nursing requirements. Before treatment oculogyric crises occurred about twice a week in three patients. After 2 weeks on L-dopa, the nursing staff reported that these crises had stopped, and they did not return until 5 weeks after withdrawing treatment. (p. 746)

Pertaining to adverse responses, Calne et al. (1969) reported that involuntary movements of a choreoathetoid nature developed in ten patients, whereas three patients had exacerbations of prior involuntary movements. Dyskinesias developed

primarily in the tongue, lips, face, neck, and limbs. Three patients became pathologically restless, and five showed overactivity when no previous psychiatric disturbances were noted.

A year later, two other reports were published detailing the use of L-dopa in
PEP patients. In the November 1970 issue of *The Lancet*, Krashner and Cornelius
reported results for PEP patients who had had symptoms for 10–49 years. The
dosages used ranged from 750 to 4,500 mg/day. Of the 12 patients who received
the drug, therapy had to be withdrawn in eight because of side effects, and seven
patients showed no favorable responses. Three showed substantial improvement,
and two showed moderate improvement. The authors noted that, in the three
patients who had benefited the most, the treatment had to be stopped because of
the adverse effects. The article concluded that the poor tolerance for L-dopa
shown by these patients called for additional study.

In a December 1970 issue of *The Lancet*, Hunter et al. also published a short
letter on using L-dopa with PEP patients. Based on their 24-week study, they concluded that PEP patients tolerated L-dopa poorly and that only a minority gained
useful and enduring benefit. Their dosages ranged from 250 to 1,750 mg/day.

Other than the work of Oliver Sacks, the final article that specifically pertained to using L-dopa in PEP patients was published in 1972 by Duvoisin et al.
In contrast to some of the prior studies, these researchers reported optimistic
results. Thirty-three patients were treated with L-dopa, of whom seven had their
treatments terminated because of adverse reactions or insufficient benefits. The
average daily dose was 2.8 g. Duvoisin et al. noted that oculogyria and drooling
were appreciably improved, whereas choreoathetoid dyskinesias were aggravated
by the drug. In general, these authors found that more than two-thirds of their
patients showed significant improvement over a prolonged period, which is similar to the outcome in patients with idiopathic PD. However, in agreement with
previous findings, they noted that involuntary movements occurred at a lower
dosage of L-dopa in PEP patients than in PD patients (in the latter, they noted
that the average dose used was 5.5 g/day). Finally, they noted that it was surprising
that PEP patients respond to lower dosages of L-dopa than did PD patients,
because it would be expected that the former patients would have fewer surviving
dopaminergic neurons. Presumably, this result reflects differences in the pathoge-
netic mechanisms of dopaminergic neuronal dysfunction in these two forms of
parkinsonism.

OLIVER SACKS AND *AWAKENINGS*

In *Awakenings*, Oliver Sacks related his experience at Mount Carmel Hospital in
New York City (this name was a pseudonym: the actual name of the hospital was
the Beth Abraham Hospital), which was opened shortly after World War I for veterans with neurological problems and for the expected victims of the EL epidemic.

When Sacks arrived in 1966, approximately 80 PEP patients were housed there. He stated that about 50% of these were virtually speechless and motionless, requiring total nursing care; the other half were less disabled, less dependent, and less isolated, and could take care of some of their own basic needs.

In the Foreword to the 1990 edition of his book, Sacks described his initial work with L-dopa and the reactions of his patients (Figs. 8.1 and 8.2) as follows:

> In the spring of 1969, in a way which he [von Economo] could not have imagined, which no one could have imagined or foreseen, these "extinct volcanos" erupted into life. The placid atmosphere of Mount Carmel was transformed— occurring before us was a cataclysm of almost geological proportions, the explosive "awakenings," the "quickening," of eighty or more patients who had long been regarded, and regarded themselves, as effectively dead. (p. xxv)

Sacks initially conceived of his study as a 90-day double-blind study, but he quickly abandoned this approach because the beneficial effects of L-dopa were obvious, and he could not imagine either stopping the treatment after 90 days or withholding the treatment from half of his patients. He furthermore felt that no quantitative presentation of the effects of L-dopa could do justice to the wide variety of complex responses he observed. "Thus I was impelled, willy-nilly, to a presentation of case histories or biographies, for no 'orthodox' presentation, in terms of numbers, series, grading effect, etc., could have conveyed the historical reality of the experience," (p. xxx). Sacks then wrote the first nine case histories. He also wrote letters to the editors of *The Lancet* and the *British Medical Journal* in order to convey the "wonder" of the clinical experience in a way that would have been quite impossible in a formal medical article.

In the summer of 1970, Sacks also reported his findings in a letter to the *Journal of the American Medical Association* (JAMA). He described the total effects of L-dopa in 30 PEP and 30 PD patients whom he had maintained on L-dopa for a year (Sacks et al., 1970). Sacks and his co-authors stated that the period of benefit from L-dopa was limited, and that it was followed in all cases by adverse effects. They specifically noted that, with the restoration of mobility, some of the patients suffered falls because there was no restoration of postural reflexes, and the patients showed weakness due to prolonged immobility. Additionally, they called attention to psychiatric or psychosocial problems, which they suggested had been generally neglected. Other reactions occurred including festination, freezing, multiple tics, and especially respiratory and oculogyric crises.

Sacks et al. (1970) noted that in some cases, these effects persisted for months following discontinuation of the drug. They suggested that perhaps the most serious were "akinetic episodes," which were associated with stupor. They also reported profound withdrawal signs, such as tremor of the whole body, rigidity, stupor, and akinesia. Finally, the authors also reported adverse emotional reactions, such as despair, after the drug was withdrawn. Sacks and colleagues called for a deeper understanding of the effects of the drug. They concluded by expressing

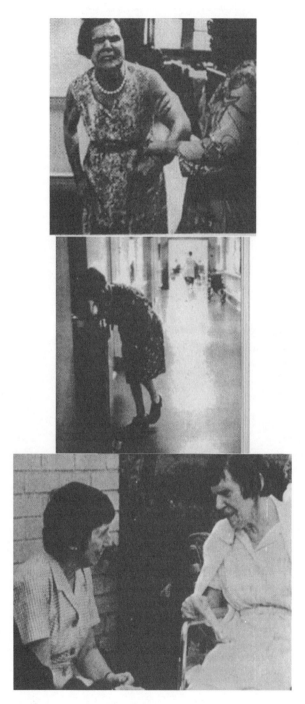

Figure 8.1 One of Sacks' patients, Margaret H. (Table 8.1), "driven by the combined effects of disease, L-dopa, and institutionalization, into a state of panic and rage, and into perpetual, compulsive water-drinking [*top* and *middle*]. In contrast, both her parkinsonism and her neuroses all but disappear in more human conditions—for example, in the hospital garden and, all above all, when visited by her much beloved sister [*bottom*]."

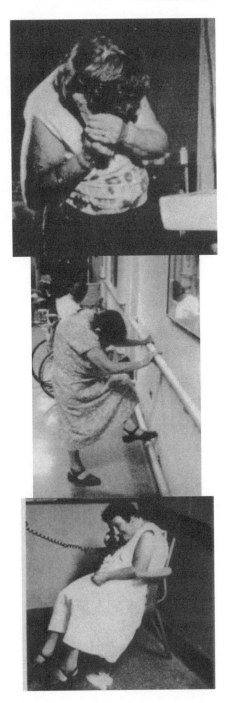

Figure 8.2 A second of Sacks' patients (Hester Y., Table 8.1), "who had been in a state of virtual standstill for more than 20 years, 'awakened' by L-dopa: now alive to her appearance, she is seen doing her hair [*top*](... she is using her left hand to unlock her 'transfixed' right hand); we see her assiduously exercising her long frozen limbs... [*middle*] and laughing as she speaks to her daughter on the phone... [*bottom*]."

concern over the release of L-dopa as a drug for parkinsonism at that time because the long-term safety had not been established.

The letter by Sacks et al. produced a strong reaction, resulting in three published responses in the December 14, 1970 issue of *JAMA* from Drs. Ryan, McDowell and Lee, and Monen. All of the letters protested against the view expressed by Sacks et al., with one suggesting that publishing the original letter did a disservice to physicians and patients. All of the letters suggested that Sacks et al.'s results might have been specific for his very disabled group of patients, who undoubtedly had underlying psychiatric issues possibly unrelated to their PEP. They also suggested that L-dopa was a very beneficial medication for parkinsonian patients, in whom the side effects can be relatively well controlled. Moreover, the withdrawal signs observed by Sacks et al. were not found by these clinicians in their patients.

In the Foreword to the 1990 edition of his book, Sacks also related how he then thought that perhaps his letter to *JAMA* had been too brief, and that he needed to publish an extended article. He thus put all of his data in proper form, with figures and tables, and submitted the article to several medical journals, all of which rejected it. "This confirmed my feeling that a deep nerve had been struck, that I had somehow elicited not just a medical, but sort of epistemological, anxiety—and rage" (p. xxxii).

Finally, in 1972, the editor of *The Listener* invited Sacks to write an article about his experiences. *The Listener* was not a medical journal, but a weekly intellectual magazine established by the British Broadcasting Corporation (BBC) in 1929 (it ceased publication in 1991). It was primarily a medium for the discussion of broadcast presentations, although it did include a small number of original contributions, and Sacks' article fitted into that category.

In *The Listener*, Sacks (1972) stated that he had observed thousands of complex and variable side effects in PEP patients. He noted that his patients did not respond to L-dopa in a dose-related manner, but rather in an all-or-none manner, and many aspects of their behavior were affected. He wrote that these patients were often immobilized not only physically but also mentally. For example, they might have no idea of the passage of time. And, as he had advocated in the *JAMA* editorial, he again proposed that the adverse effects of L-dopa should not be regarded as side effects, but rather be divided into kinematic disorders, dynamic disorders, and referential disorders.

It is clear that Sacks' findings were not well regarded by the medical community of the time and, indeed, often differed from peer-reviewed published findings; in this connection, it is important to emphasize that Sacks' perspective is very different from that of almost all other academic neurologists. This difference was well described in an article by Alan G. Wasserman, "Toward a Romantic Science: The Work of Oliver Sacks," that appeared in the September 1988 issue of the *Annals of Internal Medicine*. Wasserman highlighted Sacks' belief that disease has a much closer relationship to the personal being of the patient than was typically thought. Sacks suggested that the patient's presentation represents in part how the patient's identity reacts to his illness, and this reaction cannot be described simply in terms of numerical data. Wasserman noted that most scientists do not enter this realm because they feel we simply do not have sufficient understanding of the brain to explain it. Wasserman concluded by stating that Sacks' goal was not only to humanize medicine, but also to humanize disease.

All but three of Sacks' 20 patients showed an "awakening" when given L-dopa. He noted that PEP patients' responses to L-dopa tended to be quicker and more dramatic than those of patients with idiopathic PD. He also noted that some PEP patients showed an almost a complete recovery with L-dopa that could not be explained simply as a physiological response to the drug. "For a certain time, in almost every patient who is given L-dopa, there is a beautiful, unclouded return to health; but sooner or later, in one way or another, almost every patient is plunged into problems and troubles" (p. 243). In general, patients with the greatest disabilities initially showed the greatest untoward reactions to the drug. He stated that, "All patients, then, move into trouble on L-dopa; not into 'side-effects,' but into *radical trouble*: they develop, once more, their 'propenseness to diseases,' [quoting the poet John Donne] which can sprout and flower in innumerable forms" (p. 246).

As noted, Sacks did not believe that the reactions of his patients to L-dopa could be easily presented in chart form, because he viewed each individual's response as being unique. However, he now has kindly agreed to placing the patient data embedded in the *Awakenings* text into tabular form (Table 8.1). For this table, we have included data from the original 1973 book, as well as from the later editions (information from these later editions is in italics). Where data are missing from the table (e.g., L-dopa dosages), it is because they are not available.

Although it was not stated in the 1973 edition of *Awakenings*, two of the described cases had idiopathic PD, not PEP (Aaron E. and George W.; this is made clear in the later editions). Thus, although we have included the data for these patients in the table, they are separated and placed at the bottom of the columns. Similarly, in the later edition, Sacks indicated that Cecil M. was not actually one of his patients, but one of his father's patients in London.

The 1973 edition of *Awakenings* (and certainly the 1990 movie), as well as the articles published by Sacks mentioned above, may leave some readers with the view that, on balance, L-dopa was ultimately not a beneficial treatment for PEP patients. This would be in agreement with some of the other studies from the period (see above) but not in agreement with others (e.g., Duvosin et al, 1972). Furthermore, in the 1982 edition of his book, Sacks said, "I have become much more optimistic than when I first wrote *Awakenings*, for there have been a significant number of patients who, following the vicissitudes of their first years on L-dopa came to do—and still do—extremely well. Such patients have undergone an enduring awakening and enjoy the possibilities of life which had been impossible, unthinkable before the coming of L-dopa" (p. 278). The evidence supporting this

Table 8.1 Symptoms, Treatment, and Outcome for the 20 Patients Described in Oliver Sacks' *Awakenings**

Patient	Birth	Acute EL	PEP development	PEP@L-dopa Trial	Initial Effects	Effects & Outcome
Postencephalitic Parkinsonism Patients						
Frances D.	1904	1919; Hyperkinetic form; insomnia (sleep reversal), restlessness for 6 months	Respiratory crises immediately after EL; OCs 1924, sole symptom until 1949; rigidity, tremor developed; considered PEP in 1964	Kyphotic posture; masked facies; tremor, bradykinesia; rigidity; festination	1969; 5 days at 0.5 g; tachypnea; oral dyskinesias; 1 month later 2.0 g/day; walking improved but violent inspirations and more oral dyskinesias; dosage decreased to 1.5 g but dyskinesias much worse; dosage decreased to 0.9 g but OCs returned after lapse of 3 years; after 2 months, massive respiratory crisis and trial terminated	Parkinsonism initially worse than before L-dopa; but L-dopa started again after 5 months and continued for 3 years with good results—parkinsonian less severe than before L-dopa; remained this way until 1976 with some "drug holiday" periods; responses modest; died of pneumonia in 1976
Magda B.	1900	1918; Somnolent-ophthalmoplegic form (no details)	1923; Apathy; sialorrhea; "flapping tremor"	Extreme akinesia; masked facies; ophthalmoplegia; virtually aphonic; extreme bradykinesia	1969; 2 g, after 1 week, spoke; 3 g enabled movements; by 1 month, could walk across room and feed herself; continued for 2 years with good results	Died 2 years after initiation of L-dopa; response considered "excellent"

(Continued)

Table 8.1 continued

Patient	Birth	Acute EL	PEP development	PEP@L-dopa Trial	Initial Effects	Effects & Outcome
Rose R.	1905	1926; nightmares; catatonia; aphonic	Immediately after EL developed OCs; signs of parkinsonism	Akinesia; masked face; profuse drooling; rigidity; wheelchair-bound; coarse tremor; almost continuous OCs	1966; 1.5 g; OCs stopped; reduction in rigidity after 2 weeks; 4 g with continued improvement but then hypomanic behavior after 3 weeks; 3 g, OCs returned, delusions; gradual worsening over next month; L-dopa stopped	During next 3 years, tried 3 g five different times with only minor positive results; continued on L-dopa with moderate results but with OCs; died 1979 after OC episode while eating (aspirated chicken bone)
Robert O.	1905	1922; Somnolent form; intensely drowsy for 6 months; fits of yawning; narcolepsy; somnambulisms	1928; Fine tremor of fingers and tongue; masked face	Cogwheel rigidity in all limbs; festination; masked face; unable to look up; flat affect; thought disorder	1969; progressive increase in dosage over 10 days to 4 g; then raised to 6 g; rigidity decreased but marked increase in grimacing and tongue protrusion; L-dopa stopped after 1 month	Condition deteriorated over the next 2 years; L-dopa tried again in 1971, with minimal positive results, continued thought disorder; died

Name	Year				
Hester Y.		At 29, paroxysmal arrests of activity; became trance-like	Parkinsonian signs by age 32; immobile and mute at 35	Catatonia or trance impeding all movement, speech and thought; severe akinesia	1969; 4 g by 10 days; could walk unaided across room; 3 days later, generalized chorea and manic behavior; L-dopa stopped and reverted to akinetic state	L-dopa resumed at .75 g; multiple on-off periods with tics; brief periods of normalcy; continues with yo-yo patterns; comatose without L-dopa; disease static; walking difficult; died 1984
Rolando P.	1917	1919; 30 months of age; "virulent attack" of EL; fever and influenzal symptoms	After acute phase immediately developed masked face and great difficulty moving; loss of balance and sialorrhea	Admitted to chronic hospital at 19 years; intense rigidity; cogwheeling; severe akinesia; loss of balance; seborrhea; sialorrhea; voice almost inaudible; at age 41 had left chemopallidotomy	3 g by 10 days; voice clear; could walk about ward, although balance problems remained; at 13 days restlessness; dosage decreased to 2 g; chorea, chewing movements; 1 month, constant movement; palilalia; erotic dreams coprolalia; forced grasping; on 1.5 g was excited, akathisic, and insomniac	Continued on 1 g 1969–1972; yo-yos between excited (explosive) and akinetic states; if misses a day, lapses into stupor

(Continued)

Table 8.1 continued

Patient	Birth	Acute EL	PEP development	PEP@L-dopa Trial	Initial Effects	Effects & Outcome
Miriam H.	1914	1926; "Severe attack" of EL; slept for days; narcolepsies; sleep paralyses; nightmares; daymares; sleep-talking	OCs in 1928; counting crises in which had to count to a specific number; hospitalized at age 18	Obese, slumped in wheelchair; speech irregular; seborrheic dermatitis; speech decays into aphonia; rigidity and tremor, greater on left; intense axial rigidity	1966; 2 g, more alert and cheerful; at 2 weeks on 3g could read and keep diary; at 4 g after 3 weeks, rigidity decreased, hand movements but impatient and demanding; chewing movements; on 4 g at 2 months hiccups, nervous cough; severe respiratory crisis, parkinsonism, OCs; L-dopa stopped after 6 months	Parkinsonism returned; L-dopa tried twice more in 1970 at 4 g with mixed effects; tics developed but can read and write; continued on 825 mg q.i.d. and is helped; occasional strange obsessions, mild OCs; died 1984
Lucy K.	1924	1926; Paralysis and strabismus of the left eye for 6 weeks	1935; Parkinsonism; stiff walking; masked facies; by age 27 confined to wheelchair	Plastic rigidity, more on left; cogwheeling; dystonia; flapping tremor; myoclonic jerks; sialorrhea	1970; increasing dosage to 3 g; at week 4, patient animated and sitting upright; regressed to mutism and parkinsonism; dosage increased to 7 g with no effect; stopped after 7 weeks	Patient died in 1972

| Margaret A. | 1908 | 1925; Sleepiness and depression; slept 10 weeks | 1927; Gross tremor of hands, slowness of gait and impaired balance; OCs in early 1930s; festinating gait developed | Thin, masked face; seborrhea, sialorrhea, resting tremor of lips; voice monotone and low; extreme axial rigidity; festination | 1960; dosage 3 g by 1 week; nausea; mouth openings; after 2 weeks, posture upright, rigidity reduced; at 10 days 4 g, more improvement, could walk corridor; but restless movements of legs, anxiety, and compulsive activity; manic behavior – letdowns 3 hours after each dose; chorea; dosage reduced to 2 g at 20 days; palilalic repetition of phrases, tic-like compulsions; 1.5 g but festination with falls; OCs; L-dopa stopped and patient intensely rigid, almost aphonic; after 45 days, L-dopa started again with limited and stable improvement | 1969–1972; continued on L-dopa with reasonably good results; very dependent on L-dopa; decline during last 3 years; very sensitive to L-dopa and in crucial need of it; 1976 died of complications associated with hip fracture |

(Continued)

Table 8.1 continued

Patient	Birth	Acute EL	PEP development	PEP@L-dopa Trial	Initial Effects	Effects & Outcome
Miron V.	1908	1918; Influenza; no signs that were recognized as EL at the time	1947; Tics, impulsiveness; hyperactive, periods of trance-like behavior; admitted to hospital in '1955; intense parkinsonism and catatonia; speechless and motionless	Almost completely immobile; some tics and throat-clearing noises; could not rise or walk unaided	1969; After 1 day on L-dopa regained almost normal speech and movement pattern; within 2 weeks became impulsive, hyperactive, hypomanic and amorous; many falls with hip fracture; was able to walk about hospital and perform cobbler's work (his profession)	Relatively good outcome; was able to go home for weekends; considered to be best responding patient; hospital closed industrial workshop and subsequently L-dopa even at 6 g had no effect; parkinsonian with catatonia; died 1980 due to pneumonia

Gertie C.	1908	No documentation that patient had acute EL or influenza	1946; Violent shaking of both hands; rigidity akinesia, profuse sweating and sialorrhea; developed; pulsions; by age 44 totally immobile and speechless	Dystonic contractures of all extremities and virtually speechless	1969; 1 g; showed striking reduction of rigidity and salivation; on 1.5 g could feed herself and normal voice; after 4 weeks, reversion to parkinsonism plus depression and somnolence; L-dopa stopped and then restarted with hallucinations and violent head movements; screaming and tic-like eye movements; L-dopa stopped again; tried 5 months later at 0.25 g with restoration of voice but chorea, tic-like movements and delirium; L-dopa stopped	Hallucinations persisted for 5 months after stoppage of L-dopa; became less rigid; L-dopa again in 1974: on-off reactions; maintained for 7 years with no additional adverse effects; 6/24 good hours/day on 4 g—no better with more and worse with less; died 1984

(Continued)

Table 8.1 continued

Patient	Birth	Acute EL	PEP development	PEP@L-dopa Trial	Initial Effects	Effects & Outcome
Martha N.	1908	1918; Influenza (almost died)	1929; Parkinsonian signs; static until 1951; rigidity and tremor, inability to walk; hospitalized in 1954	Severe torticollis; immobility of legs; soft voice; immense salivation; OCs; showed remarkable improvement on Easter Sundays	1969; Initial response to L-dopa was in-sucking of tongue; restarted 1 month later at 0.75 g with great improvement; almost no rigidity or akinesia; but then had respiratory crisis, incessant palilalia, and then stupor; L-dopa stopped with recovery in 10 days; again L-dopa tried with initial good results followed by hallucinations; L-dopa stopped	Only derived minimal benefits from L-dopa overall that were overshadowed by psychotoxicity and dyskinesias; restarted on L-dopa 1974—hallucinations; audible voice, good swallowing, OCs, reduced rigidity, and salivation; torticollis; hallucinations prevent interactions with others; L-dopa stopped in 1981 and with it psychosis but became parkinsonian; and subsequently died in that year

Ida T.	1901	1921 (in Poland); Sudden onset of impatience; irritability; impetuosity; increased appetite and violent temper	Within year, parkinsonian signs with stiffness and bradykinesia; became catatonic and was hospitalized in catatonic state for 48 years	Complete immobility with dystonic deformities of hands and feet; virtually aphonic	1969; L-dopa increased daily and at 4 g rigidity disappeared; voice louder and fluent	After 3 years, some rigidity, but patient was still doing very well; responses then deteriorated with return to rigidity; died of malignancy in 1977
Frank G.	1910	1923; 9 weeks in a deep stupor; had to be tube-fed; recovery incomplete with persisting mental signs	1945; Bradykinesia and slow speech; agitated depressed; hospitalized 1950; was independent but would stare and hallucinate for hours daily	Showed flapping tremor; some rigidity and flexion of neck; bilateral ptosis; profuse sweating; mild akinesia	1969; dose slowly raised to 2 g; exacerbation of tremor, hurrying of gait; myoclonic jerks; effects subsided; after 3 months developed violent out-thrusting of tongue, which then stopped; remained static for 6 months; then became irritable and masturbated almost continually; OCs	Derived virtually no benefit from L-dopa; died 1970

(Continued)

Table 8.1 continued

Patient	Birth	Acute EL	PEP development	PEP@L-dopa Trial	Initial Effects	Effects & Outcome
Maria G.	1919	1927; Month-long delirium, fever, hallucinations, extraordinary movements; scarcely slept and could not be sedated	1932; Deeply parkinsonian; hospitalized 1969	Parkinsonian and catatonia; profuse salivation; ocular palsies, akinesia; violent flapping of right hand; soft voice; OCs; sometimes violent rages	1969; at 1.2 g great surge of energy and strength; abolition of rigidity; no sialorrhea; after 2 weeks, violence and mania with paranoid delusions; outbursts of fury; after 1 month 1.0 g with return of parkinsonian state; after 4 days, 1.1 g murderous fury, outthrusting of tongue; L-dopa stopped	Developed strange mannerisms—biting and kicking herself— very sensitive to small changes in dosage; died 1970
Rachel I.	?	No detailed information provided; may not have had EL during the epidemic period	Developed progressive parkinsonism (date unspecified)	Completely immobilized with intense rigidity and dystonia of trunk and extremities; but speech almost normal; peculiar attacks of generalized pain and deterioration of recent memory	1970; 1 g; after 10 days became intensely excited, delirious, had visual hallucinations, and became echolalic; after 3 weeks became comatose (also given sedatives); when awoke was "functionally decorticate"	Died after 7 weeks of pneumonia

Cecil M.	1905	Developed EL during the epidemic period with full recovery	1940: Megaphonia, tendency to grunt, grind, and clench teeth (trismus); (not an in-patient and not in NY; patient of father's in London)	Parkinsonian syndrome; balance impairment, festination; freezing during gait	1970: Initially felt rejuvenated; rigidity disappeared but by 16th day, intense trismus; parkinsonian signs returned and L-dopa stopped	Good results on L-dopa continued; died 1989
Leonard L.	Not provided	No information provided	At age 15 stiffness in right hand	Completely speechless and virtually without voluntary motion; extreme rigidity of neck, trunk, and limbs; marked dystrophic changes in hands; masked facies; OCs	1969: 5.0 g reached after 2 weeks; rigidity vanished, could write and type, rise from a chair and speak with clear voice; after 1 month became maniacal, with odd movements; made sexual advances to nurses; palilalia; tics developed and on-off reactions; dosage reduced to 0.75 g with no effect; L-dopa stopped; resumed 6 months later at 50 mg with no therapeutic response	Reversion to former state; started L-dopa again in 1974 after gap of 4 years; as before showed great sensitivity to L-dopa; tics, tension, blocking of thought; L-dopa stopped; tried again in 1980 and worked well; became stronger with a good voice; then died

(Continued)

Table 8.1 continued

Patient	Birth	Acute EL	PEP development	PEP@L-dopa Trial	Initial Effects	Effects & Outcome
Idiopathic Parkinsonism Patients						
Aaron E.	1907	Had excellent health; no documentation of EL/influenza	1962; Tremor of hands	Severe parkinsonism with little spontaneous speech or movement; walked with freezing, festination; stooped; masked face; moderate rigidity; tremor	1969; Dosage slowly raised to 4.0 g over 3 weeks; walked erect with arm swing; 5.5 g resulted in "virtual normalization;" did well for 9 months; in 13th month chorea in face, restless and irritable; on 3.5 g reverted to parkinsonism; after subsequent stops and starts became choreic on very small dosages (250 mg); after 6 months off-on response even to 5 g; but again started in 1971 with moderate success	Regressed since 1972; feebler reactions to L-dopa; by 1976 severely disabled; died of malignancy in 1977

| George W. | 1913 | No information provided | 1963; Tremor in hand; right-sided stiffness; not an in-patient | Rigidity and akinesia on right side; no right arm-swing and tendency to drag right foot during gait | 1971; Initially developed transient parkinsonism on normal left side; right side virtually normal after 3 wks on 3.5 g; in week 4, restlessness, chorea, rigidity, stuttering; side effects disappeared and patient remained on L-dopa thru 1972; almost normal | L-dopa until 1979 with good results |

* Data from the original 1973 book, as well as later editions.

view is apparent in Table 8.1. Of the 18 patients considered to have PEP, 13 seemed to have had substantial or moderate benefit from L–dopa, and some of the others may have died before the beneficial effects could be noted.

In accordance with our suggestion that the relationship between EL and PEP may be less direct than currently believed (see Chapter 7), of Sacks' patients, only Frances D., Magda B., Robert O., Miriam H., Margaret A., Frank G., Maria G., and Cecil M. seem to have had EL (eight of 20). For the others, either the symptoms are not consistent with EL, or there is no documentation of any antecedent condition resembling EL. Thus, only extrapyramidal symptomatology can be used to differentiate PD from PEP, and it seems that at least some of his PEP patients may actually have had PD (i.e., Gertie C.).

As we have noted elsewhere in this volume, EL/PEP shows tremendous variability in symptomatology, and the data in Table 8.1 reemphasize this. More important for the purpose of this chapter is the enormous variability in the responses of the patients to L–dopa. This variability seems to go far beyond that typically observed among patients in response to a pharmacologic agent. Sacks considered this variability to represent both the psychological and physiological response of the patient as a whole individual to his condition and to the drug. But one could also suggest a more conventional pharmacological/pathological explanation. As described in the EL and PEP neuropathology chapter, the variability in individual patients' lesions are great, affecting many and different structures and presumably neurotransmitter pathways within the brain. Flooding the brain with dopamine via ingestion of L–dopa would not affect these pathways uniformly, and we would intuitively expect that relatively normal systems might respond by functioning abnormally. Based on the symptomatology and neuropathologic data we have presented in this volume, the variability in response exhibited by the PEP patients appears to be physiologically consistent with the variable pathology, and is, therefore, to be expected. Unfortunately, the data in the table do not seem to allow us to predict how any individual patient will respond to L–dopa, although such a prediction might be possible with additional knowledge.

CONCLUSION

Awakenings, both the book and the movie, captivated audiences and did a great service in drawing attention to EL, PEP, PD, and the treatment of these conditions with L–dopa. Whenever the primary author of this book and chapter (JAV) mentioned to a new acquaintance that he was writing a book on EL/PEP and received a perplexed expression, he then mentioned *Awakenings* and there was universal recognition. On the other hand, as noted above, the original edition of the book (and certainly the movie) left the reader (viewer) with the notion that L–dopa was ultimately not a permanent remedy. However, some of the other studies, as well as later editions of *Awakenings* (see Table 8.1), demonstrate that L–dopa had more lasting beneficial effects than originally thought. In 2009, Lees stated that PEPs show an excellent response to L-dopa, albeit with the early development of motor fluctuations with disabling chorea.

One criticism of *Awakenings* is that it presents a blend of results of a clinical trial on a very diverse and profoundly affected population of PEP patients, combined with a human drama of scientific hope and disappointment. It clearly succeeded well in the latter, but was viewed poorly by most academic neurologists in terms of the former. Part of the reason for this was that the data on the use of L-dopa were embedded in the narrative of the book, making easy extraction and comparisons with other studies difficult. Sacks did not consistently present the same data for each patient, did not typically specify whether the clinical descriptions were based on his own examination or patient charts, and did not always specify additional medications that the patients were taking. Nonetheless, as we have tried to show, the final result of Sacks' study is very much in accordance with the statement by Lees (2009) and the results of Duvoisin et al.'s 1972 study; L-dopa was considered a "miracle drug" at the time of its initial development and continues in that role today for PD patients.

REFERENCES CITED

Anonymous. (1969). L-Dopa in Parkinsonism. *British Medical Journal, 2*, 202.
Calne D. B., Stern, G. N., Laurence, D. R., Sharkey. J., & Armitage, P. (1969). L-Dopa in postencephalitic parkinsonism. *Lancet, 293*, 744–747.
Cotzias, G., Papavasiliou, P., & Gellene, R. (1969). Modification of parkinsonism – chronic treatment with L-Dopa. *The New England Journal of Medicine, 280*, 337–345.
Duvoisin R; Barrett, R., Schear, M., Hoehn, M. M., & Yahr, M. (1969) The use of l-dopa in parkinsonism. In F. J. Gillingham & I.M.L. Donaldson eds., *Third Symposium on Parkinson's Disease. Edinburgh on 20, 21 and 22 May 1968,* (pp. 185–192), Edinburgh: E&S Livingston.
Duvoisin, R. C., Lobo-Antunes, J., & Yahr M. D. (1972). Response of patients with postencephalitic Parkinsonism to levodopa. *Journal of Neurology, Neurosurgery, and Psychiatry, 35*, 487–495.
Hunter, K. R., Stern, G. M., & Sharkey, J. Levodopa in postencephalitic parkinsonism. *Lancet, 296*, 1366–1367.
Krashner, N., & Cornelius, J. N. (1970). L-dopa for postencephalitic parkinsonism. *British Medical Journal, 4*, 596.
Lees, A. J. (2009). The Parkinson chimera. *Neurology, 72*(Suppl 2), S2–S11.
Sacks, O. W., Messeloff, C. R., & Schwartz, W. F. (1970). Long-term effects of levodopa in the severely disabled patient. *Journal of the American Medical Association, 213*, 2270.
Wasserstein, A. (1988). Toward a romantic science: The work of Oliver Sacks. *Annals of Internal Medicine, 109*, 440–444.

9

ETIOLOGY

Joel A. Vilensky and Sherman McCall

Two categories of etiologic factors could plausibly have caused EL: environmental (toxicological) and infectious (viral, bacterial, etc.). Genetic susceptibility presumably would interact with both of these factors. Both possibilities were raised at the time of the epidemic, and the latter has become the preferred hypothesis since then, based on cases from the epidemic period and/or more recent cases. Some authorities of the time and more recently have especially favored an etiologic association between EL and the virus that caused the approximately contemporaneous Spanish influenza epidemic (H1N1 virus). Thus, in this chapter, the possible relationship between EL and influenza will be discussed in a separate section from that of other possible viral agents. Finally, this chapter discusses two relatively new theories advanced by Dale et al. (2004, 2009) and also a hypothesis advanced by us that EL and PEP may have multiple causality because neither is a unitary condition.

VON ECONOMO'S ORIGINAL ARTICLES

Von Economo, in his initial 1917(a) article from Vienna, speculated on the cause of the disease. He stated that he had initially considered a toxic process, such as sausage poisoning, because of the poor nutrition caused by the war. However, he dismissed this idea because of the absence of gastrointestinal disturbances. Von Economo next considered and dismissed poison gas as a cause, because the patients gave no exposure history. And there was no evidence of typhoid. He then considered whether EL might be influenzal encephalitis. Spinal fluid from patients failed to demonstrate influenza bacilli (at the time, influenza was believed to be caused by *Haemophilus influenzae*, a gram-negative coccobacillus formerly called Pfeiffer's bacillus or *Bacillus influenzae* and detectable by contemporary methods). However, von Economo believed that failure to find such bacilli did not exclude influenza as a cause of EL, and he noted that most of his cases had begun with symptoms of a cold, headache and general malaise, and possibly joint pain. Von Economo also considered polio, but noted that no polio epidemic was current in Vienna at the time. His patients had negative Wasserman tests, indicating that EL was not related to syphilis. Von Economo believed that the histological findings suggested a single inflammatory process. Furthermore, in his studies of meningeal tissue from deceased patients, he found "coccus-like" formations. Von Economo was very reluctant to ascribe meaning to this finding, however, and requested colleagues who treated subsequent fatal EL cases to send brain samples to his institute for analysis.

In his second 1917 article on EL (1917b) von Economo reported that experimental work at the Pathological Institute confirmed that a specific "infectious" virus was responsible for the disease. This statement was based on the apparent transmissibility of the disease via brain tissue (unfiltered) from a deceased patient to a monkey. He further stated that a "gram-positive diplostreptococcus" was isolated, and it also caused EL symptoms when injected into a monkey.

ENVIRONMENTAL FACTORS

In line with von Economo's initial thoughts, the early forms of EL that appeared in England were considered an unusual form of food poisoning, specifically botulism (Hall, 1918). Similar to the situation in Austria, this diagnosis gained credence due to the reductions in food quality and quantity in England during the Great War. Hall (1918) described the initial attempts to find the cause of EL (Fig. 9.1) as follows:

> Those who saw the earlier cases were faced with a similar difficulty to that which faced the courtiers in the story of Cinderella. They could not find amongst the diseases of their acquaintance a foot which would go into this newly found glass slipper. A search was therefore made amongst the diseases which, so to say, did not move in Court circles, and were not personally known to the seekers. Amongst those it was at first thought that the owner of the slipper had been found, and that her name was Botulism. After many painstaking efforts to force her foot into the slipper, it was found to be impossible, and the attempt was abandoned. Botulism was not Cinderella. (p. 461)

Botulism was eventually rejected because neuropathological analyses of the brains of EL victims revealed lesions, whereas the contemporary belief was that

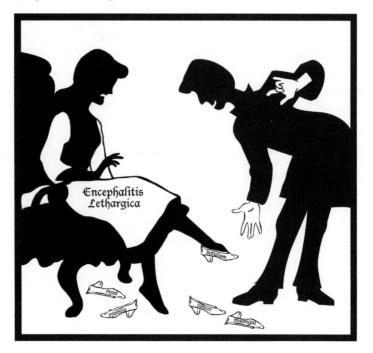

Figure 9.1 Illustration of Hall's description of search for the cause of EL (drawn by Mrs. R. Shadle).

botulism toxin could not cross the blood–brain barrier and was thus confined to the peripheral nervous system (Anonymous, 1918); however, in 1975, Boroff and Shu Chen showed that in mice the botulism toxin could enter the brain.

Furthermore, typically only single cases of EL were seen within households, some of the victims were exclusively breast-fed infants, and the disease was occurring worldwide, all of which cast doubt on an environmental etiologic agent (Matheson Report, 1929).

Despite evidence suggesting EL was an infectious disease, some slightly later reports postulated various other types of food poisoning, such as hydrocyanic acid in flour made from French beans and poisoning from chick peas (lathyrism). Nutritional deficiencies, such as vitamin B_1 (thiamine) deficiency, which is associated with the ingestion of polished rice (beriberi); or a B_3 (niacin) deficiency from over-reliance on dietary corn/maize (pellagra), were also suggested as causes of EL (Matheson Report 1929).

Although no one has postulated a toxin theory as causing EL in the post-epidemic period, there are reports advocating an environmental toxin etiology for a similar condition. In 1954, Mulder et al. described a neurological condition that the indigenous Chamorro people of Guam referred to as *lytigo-bodig*, which is now called amyotrophic lateral sclerosis/parkinsonism-dementia complex

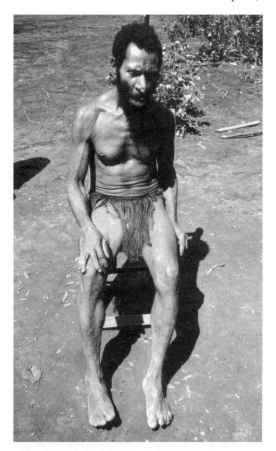

Figure 9.2 A patient from Guam with advanced Parkinson dementia complex. The man has had the disease for 5 years. At this time, he showed no dementia but a parkinsonian gait, rigidity, tremor, and masked face. (Courtesy of Dr. Drs. Ralph Garruto and Carleton Gadujek.)

(ALS-PDC) of Guam. These investigators thought the symptomatology of ALS-PDC was very similar to that of PEP (Steele, 2005; Fig. 9.2). Oliver Sacks, in his book *The Islands of the Colorblind*, writes that the catatonia exhibited by the Guam cases was similar to that in the PEP cases he described in his book *Awakenings*. We should note, however, that although the movement disorders associated with ALS-PDC may be very reminiscent of those in PEP, dementia is a much stronger component of ALS-PDC than of PEP.

In addition to the clinical features, the neuropathology of ALS/PDC is remarkably reminiscent of PEP, including the presence and distribution of neurofibrillary tangles (NFTs) (Geddes et al., 1993; see Chapter 10). Geddes et al. noted that no single pattern of pathology could distinguish PEP, progressive nuclear palsy, or ALS/PDC. They stated, "Such pathological overlap is curious, in view of the fact that each of the diseases is thought to be clinically distinct" (p. 297), although it is consistent with their finding of a lack of correlation between the severity/distribution of pathology and the clinical symptomatology. However, a more recent study of the neuropathology of ALS/PDC (Miklossy et al., 2008) found, in addition to tau (τ) pathology, other protein deposits and Lewy bodies in the brains of ALS/PDC cases; thus, the similarity to PEP now is probably no greater in terms of neuropathology than to Alzheimer or Parkinson diseases.

In 1963, Margaret Whiting suggested that ALS-PDC was due to large amounts of beta-*N*-methylamino-L-arginine (BMAA) in traditional cycad flour consumed in Guam (see also Steele & McGeer, 2008). Although data based on animal experiments initially suggested that the doses necessary to produce neurologic disease were too high to be realistic, Cox and Sacks (2002) suggested that biomagnification of the toxin might have occurred because the Chamorro ingested the meat of flying foxes which, in turn, had ingested the seeds. However, Borenstein et al. (2007) found no correlation between the ingestion of such bats and the disease. Similar to EL, the incidence of ALS-PDC has declined greatly (Steele & McGeer, 2008).

BACTERIAL/VIRAL AGENTS

During the epidemic period, a massive search was undertaken for the putative organism that was causing EL. Tissues (typically brain) and fluids (cerebrospinal fluid [CSF], blood, and nasopharyngeal washings) from EL victims were injected into the brains of a large variety of animal species (especially rabbits) in attempts to develop an animal model of the disease and isolate the causative agent—either a bacteria that could be cultured or a "filterable" virus that could pass through the smallest pores of available filters (viruses were not actually identified as structures until 1935, following the invention of the electron microscope).

Van Rooyen and Rhodes in their 1948 textbook, *Virus Diseases of Man*, said of the bacterial work, "Many [of the investigators] were undoubtedly working with contaminants which either gained access during the postmortem in the case of the brain, or else were present in the nasopharynx quite apart from the encephalitis. Certain workers were also unaware of the existence of spontaneous encephalitis of rabbits" (p. 1072). On the viral experiments, they commented: "The experiments were usually very inconclusive, however, and no recognized strain of virus emerged. The effects noted were probably in the main nonspecific, or else due to an unrecognized bacterial contaminant or to spontaneous encephalitis" (p. 1073). They also noted of the work proposing EL to be a herpes viral infection, "In general, however, herpetic encephalitis, as it is presently observed, appears not to resemble encephalitis lethargica very closely" (p. 1073). Nevertheless, the authors continued to believe that recent evidence had strengthened the view that EL is caused by herpes (although they did not detail the recent evidence).

Simon Flexner, first Director of the Rockefeller Institute for Medical Research, came to a similar conclusion in 1923. He noted that approximately 50% of nonexperimental rabbits show spontaneous brain lesions virtually identical to those reported following intradural or intracerebral injections with encephalitic or herpetic tissues from diseased patients.

As already mentioned, in 1917, von Economo had largely dismissed the hypothesis that EL was caused by the polio virus. Similarly, in 1918 England, James reported that the distributions of cases of polio and EL were quite different, suggesting that the two diseases were unrelated. However, four years later, in 1921, Neustaedter et al. reported that it had not yet been definitely shown that EL was not a different stage of epidemic poliomyelitis. To study this issue further, they injected monkeys with serum from EL victims and virus elements from polio victims because it had been shown previously that such polio serum protects monkeys from developing polio. They found that the monkeys injected with EL serum were similarly protected from developing polio. Furthermore, they did control experiments in which the monkeys were injected with the same polio viral elements together with saline or an equivalent control solution, in place of EL serum, and these monkeys usually developed polio. Due to sera cross-reaction, these results are consistent with a polio etiology for EL or some other enterovirus.

Neal, in 1942, also dismissed the earlier experimental work, saying that EL was probably caused by an unidentified virus. Details of the bacterial/viral studies are thoroughly presented in the three Matheson survey reports (1929, 1932, 1933; see below) and because all of the work is, unfortunately, unreliable for various reasons, we have chosen not to repeat such details here. We will however discuss the focal (bacterial) infection theory advanced by Dr. E.C. Rosenow of the Mayo Clinic because of its historical interest and the EL vaccine trials associated with the Matheson Commission. We will also review post-epidemic EL cases/articles relevant to EL etiology.

MATHESON VACCINE TRIALS/ROSENOW THEORY

William J. Matheson was a wealthy businessman who was diagnosed with EL during the epidemic period. He subsequently used some of his vast fortune to finance research designed to find a cure for EL. Beginning in 1927, he donated $10,000 annually to a "Commission" located at Columbia University in New York: *The Matheson Commission for the Study of Epidemic Encephalitis*. After Matheson's death in 1930, his heirs only funded the Commission until 1932. It continued, using other donations, until 1940. Appointed to direct the survey of the literature on EL, and later the clinical trials, was a woman physician, Josephine B. Neal. Dr. Neal was a neurologist with expertise in bacteriology and had been Assistant Director of the New York City Health Laboratories—she became a world expert on EL (Kroker, 2004). Matheson believed this Commission would find a cure for EL in 2 years and then proceed to find a cure for polio. The Commission produced three significant reports on the disease (1929, 1932, and 1939), all published by Columbia University Press. Neal edited what may be considered a fourth and final report in 1942.

Neal noted in that final report how difficult it was to prove the efficacy of a treatment for EL because of EL's course of natural remissions and progressions. Nevertheless, she argued for vaccine development because it was believed that the chronic stage of the disease was caused by a persistent infection. Neal hoped a vaccine might produce sufficient immunity to reduce or eliminate the infection. In relating the following description of the development and testing of vaccines to treat EL, we want to emphasize that these studies are easy to dismiss because the methods contained no controls to assure that the putative vaccines actually contained any of the viral/bacterial elements associated with their names (i.e., there is no evidence provided, and really could be no definitive evidence at the time that the "herpes" vaccine actually contained any herpes material); nevertheless, the trials were conducted using the standards of the time and, as such, are interesting from a historical perspective may contain some biologically useful information.

The Matheson Commission's vaccine research was guided by two main theories: that EL was a form of herpes (Levaditi & Harvier, 1920); or that it was a focal infection resulting from a neurotropic form *Streptococcus viridans* (Rosenow, 1922). A "herpes" vaccine (Vaccine C) was initially developed by Dr. Frederick Gay of the Department of Bacteriology at Columbia University by injecting a putative neurotropic herpes virus (Le Févre strain; this strain was believed not to have dermatotrophic properties) from a morbid case of EL (obtained from the laboratory of Dr. Levaditi) intracerebrally into rabbits. Some rabbits died from these injections, whereas others survived after showing signs of encephalitis. The brains of the surviving rabbits were emulsified and became a "vaccine." This vaccine was, however, only used for a short time because of a loss of virulence (i.e., rabbits no longer died). Thus, a second herpes vaccine was developed by Dr. Gay (Vaccine X). This one was created by repeatedly injecting rabbits with putative herpes virus derived from an EL victim. The brains of those rabbits found to be immune to injections of the solution were used to make a vaccine that Dr. Gay considered to be a "hyperimmune rabbit brain vaccine" (Neal, 1942). The latter rabbits were also bled, and a serum was developed and used to treat acute EL; however, this was soon discontinued because patients developed serum sickness (a reaction to proteins in antiserum developed from an animal source). A third herpes vaccine was created in 1933. For this vaccine, Dr. Gay formulated a formalized herpes virus vaccine (Vaccine F) based on suspensions of virulent rabbit brains that were inactivated with 0.075% formaldehyde solution (Neal, 1942; Louis, 2002).

Rosenow believed he had found a strain of *Streptococcus viridans* in the brains of EL patients who had died, and that these bacteria had caused the encephalitis

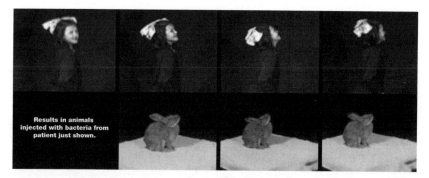

Results in animals injected with bacteria from patient just shown.

Figure 9.3 Sequential images from a film made by Rosenow showing a 3-year-old girl who developed encephalitis lethargica–associated flexion and extension movements of the head and neck. Rosenow extracted fluid from her tonsils that was subsequently injected intracerebrally into a rabbit, producing the same type of unusual head movements. The original film clip showed the same concordance between the abnormal movements in two other EL patients and rabbits injected with their respective bacteria. However, as noted in the text, the movements shown by the rabbits are not uncommon in poorly cared-for laboratory rabbits. Two of the patients presented in the filmstrip were described in detail by Parker (1922). The unusual head movements in this 3-year-old were associated with abnormal breathing so that maximum inspiration occurred with maximum head extension.

that had killed them. Furthermore, Rosenow believed that he could culture the bacteria from specimens taken from the teeth, throats, and nasopharynges of EL patients (Rosenow, 1922) and that the oral cavity was in fact the source of the infection. Rosenow developed both a vaccine and a horse antiserum for treating EL patients (Fig. 9.3).

Rosenow's belief that EL was caused by bacterial spread from the oral cavity to the brain was part of the early 20th-century "focal infection theory." This theory hypothesized that bacteria in the mouth could, through lacerations, enter the bloodstream and cause severe infections in distant parts of the body. Many diseases were thought to be associated with "focal infections," including arthritis, duodenal ulcers, and heart disorders. To reduce further spread of the infection, patients often had all or some of their teeth extracted. Rosenow's work led directly to Henry Cotton's disastrous early 20th-century experimental surgeries on mentally retarded patients in which he surgically removed previously filled teeth, tonsils, sinuses, colons, and uteri. In one year, he claimed an improvement rate of 77% (Kushner, 2005). Rosenow produced a remarkably convincing film depicting patients with specific types of EL who subsequently died; he then showed rabbits with similar signs who had been injected with extracts from the respective patient's brains (Fig. 9.3) However, a laboratory veterinarian who recently viewed the video for us said that the signs shown by these rabbits may also be seen in poorly cared-for laboratory rabbits. Thus, Rosenow's results are not as convincing as they appear.

When the vaccine trials began, a control group of chronic EL patients received injections of normal rabbit brain in a "blind" study versus an experimental group that received the hyperimmune vaccine. However, after a year, such a marked difference was noted between the groups in favor of the hyperimmune vaccine that the Commission voted to discontinue the control group (unfortunately, the actual numerical data are not presented; Neal, 1942). Neal also compared 93 acute EL patients treated with the hyperimmune vaccine with 293 untreated cases recorded by the New York City Health Department. The mortality among the treated cases was less than half that of the untreated cases (11/93 treated patients died, whereas 72/293 untreated patients died). Forty-two subacute patients were treated with the hyperimmune vaccine, and Neal reported that 59.5% showed complete recovery, which she believed was a quite high proportion, although comparative data were not provided.

Also, as part of the vaccine trials, chronic EL patients were treated with either the Rosenow or herpes vaccine. However, it soon became apparent that those patients receiving the Rosenow vaccine were getting worse, not better (of 134 cases, 113 showed exacerbations of symptoms; the symptoms that were especially evaluated included rigidity, tremor, gait, posture, facial expression, speech, difficulty in swallowing, sialorrhea, oculogyric crises, disturbance of sleep, fatigability, mental depression, emotional instability, and disorders of behavior). The Rosenow vaccine was thus discontinued as therapy, but these patients were considered "so far as possible" a placebo group, because Neal believed it was necessary to develop a control group under observation for an extended period of time (1942, p. 283).

Based on her findings, Neal (1942) concluded that, "After a consideration of the results in the acute, subacute, and chronic stages of encephalitis of the treatment with vaccine F, it is difficult to avoid the conclusion that this method of therapy had merit" (p. 284). She also stated, "I realize that the weight of scientific opinion is against the herpes virus being the cause of epidemic encephalitis... . What, then is the reason for its apparent beneficial effect? It can hardly be the action of the foreign protein. Otherwise, the results with Rosenow's vaccine, or with 'X,' should be equally good. For the same reason, it cannot be a psychological effect. Moreover, the improvement in the great majority of patients in the chronic stage took place after the vaccine had been given for several months and not immediately, as would have been the case were it on a psychological basis" (p. 286).

Neal clearly was aware that the weight of scientific evidence at the time was against the herpes hypothesis. Gay and Holden published two articles (1933a,b) advocating the hypothesis, but two discussants to their presentation (Drs. Evans and Rivers) noted that one of the two adult EL cases from which they isolated herpes did not appear to be an EL case at all, but rather a case of generalized herpetic infection (the man became ill after having been bitten by a monkey). The three pediatric cases all followed measles, which in itself would argue against herpes causing EL. Furthermore, herpes simplex encephalitis typically causes necrotic lesions in the temporal lobes of the brain (Booss & Esiri, 2003), and such lesions typically do not occur in EL (see Chapter 10).

Today, the idea of using a "vaccine" in patients with active disease is generally perplexing, although the theoretical basis of immunotherapy for treating cancer is quite similar. Neal and her collaborators were presumably hoping that the vaccine would act in an analogous manner to the previously developed rabies vaccine. (Pasteur had demonstrated in 1885 that injecting the dried spinal cords of rabbits that had been infected with rabies could, if given soon enough after a person had been bitten by a rabid animal, prevent central nervous system [CNS] manifestations of the disease and death.) Contemporary investigators did not know that the rabies vaccine was effective because of the extended time the virus required to travel through nerves to the brain (thus, the vaccine could induce an immune response before the virus infiltrated the CNS). The clinicians of the time further believed that the herpes and rabies viruses reached the CNS in the same manner (Rivers, 1932) and that EL patients had a reduced number of antibodies to herpes (Gay & Holden, 1929).

Although Neal's work was carefully done for the time, it suffers from the contemporary shortcomings in scientific methodology. Her data are qualitative, and she failed to describe precisely how patients were evaluated (i.e., what type of scales were used to measure improvement or deterioration in signs and symptoms). In 2002, Louis published an article on the vaccine trials in which he suggested they were not successful and described problems with the study. However, in some respects, he seemed to rely for his original information more on a 1932 preliminary report (Neal & Bentley, 1932) of the trials than on the later 1942 analysis. Specifically, Louis indicated the lack of a placebo group, when it is clear from the 1942 report that, at least initially, there was such a group. Louis also correctly indicated that the investigators did not have the statistical methods to evaluate outcomes in longitudinal studies of diseases with waxing and waning courses. However, Neal and Bentley stated, "The estimation of improvement in cases of chronic encephalitis is extremely difficult because of the marked irregularity of the natural course of the disease.... We have observed that most patients show a temporary improvement with any method of treatment... We have tried to be particularly conservative in classing patients as improved and have disregarded slight changes for the better in a single symptom. In several patients, there has been evidence of marked improvement in many symptoms, but the extension of tremor to a part not heretofore involved has indicated the disease was progressing" (p. 905).

Louis also correctly indicated that relatively few acute EL patients were treated and suggested that this hindered the value of the vaccine trials. However, as already noted, it was believed at the time that the chronic disease resulted from continued infection, so, as stated by Neal and Bentley, "measures aimed at the destruction of this agent would be applicable at all stages" (p. 899). Last, Louis reported that little attempt was made to control the use of antiparkinsonian medications (anticholinergic agents). However, Neal and Bentley specifically stated that they avoided prescribing drugs of the scopolamine group in patients under their control and endeavored to persuade other patients to cease taking the medications or at least to reduce their dosage.

The results from the Matheson trials cannot be easily evaluated. The available reports don't give important details of the statistics, subject and control group selection, case definition, blinding, and clinical evaluation. Nevertheless, the positive results from the "herpes" vaccines suggest that some aspect of the injected materials, perhaps nonspecifically, had some benefit for some of the patients.

VIRAL AND BACTERIAL TESTING IN POST-1940 CASES OF ENCEPHALITIS LETHARGICA

Many of the post-1940 case reports of putative EL have incorporated testing serum or CSF for possible viral or bacterial agents. Details are presented in Tables 9.1 and 9.2 and are discussed next. However, we leave the discussion of the potential relationship between influenza and EL to a subsequent section that is devoted solely to this issue.

The bacterial data (Table 9.1) do not appear significant because most of the studies were negative and involved so few cases. The four-fold increase in *Mycoplasma pneumonia* reported by Al-Mateen et al. is interesting, but again very limited because it is only a minimal elevation in a single case. Similarly, the viral studies detailed in Table 9.2 are very inconsistent and inconclusive. The question also remains whether these patients had the same disease that existed during the epidemic period (see Chapter 5).

ENCEPHALITIS LETHARGICA AS AN AUTOIMMUNE DISEASE

In 2004, Dale et al. published an intriguing article in the journal *Brain*, in which they described 20 patients with an EL-like phenotype, all of whom had had a preceding pharyngitis. The authors investigated the possibility that this disorder could be a postinfectious autoimmune CNS disorder, with an etiology similar to that of Sydenham chorea. Sixty-five percent of the patients showed elevated antistreptolysin-O titers, and 95% had autoantibodies reactive against basal ganglia antibodies in their CSF; such antibodies were only present in 2%–4% of a control group. The authors thus hypothesized that EL may be secondary to autoimmunity against deep gray nuclei and may be a pediatric autoimmune neuropsychiatric disorder associated with streptococcal infection (PANDAS) disease.

In 2005, McKee and Sussman described a 17-year-old male with putative EL who, similar to most of the Dale et al.'s cases, had had a preceding episode of

Table 9.1 Results of Tests of Post–Epidemic Period Cases of Putative EL/PEP for Bacterial Infection

Reference	Cases	Agents and Results
Al-Mateen et al. (1988)	1 EL case	Paired serum levels for *Mycoplasma pneumoniae* on 3rd and 11th hospital days were 1:512 and 1:2,048
Mellon et al. (1991)	1 EL case	Serum antibodies to *M. pneumoniae* and *Borrelia burgdorferi* were negative
Blunt et al. (1997)	2 EL cases	One case tested for Lyme serology, negative; blood cultures, negative; autoantibody screen, negative; both cases showed negative serology for *M. pneumoniae* and Q fever Ph2
Kiley and Esiri (2001)	1 EL case	Cerebrospinal fluid (CSF) cultures, negative; antineuronal antibodies not detected
Dale et al. (2004)	20 EL cases	Bacterial culture, negative; mycoplasma, negative
Dale et al. (2007)	2 EL cases	Culture for mycoplasma and streptococcus, negative
Ragdev et al. (2007)	3 EL cases	Antineuronal and antistreptolysin-O titre, negative
Sridam and Phanthumchinda (2006)	1 EL case	Serum ANA, C3, CH50, AFP, and B-HCG within normal limits
Basheer et al. (2007)	2 EL cases	No growth from pharyngeal culture for bacterial pathogens
Dale et al. (2009)	20 EL cases	Negative for mycoplasma

AFP, α-fetoprotein; ANA, antinuclear antibodies; B-HCG, β-human chorionic gonadotropin; C3, complement C3; CH50, total hemolytic complement.

pharyngitis and who showed an elevated serum antistreptolysin titre, and raised anti–basal ganglia antibodies. In 2009, Lopez-Alberola described seven new cases of putative EL, four of whom showed elevated anti–basal ganglia antibodies in their CSF but only one of whom had a positive streptococcal serology. However, fluorodeoxyglucose positron emission tomography (FDG-PET) studies found abnormal patterns of cerebral metabolism of 4/7 patients, with the most frequent pattern being an increased glucose metabolism in the basal ganglia.

In the same issue of *Brain* that contained the Dale et al. article, Vincent (2004) published an editorial that raised doubt about the hypothesis that EL is a PANDAS disease. She began by suggesting that the acute "fulminating" form of EL that was apparent during the epidemic period is no longer manifested in the sporadic cases that still occur. She noted that 60% of Dale et al.'s patients did not have magnetic resonance imaging (MRI) data to document basal ganglia disease, and 35% did not have antistreptolysin-O elevation. Furthermore, the putative anti–basal ganglia antibodies detected were not documented to cross-react with streptococcal

Table 9.2 Results of Tests of Post–Epidemic Period Cases of Putative EL/PEP for Viral Infections

Reference	Cases	Agents and Results
Espir and Spalding (1956)	3 EL/PEP cases (two acute)	Specimens of blood, feces, cerebrospinal fluid (CSF) failed to show antibody reactions to known viruses, including polio; attempts at virus isolation via inoculation into mice, monkey kidney, and eggs were all negative
Gamboa et al. (1974)	6 PEP cases	Influenza A antigens detected in hypothalamus and midbrain of all six; herpes not detected in any
Bonduelle et al. (1975)	1 EL case	Coxsackie B elevated in serum (1/32; 2 weeks later, 1/16); herpes, influenza, as well as other viruses were negative or showed no change
Martilla et al. (1977b)	20 PEP cases	No difference from idiopathic PD with regard to influenza antibodies
Martilla et al. (1977a)	441 PEP/PD subjects (no information provided on how many of each)	Higher herpes simplex titre in PD/PEP vs. control (1% higher, but significant because of large patient groups); no differences between PD and PEP; no significant difference between PD/PEP and controls in any other of 15 virus serum antibody titre
Pilz and Erhart (1978)	1 EL case	Herpes simplex titre was increased 16-fold at the beginning of the infection, compared to 6 months later; but rapid decrease suggests not herpes encephalitis; parainfluenza II increased four times over first 3 weeks
Elizan et al. (1978)	29 PEP	Serum tested against 17 arboviruses; no differences between PEP and controls
Elizan and Casals (1979)	29 PEP	Serum tested against LCA virus; no difference from controls
Esiri and Swash (1984)	1 EL case from 1920	No evidence of herpes simplex antigen in brain slice
Elizan et al. (1989)	27 PEP	Serum tested against herpes simplex, cytomegalovirus, measles, rubella, and influenza; not consistently elevated compared to controls
Elizan and Casals (1989)	2 PEP cases	No antigens found in brain slices to influenza, Japanese, rubella, cytomegalovirus, measles, and mumps viruses

Table 9.2 continued

Reference	Cases	Agents and Results
Mellon et al. (1991)	1 EL case	Antibody titre to measles was elevated (1:160 at time of rash; 1:80, 3 weeks later [this is probably not a significant finding because of time frame]); antibodies to mumps, influenza, Coxsackie, varicella-zoster, herpes simplex, Epstein-Barr, adenovirus all negative
Motta et al. (1994)	1 EL case	Negative findings to "full" virological investigation
Isaacson et al. (1995)	7 PEP cases	No influenza RNA detected in brain sections
Blunt et al. (1997)	2 EL cases	No elevation of antibodies to adenovirus, influenza, mycoplasma, cytomegalovirus, mumps, measles, herpes simplex, varicella-zoster, coxsackie; viral PCR all negative
McCall et al. (2001)	5 EL and 2 PEP cases	No influenza RNA in brain slices
Dale et al. (2004)	20 EL cases	Patients tested for many virus antibodies, although not every patient tested for each; all tests negative
Dimova et al. (2006)	1 EL case	Negative serological investigation of serum and CSF for influenza, parainfluenza, entero- and herpes simplex viruses; serum tested positive for Epstein-Barr virus
Dale et al. (2007)	2 EL cases	CSF culture and PCR for enterovirus and herpes simplex negative; serology for herpes simplex and Epstein-Barr virus, negative
Ragdev et al. (2007)	3 EL cases	CSF and blood viral tests negative, except for arborvirus B; serology positive at low titre in one patient (suggested that occurred due to past infection)
Sridam and Phanthumchinda (2006)	1 EL case	Serum PCR for HIV-RNA negative
Basheer et al. (2007)	2 EL cases	Herpes zoster, herpes simplex, Epstein-Barr, cytomegalovirus, all negative
Lopez-Alberola et al. (2009)	7 EL cases	Patients negative for known, "infectious, inflammatory and metabolic" cerebral disorders
Dale et al. (2009)	20 EL cases	Patients negative for herpes and Epstein-Barr

antigens, and they varied in specificity among patients, thus suggesting that they might be secondary to an immune condition rather than causative.

Additional criticism can be found in a report by Singer et al. (2005), who took serum from patients in three groups (PANDAS, Tourette syndrome patients, and age-matched controls). Enzyme linked immunosorbent assay (ELISA) and Western blots against crude soluble extracts of postmortem brain regions, as well as Western blots against putative antigens, were performed. Antibodies were found for all groups, and there were no differences in antibody frequencies between patient groups and controls. According to Vernino (2005), these results cast doubt on a role of neurologic antibodies in these pediatric neuropsychiatric movement disorders, but do not exclude an immune-mediated (or even antibody-mediated mediated) etiology for these diseases (and presumably for EL). Similarly, Basheer et al. (2007) described two children with parainfectious encephalitis of a similar phenotype to EL with serologically detectable anti–basal ganglia antibodies. However, the two cases had different associated pathogens, β–hemolytic streptococcus and herpes zoster. They suggested that, whereas anti–basal ganglia antibodies may contribute to the etiology of EL, their presence may be a general complication of inflammatory encephalopathy of the basal ganglia and brainstem, and thus not specific to *streptococcus* infections.

Finally, PANDAS, by definition, must have a pediatric onset, but three of Dale et al.'s original patients were above age 35. Also, EL during the epidemic period was never considered a pediatric disease.

Interestingly, in a very recent report, Dale et al. (2009) seemed to rescind the PANDA theory on EL and suggested instead that at least the dyskinetic form of EL is due to the development of autoantibodies to the extracellular domain of NR1/NR2 subunits of the N-methyl-D-aspartate receptor (NMDAR$_{Ab}$). Sera from 10/20 pediatric patients with putative EL were found to be NMDAR$_{Ab}$ positive with dyskinesias, parkinsonism, and somnolence. The authors refer to recent studies that have identified EL-like features in young females with ovarian teratomas who also were serum and CSF positive for NMDAR$_{Ab}$. They concluded that the dyskinetic (hyperkinetic) form of EL is an NMDAR$_{Ab}$ encephalitis that can affect very young children.

As with the PANDA hypothesis, this one is open to question. For example, does the Dale et al. (2009) finding mean that the different forms of EL had different etiologies? Were adults who had the hyperkinetic form of EL also infected with NMDAR$_{Ab}$ encephalitis? Why were there more males affected than females during the epidemic period if this is the cause? And, children with EL during the epidemic period typically became very antisocial (see Chapter 2); there is no indication that this occurred with Dale et al.'s patients.

Despite the apparent inconsistencies, it is important to highlight that Dale et al.'s ideas for the etiology of EL were presented as hypotheses, which represent the first new frameworks within which to view this syndrome almost since the epidemic period. And, in that sense, they make a very important contribution to the EL literature.

INFLUENZA AND ENCEPHALITIS LETHARGICA

In his original 1917 article, von Economo (1917a) considered the possibility that EL was an influenzal encephalitis, primarily because encephalitis had been associated with earlier influenza epidemics. His tests to identify the "influenza bacilli" in the spinal fluid of his patients were negative, but he insisted that this did not exclude influenza as a cause of EL. Von Economo believed that the synchrony in the seasonality of the two conditions supported the idea that they were related, and also reported that he had seen many "grippe" cases in Vienna. Furthermore, he reported that most of the EL cases had begun with feelings of a cold, headache, general malaise, and possibly joint pain.

In his 1929 monograph on EL von Economo devoted an entire section to this question, "Influenza, Influenza encephalitis and Encephalitis Lethargica". He began by noting that the neuropathology of EL differs from that of influenza encephalitis (patients who died from influenza may show some capillary hemorrhages in the brain but not the inflammatory processes evident in EL; see Chapter 10). However, he also stated that, despite this difference, it would be equally futile to deny any epidemiological connection between EL and influenza: "A connection is obvious not only from the recrudescence of the encephalitis epidemics in the wake of the influenza pandemic of 1918–1921 and its simultaneous subsidence in the years 1922–1925, but also from historical considerations" (1931, p. 98). He thought that perhaps influenza paved the way for the assumed virus of encephalitis lethargica. Similar to von Economo, many of his contemporaries believed influenza might "predispose to infection with the virus of encephalitis lethargica" (e.g., Wilson-Smith, 1920; Symonds, 1921; Flexner, 1923; Kramer, 1924).

In more recent times, data and articles have appeared both supporting and refuting the influenza etiology. Ravenholt and Foege, in 1982, published two sets of epidemiological data supportive of the idea that influenza caused EL. For Seattle, Washington, from 1918 to 1926, they showed that peaks in influenza deaths occurred consistently about 1 year prior to peaks in EL deaths. Based on this relationship, they assumed a common etiology. However, although the number of deaths per month for influenza during 1918–1919 reached 400, the maximum number of deaths per month for EL was eight, so that assuming similar causality would seem to be highly speculative and probably unjustified. Reid et al. (2001) also criticized these data, stating that the pattern reported for Seattle was not observed globally; they suggested that all these data show is that both diseases peaked in late winter.

Ravenholt and Foege's second set of data is from are from Samoa. In Western Samoa, following the importation of the influenza virus there via passengers on a ship arriving on November 7, 1918, approximately 20% of the population died from influenza and there were many cases of EL, which had not been reported to previously be there. In contrast, American Samoa (just 70 km away), which maintained a strict quarantine, at least for a number of years during the epidemic

period, did not have any cases of influenza or EL. This data set is strongly suggestive of a direct relationship between EL and influenza, and Ravenholt and Foege
seem to have made every effort to ensure the accuracy of the data; nevertheless,
the validity of the data is very hard to assess. For example, Ravenholt and Foege
interpreted deaths between 1919 and 1922 due to *fa-aniniva* (interpreted as fatal
diseases of the head) as being due to EL, although clearly this is a post hoc diagnosis. Furthermore, no other study has replicated these findings in any way, and
some of the source data do not appear to be accessible (e.g., letters; for many years
we tried to obtain supportive material from the Samoan government but failed to
receive any responses to our requests).

Following Ravenholt and Foege's article, in 1989 Maurizi published an article
entitled "Influenza Caused Epidemic Encephalitis (Encephalitis Lethargica): The
Circumstantial Evidence and a Challenge to the Naysayers." After noting that all
evidence in favor of an influenza etiology is circumstantial, Maurizi addressed the
common arguments against the influenza hypothesis and then asked the "naysayers" to propose another known viral agent that fits the data better than the influenza virus.

Maurizi addressed the common arguments against the influenza virus hypothesis as follows:

1. *Not all cases of EL had a history of preceding influenza.* Asymptomatic
   serum-identified viral infections are well-documented; and, mild
   clinical influenza could easily have been misdiagnosed as a cold.
2. *Most epidemics of influenza were not associated with EL.* Successive waves
   of influenza were due to different variants of influenza virus and
   thus only some variants presumably caused EL.
3. *A delay occurred between influenza and EL epidemics.* It is not unusual
   for mental symptoms of diseases to follow physical symptoms after a
   period of days, weeks, or even months.
4. *The earliest cases of EL were seen in Europe before the 1918 influenza
   pandemic.* Earliest EL cases could have been caused by a primarily
   neurovirulent species of influenza.
5. *Influenza and EL have differences in prevalence, clinical features, infectivity,
   and sequelae.* The same is true of primary syphilis and tertiary
   syphilis, and measles and acute sclerosing panencephalitis.

Maurizi's arguments are reasonable, but not convincing; "absence of evidence"
of another agent is not sufficient reason to conclude that there wasn't one
("evidence of absence"). Furthermore, Maurizi's explanations require making
assumptions that do not seem reasonable (e.g., that the strain of influenza that
could cause EL continually appeared and disappeared during the epidemic period).
However, relative to his argument Oxford (2000) reviewed respiratory disease
outbreak reports from World War I and concluded that sporadic influenza
outbreaks occurred in Europe in 1916 and 1917 that might have represented early
limited circulation of the pandemic influenza virus. These outbreaks would have

been roughly contemporaneous to the first reported EL cases. An earlier review, however, suggested that they were the final presentations of the preexisting influenza subtype (Jordon, 1927).

Maurizi did not discuss another common argument against the influenza hypothesis: Although the influenza pandemic apparently spread from North America to Europe in 1918, EL appears to have spread from Europe to North America (see Chapter 3). However, it is conceivable that a variant influenza virus spread from east to west during the early phase of the pandemic, or that pandemic influenza circulated early, at least at low levels, in Europe. Furthermore, EL may have existed in North America prior to its recognition there as a nosological entity. This is plausible due to poor information exchange between World War I belligerents, censorship, only annual indexing of the medical literature, and the publication of initial case reports in German and French.

Reid et al. (2001) also addressed the issue of the relationship between EL and influenza based on some historical information and on published biochemical/molecular data. The latter information is also evaluated in the article that we wrote on this relationship (McCall et al., 2008), and is discussed below. Reid et al.'s historical analysis suggested that most clinicians of the epidemic period rejected the idea that the influenza virus was directly responsible for EL, but that later the two diseases began to be regarded as having a similar etiology. This may not be an accurate evaluation of the historical data, because Reid's et al.'s historical analysis was very limited, considering the approximately 9,000 books/articles on EL that appeared during the epidemic period (Peng, 1993). For example, in 1927, Jordan, in an excerpt from his monograph on influenza that was also published that same year, listed some of the clinicians of the period who were greatly "impressed" with the connection between influenza and EL, including Bonhoeffer (1921), Hagelstam (1925), Tucker (1918), and Ebaugh (1924).

And, pertaining to the relatively few post-epidemic period nonexperimental studies that specifically addressed this issue, only Ravenholt and Foege (1982) and Maurizi supported this relationship, whereas Neal and Wilcox (1937) and Blattner (1956) argued against such a relationship, and virtually all of the recent biochemical/molecular experimental studies found no data supporting such a relationship.

Next, we summarize some of the data from our 2008 review paper in *Neurovirology* (McCall et al.) that provides support for and against the influenza hypothesis, emphasizing the clinical and biochemical/molecular information.

INFLUENZA AND ENCEPHALOPATHY/ENCEPHALITIS

Influenza-related encephalopathy is mainly observed in pediatric populations in Asia. It can occur at the peak of viral illness and may be fatal (Mizuguchi et al., 2007). The influenza virus has been reported to have been found at low titers in extrapulmonary tissues, including meninges (Hoult & Flewett, 1958; Delorme & Middleton, 1979). A more serious condition, acute necrotizing encephalopathy, has also been linked to influenza virus infection and other viral pathogens (Mizuguchi et al., 1995; Weitkamp et al., 2004).

Postinfluenzal encephalitis syndrome is extremely rare and, in contrast to encephalopathy, occurs 2–3 weeks after recovery from influenza. The CSF shows inflammatory changes, and recovery is typical. Influenza virus RNA has been identified by reverse transcription polymerase chain reaction (RT-PCR) of the CSF, and initial serology may already reflect a rising titer (Hoult & Flewett, 1958; Hayase & Tobita, 1997).

Frankova and Jirasek (1974) reported the detection of influenza virus by immunofluorescence in the brain tissue of patients infected with the H3N2 virus. However, an 11-year study of over 22,000 cultures of CSF samples in meningoencephalitis recovered 1,270 viral isolates, but not a single case with influenza (Polage & Petti, 2006).

BIOCHEMICAL/MOLECULAR STUDIES

Experimental studies pertaining to the influenza hypothesis are presented in Table 9.3. They are arranged by type: (1) serology, which examined antibodies against influenza present in the serum of patients; (2) RT-PCR, which tests for influenza viral RNA in brain tissue samples; and (3) antigen (immunohistochemistry), which utilizes anti-influenza antibodies to search for influenza proteins still present in brain tissue samples. In our compilation of data for Table 9.3, we did not include studies of purported modern EL patients because diagnosis outside the epidemic period is especially tenuous (see Chapter 5).

Despite the strong apparent weight of direct evidence against the influenza hypothesis (all but one of the listed studies in Table 9.3 report negative results), the studies are all limited by the extreme rarity of acute EL material and by the difficulty of retrospective confirmatory diagnosis of acute EL. For example, in the Lo et al. study, the 3-day case was a 4-month-old infant, and diagnosis of EL in such a patient seems questionable. Similarly, the meaning of "fulminating EL" in the 1916 London case is unclear, and that patient died before the first published report of EL in 1917 in Vienna.

Presumably as a means to compensate for the shortage of EL brain tissue, many studies used more readily available PEP tissue or serum. However, we believe that the relationship between EL and PEP is not entirely clear (see Chapter 7).

The two serological studies found PEP patients no more likely to have influenza exposure than were PD patients. However, differences in circulating influenza strains detectable in the employed hemaglutination-inhibition tests usually occur after only 2–5 years of antigenic drift (Wright et al., 2006). Therefore, these studies perhaps used influenza strains that would not have cross-reacted with the 1918 strain, and so their findings may be questionable.

Table 9.3 Experimental Studies of the Influenza Hypothesis

Source	Type	Findings	Clinical Details	Comments
Marttila et al. (1977a)	S	No difference between 23 PEP and 421 PD patients, and controls for antibodies to influenza strain PR/8/34	No details provided on how PEP was distinguished from PD (but see below)	Authors indicate results do not support the findings of Gamboa et al. (1974)
Marttila, et al. (1977b)	S	No significant differences among 20 PEP, 55 PD patients, and matched controls in antibodies to influenza strains PR/8/34 and Sw/1976; same PEP patients as Marttila et al. 1977.	PEP patients either had reliable history of encephalitis or oculogyric crises (OCs)	Authors indicate results not supportive of viral etiology for PEP
Isaacson et al. (1995)	R	Could not detect influenza RNA in 7 PEP patients	No clinical data provided	Implies that influenza virus may have been detectable during the EL phase of disease
McCall et al. (2001)	R	Detected β2-microglobulin mRNA from 2 EL, 3 possible EL and 2 PEP cases but unable to detect any influenza RNA fragments	Only 1/5 EL patients had ocular signs; lethargy definite in 3/5; clinical diagnosis in only one case	Authors note the possibility that secondary effects of influenza, e.g., autoimmunity was responsible for EL
Lo et al. (2003)	R	Detected mRNA of the β-actin gene in 8 EL brains but unable to detect influenza RNA	Little clinical information provided; 2/8 EL cases from 1916; 1 patient died in 24 hrs.; another died of influenza; one was 3-month-old infant	One of the authors (Oxford, 2000), suggests the PCR technique utilized may have lacked sensitivity to detect influenza RNA
Gamboa et al. (1974)	A	NWS and WSN antigens detected in hypothalamus and midbrain in 6 PEP patients, but not PD patients	4/6 PEP had OCs; all had encephalitic features consistent with von Economo	Authors state results are not conclusive proof of the influenza etiology of EL
Elizan & Casals (1980)	A	Negative immunostains for several influenza strains including WS/33, Sw/1976 and NWS in one acute EL and one PEP brain	PEP had OCs; EL case was 20-year-old male who died one week following headache, drowsiness, fever and coma	Authors suggest negative results possibly because antigen detection not sensitive enough, proper antigen not tested for, or virus not present at death

S, serology type study; R, RT-PCR type study; and A, antigen type study.

A possible flaw in the RT-PCR studies listed in Table 9.3 is primer mismatch due to influenza viral mutation between 1918 and the later sequences against which primers were designed. The McCall et al. (2001) primers were matched to A/Puerto Rico/8/34 (H1N1) virus DNA and preliminary 1918 sequence information. The Lo et al. (2003) work was also performed before publication of the most relevant 1918 genetic sequences. The 1918 influenza virus (A/South Carolina/1/18 and A/Brevig Mission/1/18) was sequenced from 1997 to 2005 and has now undergone a remarkable laboratory anabiosis (Taubenberger et al., 1997; Reid et al., 1999; Reid et al., 2000; Taubenberger & Reid, 2002; Reid et al., 2002, 2003a,b, 2004; Tumpey et al., 2004; Taubenberger et al., 2005a,b).

The Lo et al. study used a control of mouse brains infected with influenza virus A/NWS/33 by intracerebral inoculation. Unlike the 1918 condition, however, the Lo et al. control was harvested at an optimal time of 3 days post infection. Considering their small size, the mouse brains were also rapidly and efficiently fixed after having been removed from the skull under 70% formal saline. Victims in 1918 died at various phases in the disease course, with variable postmortem intervals at room temperature before autopsy, during which time autolysis occurred. Refrigeration did not become common in morgues until after chlorofluorocarbons became available in the 1930s.

Thus, the Lo et al. control may have suggested a sensitivity that their assay did not possess in historic clinical material. In contrast, the McCall et al. primers were retested against actual 1918 flu material at the conclusion of the testing to prevent the generation of 1918 PCR product.

Another issue is that both the McCall et al. and Lo et al. studies were limited by failure to test non-CNS material, especially lung, and thus cannot rule out a remote effect of influenza.

Only the Gamboa et al. immunohistochemistry study listed in Table 9.3 yielded experimental support for the influenza hypothesis. However, their detection of A/WSN/33 and A/NWS/33 influenza viral antigens is inconsistent with the fact that A/PR/8/34 and A/WS/33 influenzal viral antibodies (one known to cross-react with 1918 influenza, and the second, the virus from which A/WSN/33 and A/NWS/33 were derived) did not react at all. In addition, all of Gamboa et al.'s material was obtained from PEP patients more than 45 years after EL onset. Viral detection after half a century suggests chronic influenza infection rather than an acute infection associated with EL.

These authors did not consider their study to be conclusive, and their findings could not be replicated (Elizan & Casals, 1989).

INFLUENZA CONCLUSIONS

Pertaining to the influenza hypothesis, it must be emphasized that it is impossible to prove a negative. Furthermore, as discussed here and in our article, many technical limitations potentially could have caused experimental false negatives. Additionally, epidemic-period morgues were not refrigerated, so that autolysis likely caused viral degradation and difficulty in fixation. In addition, formalin fixation is suboptimal for molecular studies. Finally, most available cases from which neural tissue had been taken had had long clinical courses, so that an acute viral infection might no longer be detectable.

Influenza causation would provide a convenient explanation for EL's disappearance, because the 1918-like influenza strains ceased human circulation sometime before 1933, when the first human influenza strain was cultured (Taubenberger, 2006). Empirical studies provide little evidence of influenza causation, but technical limitations and the shortage of appropriate material for testing limit the degree of confidence. Therefore, unless another cause of classical EL is positively identified, its return in the context of another influenza pandemic remains formally possible. Accordingly, a very recent article by Jang et al. (2009) determined the infectivity of an H5N1 influenzal viral strain in mice and found that the virus could travel from the peripheral to the central nervous system. Furthermore, once in the CNS, the virus reached the substantia nigra with resulting symptomatology and neuropathology resembling parkinsonism (see Chapter 10). Although the abnormal protein pathology resulting from this specific influenza virus differed from that in PEP, the authors concluded that viruses (influenzal) may be important in the etiogenesis of neurodegenerative diseases.

ADDITIONAL THEORIES ON CAUSATION

In 1980, Elizan et al. presented data suggesting a strong genetic component to PEP susceptibility based on an analysis of human leucocyte antigens (HLA). They typed 18 Jewish PEP patients for HLA-A, HLA-B, and HLA-C antigenic determinants and compared the results with 147 Jewish control subjects. HLA-B14 antigen was statistically significantly increased in the PEP group; however, these findings were not confirmed in a similar study (although not using Jewish patients) by Lees et al. (1982).

Cernack and Jean (1990) highlighted similarities between acquired immune deficiency syndrome (AIDS) dementia complex and EL, such as common stages, neurotropisms, premature psychological disorders, mononucleosis-like symptoms, similar somatic manifestations, and terminal dementia; they suggested that EL could have been caused by a sexually transmitted retrovirus. Similarly, Elizan and Casals (1991) noted that marked general astrogliosis was observed in the frontal and temporal white matter from a case of EL/PEP. They suggested that the marked astrogliosis in areas distant from the primary lesions seemed to indicate extensive pathological involvement, similar to concurrently studied cases of encephalitides caused by human immunodeficiency virus (HIV).

In Chapter 7 we delineated our arguments against a simple relationship between EL and PEP. Although we think EL is probably a factor in the development of

PEP, it is probably not the only factor. Further, we also suggested there and repeat here that part of the complexity surrounding EL and PEP may result because they are not unitary entities. Considering the incredible breadth of symptomatology characterizing EL and the issues pertaining to PEP, these may be phenotypically related conditions but with differing etiologies (see also the discussion of Dale et al. [2009] above). This was also suggested by others for PEP. Jakob (1923; cited in Neutstadler & Liber, 1937) concluded that, clinically and anatomically, two types of PEPs exist. The most common form is anatomically characterized by simple gray matter degeneration, with rarely any infiltrative lesions. In these cases, the substantia nigra is uniformly affected, as is typically the globus pallidus, but rarely the striatum. The second type is characterized by repeatedly febrile episodes, and the pathology is typified by a polymorphous and progressive syndrome of focal processes with diffuse infiltration phenomena. In these cases, the substantia nigra, as well as many other brain structures and regions are affected, and pronounced akinesia and hypertonia is present. Similarly, Forno and Alford (1971) thought that perhaps PEP patients with and without a history of EL might represent different forms of parkinsonism.

CONCLUSION

The herpes vaccine trial data presented by Neal are intriguing, but inconsistent with a modern understanding of herpes encephalitis. Influenza seems very unlikely as the cause of EL, but cannot be ruled out. The PANDAS hypothesis based on modern cases is also intriguing, but seems inconsistent with many aspects of the epidemic-period disease. No known agent accounts for all the features of EL and PEP; thus, our reiteration of earlier suggestions that perhaps EL/PEP is not a single entity. And this would be in agreement with Dale et al.'s (2009) hypothesis relative to the hyperkinetic forms of EL.

Pertaining to the viral etiology of EL/PEP, the idea that PD was similarly due to a viral agent was not generally thought credible by most neurologists. However, in 2007, Hawkes et al. proposed the "double hit" theory of PD causation, which hypothesized that a transmissible agent, most likely a neurotrophic virus, entered the brain through the nose and at the same time, was swallowed via nasal secretions and transported from the gut to the medulla via retrograde transport in the vagus nerve. EL/PEP is similarly thought to be caused by a neurotrophic virus and, remarkably, most of the early 20th-century clinicians believed it similarly entered the brain via the nose and nasal secretions (e.g., von Economo, 1929). If the theory is true, it might indicate that "idiopathic PD" and EL/PEP are very similar in etiology.

Unfortunately, it is possible that, unless a future EL epidemic occurs or better techniques for analyzing existing specimens (or additional specimens) are found, we may never learn the actual cause of EL/PEP. This is a frustrating conclusion to almost 100 years of research on this condition.

REFERENCES CITED

Al-Mateen, M., Gibbs, M., Dietrich, R., Mitchell, W. G., & Menkes, J. H. (1988). Encephalitis lethargica-like illness in a girl with mycoplasma infection. *Neurology, 38,* 1155–1158.

Anonymous. (1918). Combined sections of medicine, pathology and epidemiology, encephalitis lethargica. *Lancet, 2,* 557.

Basheer, S. N., Wadsworth, L. D., & Bjornson, B. H. (2007). Anti-basal ganglia antibodies and acute movement disorder following herpes zoster and streptococcal infections. *European Journal of Paediatric Neurology, 11,* 104–107.

Blattner, R. J. (1956). Encephalitis lethargica, type A encephalitis, von Economo's disease. *The Journal of Pediatrics, 49,* 370–372.

Blunt, S. B., Lane, R. J. M., Turjanski, N., & Perkin, G. D. (1997). Clinical features and management of two cases of encephalitis lethargica. *Movement Disorders, 12,* 354–359.

Bonduelle, M., Bouygues, P., Lormeau, G., & Degos, C. (1975). Case of lethargic-type hypersomnia. *Revue Neurologique, 131,* 737–739.

Bonhoeffer, K. (1921). Die encephalitis epidemics. *Deutsche medizinische Wochenschrift, 47,* 228–233.

Booss, J., & Esiri, M. M. (2003). *Viral Encephalitis in Humans.* Washington DC: American Society for Microbiology.

Borenstein, A. R., Mortimer J., Schofield E., Wu Y., Salmon D. P., Gamst A., et al. (2007). Cycad exposure and risk of dementia, MCI, and PDC in the Chamorro population of Guam. *Neurology, 68,* 1764–1771.

Boroff, D. A., & Shu Chen, G. (1975). On the question of permeability of the blood-brain barrier to botulinum toxin. *Archives of Allergy and Applied Immunology, 48,* 495–504.

Cox, P. A., & Sacks, O. W. (2002). Cycad neurotoxins, consumption of flying foxes, and ALS-PDC disease in Guam. *Neurology, 58,* 956–959.

Czermak, M., & Jean, T. (1990). The encephalitis lethargic of Von Economo-Cruchet and its reports with the infection HIV. *L'Encephale, 5,* 375–382.

Dale, R. C., Church, A. J., Surtees, R. A. H., Lees, A. J., Adcock, J. E., Harding, B., et al. (2004). Encephalitis lethargica syndrome: 20 new cases and evidence of basal ganglia autoimmunity. *Brain, 127,* 21–33.

Dale, R. C., Irani S. R., Brilot, F., Pillai S., Webster, R., Gill, D., et al. (2009). N-Methyl-D-Aspartate receptor antibodies in pediatric dyskinetic encephalitis lethargic. *Annals of Neurology, 66,* 704–709.

Dale, R. C., Webster, R., & Gill, D. (2007). Contemporary encephalitis lethargica presenting with agitated catatonia, stereotypy, and dystonia-Parkinsonism. *Movement Disorders, 22,* 2281–2284.

Delorme, L., & Middleton, P. J. (1979). Influenza A virus associated with acute encephalopathy. *American Journal of Diseases of Children, 133,* 822–924.

Dimova, P. S., Bojinova, V., Georgiev, D., & Milanov, I. (2006). Acute reversible parkinsonism in Epstein-Barr virus-related encephalitis lethargica-like illness. *Movement Disorders, 21,* 564–566.

Ebaugh, F. G. (1924). Two cases of acute epidemic encephalitis occurring in one family. *American Journal of Diseases of Children, 27,* 230–232.

Elizan, T. S., & Casals, J. (1989). No viral antigens detected in brain tissue from a case of acute encephalitis lethargica and another case of post-encephalitic Parkinsonism. *Journal of Neurology, Neurosurgery, and Psychiatry, 52,* 800–801.

Elizan, T. S., & Casals, J. (1991). Astrogliosis in von Economo's and postencephalitic Parkinson's diseases supports probable viral etiology. *Journal of the Neurological Sciences, 105,* 131–134.

Elizan, T.S., Schwartz, J., Yahr, M.D., & Casals, J. (1978). Antibodies against arboviruses in postencephalitic and idiopathic Parkinson's disease. *Archives of Neurology, 35,* 257–260.

Elizan, T. S., Terasaki, P. I., & Yahr, M. (1980). HLA-B14 antigen and postencephalitic Parkinson's Disease. *Archives of Neurology, 37,* 542–544.

Esiri, M. M., & Swash, M. (1984). Absence of herpes simplex virus antigen in brain in encephalitis lethargica. *Journal of Neurology, Neurosurgery and Psychiatry, 47,* 1049–1050.

Espir, M. L. E., & Spalding, J. M. K. (1956). Three recent cases of encephalitis lethargica. *British Medical Journal, 1,* 1141–1144.

Flexner, S. (1923). Epidemic (lethargic) encephalitis and allied conditions. *Journal of the American Medical Association, 81,* 1688–1893, 1785–1789.

Forno, L. S., & Avord Jr., E. C. (1971). The pathology of Parkinsonism. Part I. Some new observations and correlations. *Contemporary Neurology Series, 8,* 119–130.

Frankova, V., & Jirasek, A. (1974). Immunofluorescence demonstration of influenza A virus in human brains. *Acta Virology, 18,* 444.

Gamboa, E. T., Wolf, A., Yahr, M. D., Harter, D. H., Duffy, P. E., Barden, H., & Hsu, K. C. (1974). Influenza virus antigen in postencephalitic parkinsonism brain. *Archives of Neurology, 31,* 228–232.

Garruto, R. M., & Yanagihara, R. (2009). Contributions of isolated Pacific populations to understanding neurodegenerative diseases. *Folia Neuropathologica, 47,* 149–170.

Gay, F. P., & Holden, M. (1929). The herpes-encephalitis problem. *The Journal of Infectious Diseases, 45,* 415–434.

Gay, F. P., & Holden, M. (1933a). Further evidence for the presumed herpetic origin of epidemic encephalitis. *Transactions Association of American Physicians, 48,* 16–22.

Gay, F. P., & Holden, M. (1933b). The herpes encephalitis problem, II. *Journal of Infectious Disease, 53,* 287–303.

Geddes, J. F., Hughes, A. J., Lees, A. J., & Daniel, S. E. (1993). Pathological overlap in cases of parkinsonism associated with neurofibrillary tangles. *Brain, 116,* 281–302.

Hagelstam, J. (1925). Influenza and epidemic encephalitis. *Journal of the American Medical Association, 84,* 156.

Hall, A. J. (1918). Epidemic encephalitis. *British Medical Journal, 2,* 461–463.

Hawkes, C. H., Del Tredici, K., & Braak, H. (2007). Review: Parkinson's disease: A dual-hit hypothesis. *Neuropathology and Applied Neurobiology, 33,* 599–614.

Hayase, Y., & Tobita, K. (1997). Influenza virus and neurological diseases. *Psychiatry and Clinical Neurosciences, 51,* 181–184.

Hoult J. G., & Flewett, T. H. (1958). Influenzal encephalopathy and post-influenzal encephalitis. *Lancet, 2,* 11–15.

Isaacson, S., Asher, D., Gibbs, C., Gajdusek, D., & Yahr, M. D. (1995). In situ RT-PCR Detection of Influenza viral RNA. *Journal of Neuroscience, 21,* 1272.

James, S. P. (1918). Lethargic encephalitis. Note on its distribution in England. *Lancet, 2,* 837–838.

Jang, H., Boltz, D., Sturm-Ramirez, K., Shepherd, K. R., Jiao, Y., Webster, R., & Smeyne, R. J. (2009). Highly pathogenic H5N1 influenza virus can enter the central nervous system and induce neuroinflammation and neurodegeneration. *Proceedings of the National Academy of Sciences, 106,* 14053–14068.

Jordon, E. O. (1927). The influenza epidemic of 1918: Encephalitis and influenza. *Journal of the American Medical Association, 89,* 1603–1606, 1689–1779.

Kiley, M., & Esiri, M. M. (2001). A contemporary case of encephalitis lethargica. *Clinical Neuropathology, 20,* 2–7.

Kramer, P. H. (1924). Clinical and epidemiological study of encephalitis. *Geneeskundige Bladen Uit Kliniek En Laboratorium Voor De Praktijk*, *24*, 1–40.

Kroker, K. (2004). Epidemic encephalitis and American neurology, 1919–1940. *Bulletin of Medical History*, *78*, 108–147.

Kushner, H. (2005). Cutting edge psychiatry (book review). Cerebrum *7*(*3*).

Lees, A. J., Stern, G. M., & Compston, D. A. S. (1982). Histocompatibility antigens and post-encephalitic Parkinsonism. *Journal of Neurology, Neurosurgery and Psychiatry*, *45*, 1060–1061.

Levaditi, C., & Harvier, P. (1920). Le virus de l'encephalite lethargique. *Societe De Biologie*, *83*, 354–355.

Lo, K. C., Geddes, J. F., Daniels, R. S., & Oxford, J. S. (2003). Lack of detection of influenza genes in archived formalin-fixed, paraffin wax-embedded brain samples of encephalitis lethargica patients from 1916 to 1920. *Virchows Archives*, *442*, 591–596.

Lopez-Alberola, R., Georgiou, M., Sfakianakis, G. N., Singer, C., & Papapetropoulos, S. (2009). Contemporary encephalitis lethargica: Phenotype, laboratory findings and treatment outcomes. *Journal of Neurology*, *256*, 396–404.

Louis, E. D. (2002). Vaccines to treat encephalitis lethargica. *Archives of Neurology*, *59*, 1486–1490.

Marttila R. J., Arstila P., Nikoskelaninen J., Halonen, P. E., & Rinne, U. K. (1977a). Viral antibodies in the sera from patients with Parkinson disease. *European Neurology*, *15*, 25–33.

Marttila, R. J., Haloene, P., & Rinne, U. K. (1977b). Influenza virus antibodies in parkinsonism. *Archives of Neurology*, *34*, 99–100.

Matheson Commission. (1929). *Epidemic Encephalitis; Etiology, Epidemiology, Treatment*. New York: Columbia University Press.

Matheson Commission (1932). *Epidemic Encephalitis: Etiology, Epidemiology, Treatment*. Second Report by the Matheson Commission. New York: Columbia University Press.

Matheson Commission (1939). *Epidemic Encephalitis: Etiology, Epidemiology, Treatment*. Third Report by the Matheson Commission. New York: Columbia University Press.

Maurizi, C. P. (1989). Influenza caused epidemic encephalitis (encephalitis lethargica): The circumstantial evidence and a challenge to the naysayers. *Medical Hypotheses*, *28*, 139–142.

McCall, S., Henry, J. M., Reid, A. H., & Taubenberger, J. K. (2001). Influenza RNA not detected in archival brain tissues from acute encephalitis lethargica cases or in postencephalitic Parkinson Cases. *Journal of Neuropathology & Experimental Neurology*, *60*, 696–704.

McCall, S., Vilensky, J. A., Gilman, S., & Taubenberger J. K. (2008). The relationship between encephalitis lethargica and influenza: A critical analysis. *Journal of Neurovirology 14*, 177–185.

McKee, D. H., & Sussman, J. D. (2005). Case report: Severe acute parkinsonism associated with Streptococcal infection and antibasal ganglia antibodies. *Movement Disorders*, *20*, 1661–1663.

Mellon, A. F., Appleton, R. E., Gardner-Medwin, D., & Aynsley-Green, A. (1991). Encephalitis lethargica-like illness in a five-year-old. *Developmental Medicine and Child Neurology*, *33*, 158–161.

Miklossy, J., Steele, J. C., Yu, S., McCall, S., Sandberg, G., McGeer, E. G., & McGeer, P. L. (2008). Enduring involvement of tau, ß-amyloid, α-synuclein, ubiquitin and TDP-43 pathology in the amyotrophic lateral sclerosis/parkinsonism-dementia complex of Guam (ALS/PDC). *Acta Neuropathology*, *16*, 625–637.

Mizuguchi, M., Abe, J., Mikkaichi, K., Noma, S., Yoshida, K., Yamanaka, T., & Kamoshita, S. (1995). Acute necrotizing encephalopathy of childhood: a new syndrome presenting with multifocal, symmetric brain lesions. *Journal of Neurology, Neurosurgery and Psychiatry* *58*, 555–651.

Mizuguchi, M., Yamanouchi, H., Ichiyama, T., & Shiomi, M. (2007). Acute encephalopathy associated with influenza and other viral infections. *Acta Neurologica Scandinavica Supplement*, *186*, 45–56.

Motta, E., Rosciszewska, D., & Piela, Z. (1994). Diagnostic difficulties in the case of a 57-year-old. *Przeglad Epidemiologiczny*, *48*, 495–497.

Mulder, D. W., Kurland, L. T, & Iriarte, L. L. G. (1954). Neurologic diseases on the island of Guam. *U. S. Armed Forces Medical Journal*, *5*, 1724–1739.

Neal, J. B., & Bentley, I. A. (1932). Treatment of epidemic encephalitis. Review of the work of the Matheson Commission. In: I. Strauss, T. K. Davis, A. M. Frantz (Eds.), *Infections of the Central Nervous System. An Investigation of the Most Recent Advances. Association for Research in Nervous and Mental Disease, Volume XII* (pp. 302–314). Baltimore: Williams and Wilkins.

Neal, J. B. (1942). *Encephalitis: A Clinical Study*. New York: Grune & Stratton.

Neal, J. B., & Wilcox, H. L. (1937). Does the virus of influenza cause neurological manifestations. *Science*, *86*, 267–268.

Neustaedter, M., Larkin, J. H., & Banzhaf, E. J. (1921). A contribution to the study of lethargic encephalitis in its relation to poliomyelitis. *American Journal of Medical Science*, *162*, 715–720.

Neustaedter, M., & Liber, A. F. (1937). Concerning the pathology of parkinsonism (idiopathic, arteriosclerotic, and post-encephalitic). *Journal of Nervous and Mental Disease*, *86*, 264–283.

Oxford, J. S. (2000). Influenza A pandemics of the 20th century with special reference to 1918: virology, pathology and epidemiology. *Review of Medical Virology*, *10*, 119–133.

Parker, H. L. (1922). Disturbances of the respiratory rhythm in children, a sequela to epidemic encephalitis. *Archives of Neurology and Psychiatry*, *7*, 630–638.

Peng, S. L. (1993). Reductionism and encephalitis lethargica, 1916-1939. *New Jersey Medicine*, *90*, 459–462.

Pilz, P., & Erhart, P. (1978). Gibt es noch eine Encephalitis lethargic Economo? Zur Problematik virologisch-serologischer Diagnostik neurologischer Krankheitsbilder. [Is there still an encephalitis lethargica Economo? On the problems of virological-serological diagnosis of neurologic diseases.] *Wiener Medizinische Wochenschrift*, *128*, 762–763.

Polage, C. R., & Petti, C. A. (2006). Assessment of the utility of viral culture of cerebrospinal fluid. *Clinical Infectious Disease*, *43*, 1578–1579.

Raghav, S., Seneviratne, J., McKelvie, P. A., Chapman, C., Talman, P. S., & Kemster, P. A. (2007). Sporadic encephalitic lethargica. *Journal of Clinical Neuroscience*, *14*, 696–700.

Ravenholt, R. T. & Foege, W. H. (1982). 1918 Influenza, Encephalitis, Parkinsonism. *Lancet*, *2*, 860–864.

Reid, A. H., Fanning, T. G., Hultin, J. V., & Taubenberger, J. K. (1999). Origin and evolution of the 1918 "Spanish" influenza virus hemagglutinin gene. *Proceedings National Academy of Science*, *96*, 1651–1656.

Reid, A. H., Fanning, T. G., Janczewski, T. A., Lourens, R. M, & Taubenberger, J. K. (2004). Novel origin of the 1918 pandemic influenza virus nucleoprotein gene. *Journal of Virology* *78*, 12462–12470.

Reid, A. H., Fanning, T. G., Janczewski, T. A., & Taubenberger J. K. (2000). Characterization of the 1918 "Spanish" influenza virus neuraminidase gene. *Proceedings National Academy of Science U S A*, *97*, 6785–6790.

Reid, A. H., Janczewski, T. A., Lourens, R. M., Elliot, A. J., Daniels, R. S., Berry, C. L., Oxford, J. S., & Taubenberger, J. K. (2003a). 1918 Influenza pandemic caused by highly Conserved viruses with two receptor-binding variants. *Emerging Infectious Diseases*, *9*, 1249–1253.

Reid, A. H., McCall, S., Henry, J. M., & Taubenberger, J. K. (2001). Experimenting on the past: The enigma of von Economo's encephalitis lethargica. *Journal of Neuropathology & Experimental Neurology*, *60*, 663–670.

Rivers, T. M. (1932). Relation of filtrable viruses to diseases of the nervous system. *Archives of Neurology and Psychiatry*, *28*, 757–777.

Rosenow, E. C. (1922). Experimental studies on the etiology of encephalitis. *Journal of the American Medical Association*, *79*, 443–448.

Sacks, O. (1996). *The Islands of the Colorblind.* New York: Alfred A. Knopf.

Singer H. S., Hong J. J., Yoon D., & Williams, P. N. (2005). Serum autoantibodies do not differentiate PANDAS and Tourette syndrome from controls. *Neurology*, *65*, 1701–1707.

Sridam, N., & Phanthumchinda, K. (2006). Encephalitis lethargica-like illness: Case report and literature review. *Journal of the Medical Association of Thailand*, *89*, 1521–1527.

Steele, J. C. (2005). Parkinsonism-Dementia complex of Guam. *Movement Disorders*, *20*, S99–S107.

Steele, J. C., & McGeer, P. L. (2008). The ALS/PDC syndrome of Guam and the cycad hypothesis. *Neurology*, *70*, 1984–1990.

Symonds, C. P. (1921). Critical review: encephalitis lethargica. *Quarterly Journal of Medicine*, *14*, 283–308.

Taubenberger, J. (2006). The origin and virulence of the 1918. "Spanish" influenza virus. *Proceedings American Philosophical Society*, *150*, 86–112.

Taubenberger, J. K., & Reid, A. H. (2002). The 1918 "Spanish" influenza pandemic and characterization of the virus that caused it. In: C. W. Potter (Ed.), *Influenza* (pp. 101–122). Philadelphia: Elsevier.

Taubenberger, J. K., Reid, A. H., & Fanning, T. G. (2005). Capturing a killer flu virus. *Scientific American*, *292*, 48–57.

Taubenberger, J. K., Reid, A. H., Krafft, A. E., Bijwaard, K. E., & Fanning, T. G. (1997). Initial genetic characterization of the 1918 "Spanish" influenza virus. *Science*, *275*, 1793–1796.

Taubenberger, J. K., Reid, A. H., Lourens, R. M., Wang, R., Jin, G., & Fanning, T. G. (2005). Characterization of the 1918 Influenza virus polymerase genes. *Nature*, *437*, 889–893.

Tucker, B. R. (1918). Epidemic encephalitis lethargic, or epidemic somnolence, or epidemic cerebritis, with report of cases and two necropsies. *Journal of the American Medical Association*, *72*, 1448–1450.

Tumpey, T. M., Garcia-Sastre, A., Taubenberger, J. K., Palese, P., Swayne, D. E., & Basler, C. F. (2004). Pathogenicity and immunogenicity of influenza viruses with genes from the 1918 pandemic virus. *Proceedings National Academy of Sciences*, *101*, 3166–3171.

van Rooyen, C. E., Rhodes, A. J. (1948). *Virus Diseases of Man.* Thomas Nelson & Sons.

Vernino, S. (2005). Neurologic autoantibodies. *Neurology*, *65*, 1688–1689.

Vincent, A. (2004). Encephalitis lethargica: part of a spectrum of post-streptococcal auto-immune diseases? *Brain*, *127*, 2–3.

von Economo, C. (1917a). Encephalitis lethargica. *Wiener klinische Wochenschrift*, *30*, 581–585.

von Economo, C. (1917b). Neue Beitrage zur Encephalitis lethargica. *Neurologisches Centralblatt*, 5, 866–878.

von Economo, C. (1929). *Die Encephalitis lethargica, ihre Nachkrankheiten und ihre Behardlung*. Berlin: Urban & Schwarzenberg. (Published in English in 1931: Translated by K. O. Newman; London: Oxford University Press.)

Weitkamp, J., Spring, M., Brogan, T., Moses, H., Bloch, K., & Wright, P. (2004). Influenza A virus-associated acute necrotizing encephalopathy in the United States. *Pediatric Infectious Diseases Journal* 23, 259–263.

Whiting, M. (1963). Toxicity of Cycads. *Economic Botany*, 17, 271–299.

Wilson-Smith, W. A. (1920). Arsenic in lethargic encephalitis. *British Medical Journal*, 1, 655.

Wright, P. F., Neumann, G., & Kawaoka, X. (2007). Orthomyxoviruses. In Virology (Fields), Philadelphia: Lippincott Williams & Wilkins.

10

NEUROPATHOLOGY OF ACUTE AND CHRONIC ENCEPHALITIS LETHARGICA

Joel A. Vilensky, Lindsay L. Anderson, Roger C. Duvoisin,
Keith A. Josephs, and Ravil Z. Mukhamedzyanov

As described in Chapter 2, differentiation of the stages of encephalitis lethargica (EL) based on symptomatology is problematic because the acute phase may merge seamlessly into the chronic phase. It is similarly difficult to separate the neuropathology of acute EL from that of chronic EL. Nevertheless, within limits, in this chapter, we will differentiate the two because the literature is typically divided accordingly.

Before presenting the neuropathologic data, we want to emphasize that a complete histopathologic analysis of the human brain using multiple stains is an enormous project involving months of tedious analysis. Thus, to what extent each of the noted investigators analyzed the EL and postencephalitic parkinsonism (PEP) brains is often impossible to discern. Accordingly, some of the very apparent inconsistencies in the various descriptions of the neuropathology of acute and chronic EL reflect different levels of analysis by the investigators, as well as different fixatives and staining techniques.

ACUTE ENCEPHALITIS LETHARGICA

Introduction

At the time of the EL epidemic, the only methods of studying neuropathology were macro- and microscopic examination at autopsy. Such a process has significant limitations: (a) the disease characteristics within any single individual can only be characterized at one point in time, as opposed to the results of current technologies, such as various imaging modalities and sequential biopsies; (b) the very early disease processes are especially difficult to discern because patients don't typically die until the development of significant lesions in critical structures; (c) similarly, information from milder forms of the disease in which the patients don't die are not available and may be dissimilar from those that are fatal; (d) the brain and meninges are easily torn when removed from the skull, especially when swollen, so that some observed lesions may have occurred postmortem; (e) improper or delayed fixation can distort identification of abnormalities; and (f) because almost no preserved EL tissue remains available for study, we have to rely on the skill of the clinicians and pathologists who studied them at the time of the epidemic (Booss & Esiri, 2003; Fig. 10.1).

Microscopic Changes

Of the 11 cases described by von Economo in his two 1917 articles, five died. In the second article from that year, von Economo expressed the view that four of the five cases had similar microscopic lesions, suggesting a uniform pathology to the disease. The exception was case 1, in which the symptoms had disappeared,

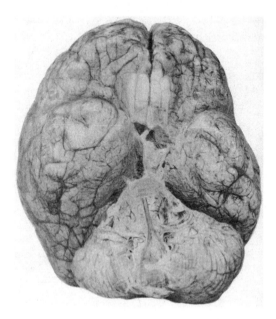

Figure 10.1 Base of a brain from a patient with encephalitis lethargica brain showing hyperemia and a moderate exudate especially in the region of the pons and medulla (from Alexander, 1921).

but the patient died 2 months later of pneumonia. The consistent microscopic changes were: (a) small-cell infiltration of the adventitia of the blood vessels, especially of the veins; 2(b) spotted small-cell infiltration of the parenchyma of the gray matter; and (c) neuronophagia of the "ganglion cells" (i.e., neurons). Von Economo then proceeded to provide details on these changes. Although he also discussed these more specific changes in his 1929 monograph on EL, the description he provided in the relatively uncited second 1917 German article (1917b) on EL is more succinct and thus will be delineated below based on the translation in the Bogaert and Théodoridés biography of him (1979):

1. *Small and medium-sized veins, and to a much lesser extent arteries, were very hyperemic, showing small-cell infiltration in their adventitial sheaths.* These cells were partly lymphocytic, and their penetration through the walls of the vessels was often apparent. Occasionally, plasma cells surrounded the blood vessel, as in a sheath, and polyblasts and polymorphonuclear cells were sometimes apparent. Typically, the blood vessels were surrounded by only a single layer of cells. Rather than being infiltrated over an entire area, the vessel infiltration was sporadic. In addition, there were many sporadic vascular petechiae, but large hemorrhages were rare.

2. *Infiltration of the gray matter similarly showed a spotty distribution.* The infiltration was predominantly by glial cells. In addition, there were lymphocytes congregated around the blood vessels, from which they seem to have originated. In some locations, polymorphonuclear cells were so densely packed that they resembled an abscess.

3. *At the areas of infiltration of the parenchyma, cells can be seen to be penetrating the ganglion cells and destroying their protoplasm.* The spaces formerly occupied by these ganglion cells are filled by small and large cells rich in protoplasm in this manner, they resemble the anterior horn cells of the spinal cord in poliomyelitis. This infiltration can be found in areas free of blood vessel infiltration. Nerve fibers and myelin sheaths tend to be unaffected by the disease process. The cranial nerves themselves are not affected by the degenerative process.

In 1920, 35-year-old J.P. Greenfield (who later would become the author of *Greenfield's Neuropathology*, which, as of 2008, is in its 8th edition) co-authored an article with E.F. Buzzard on the neuropathology of EL. They listed the following features as common to all cases they studied in the early stages of the disease (the features are listed in order of constancy):

1. Vascular congestion
2. Evidence of toxic degeneration of the nerve cells and neuronophagy.
3. Proliferation of the mesoblastic cells of the vessel walls, and infiltration of the nervous tissue by these cells

4. Small-celled infiltration of the Virchow-Robin space
5. Glial proliferation.

Buzzard and Greenfield (1920) noted that the vascular changes were the most striking pathology and that, in contrast to von Economo, all vessels were affected, including the smallest capillaries. However, in agreement with von Economo, they reported that the neuronal degenerative changes were sporadically located. They reported that the cells participating in the neuronal destruction were derived from the mesoblastic elements, closely allied to plasma cells. The cells resembled the round cells in the same field that surrounded the capillary walls. Interestingly, and in contrast to von Economo, Buzzard and Greenfield reported that dense clusters of cells, such as those that invade the anterior horn of the spinal cord in cases of poliomyelitis, were never seen. They also noted, as did von Economo that, especially in early cases, it was typical to find infiltration in the gray matter in regions in which there is little if any perivascular infiltration. However, although von Economo considered glial cell proliferation to be highly prevalent, Buzzard and Greenfield indicated that such proliferation was inconspicuous, although present.

Buzzard and Greenfield also mentioned that venous thrombosis was relatively common, more common than hemorrhage. Von Economo did not mention such thrombosis.

In an article from 1919, Bassoe and Hassin reviewed the histopathology of acute EL based on three cases and contrasted it with other conditions. They noted both parenchymal and interstitial changes and that the two were independent. Bassoe and Hassin reported that, in the absence of foci of softening, large hemorrhages, gitter cells (microglia), and polymorphonuclear elements, EL differed from other forms of encephalitis such as Wernicke polioencephalitides superior hemorrhagica, acute hemorrhagic encephalitis, influenza encephalitis, and traumatic and experimental encephalitis. On the other hand, the histological changes resembled those of African sleeping sickness, dementia paralytica, and acute anterior poliomyelitis. They also stated that the pia showed congested vessels, mainly by lymphocytes and plasma cells. In contrast to Buzzard and Greenfield, they found little perivascular infiltrations in the cortex, but an abundance of other pathological changes. Parenchymatous changes were marked in subcortical regions, basal ganglia, substantia nigra (SN), and tegmentum, although some neurons within the SN were remarkably normal. In the cortex, the parenchymatous changes predominated, whereas in other regions (peduncles, internal capsule, and lower portion of pons, medulla, and cord), interstitial changes predominated. In the basal ganglia, SN, and tegmental region of the pons, both types were equally in evidence.

Bassoe and Hassin also stated that EL neuropathology resembled African sleeping sickness, paralytic dementia, and acute anterior poliomyelitis. The resemblance to African sleeping sickness was so great that Bassoe and Hassin suggested that differential diagnosis based on histology was impossible, and suggested that

EL may have been caused by a parasite similar to a trypanosome. The resemblance of the microscopic lesions of EL to that of African sleeping sickness was also noted by Marinesco in his description of the neuropathology in the 1918 British Local Government Report (Newsholme et al., 1918).

Hall (1924) summarized some of the prior work on the histopathology of EL. In addition, he provided some details on the importance of the vascular changes. Hall noted that the amount of cuffing around each vessel was variable. In some locations, it consisted of nothing more than an elongated protrusion, whereas, when fully developed a sheath consisting of four or more rows of cells surrounded the vessel. The infiltrate occupied mainly the Virchow-Robin space and was composed of mononuclear cells. In addition to the perivascular cuffs, the affected areas were characterized by the presence of small scattered masses of loosely packed collections of round cells. Pertaining to the changes in the neurons, Hall reported that, considering the other pathological changes, the neurons showed fewer signs of degeneration than might be expected. Hall concluded that the tissue and vascular changes in EL were inflammatory in nature, with cellular remnants and later proliferative processes of a reparative nature.

In his 1929 monograph, von Economo described the microscopic pathology of EL as a "nonpurulent, and, properly speaking, non-haemorrhagic acute inflammation of the gray matter, with approximately negative macroscopic findings" (p. 69). However, he did note that, on section, the gray matter was hyperemic with a conspicuous reddening, although in hyperkinetic cases, edema was more prevalent than hyperemia.

In his 1929 monograph, von Economo provided additional information on the microscopic pathology that was similar to that presented in his 1917 articles, except that he noted some differences for the hyperkinetic type of EL(#7 below):

1. Striking perivascular infiltrations, mostly in veins
2. No relationship between vascular infiltrations and severity of the case
3. Changes in nervous parenchyma mainly of a focal infiltration, without any tendency to softening or histolysis
4. Absence of tissue necrosis, indicating a very gradual disease
5. Existence of lacunae in advanced stages of the disease; presence of "glial-nodules" where neurons once were located
6. Destruction of "ganglion" cells, similar to poliomyelitis, but occurring more slowly and in different regions
7. Pathology of the hyperkinetic cases may be different from other forms; upon acute death, brain typically simply shows signs of edema presumably, these patients died before inflammatory lesions developed (Figs. 10.2–10.4).

In 1933, Greenfield published an article on the neuropathology of encephalitis. He suggested that EL is caused by a neurotrophic virus with an affinity for neurons. He thought that EL was similar in this nature to poliomyelitis, rabies,

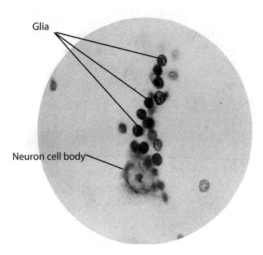

Figure 10.2 Neuronophagia in an encephalitis lethargica brain with very pale neuronal cell body surrounded by glia, which are also surrounding the apical and basal processes of the neuron (Toluidine blue stain ×100 [although the magnification is noted in the original as ×100, this is undoubtedly incorrect—we believe the magnification is about ×400]). (Modified from Bassoe & Hassin [1919].)

and herpes zoster, and to three minor veterinary conditions: Borna diseases of horses, experimental herpes encephalitis of rabbits, and "louping ill" of sheep. According to Greenfield, this class of viruses has two very distinctive properties: they reach the neurons by traveling along nerves, probably along axis cylinders; and the virus attacks the nerve cell directly, apparently by entering the protoplasm.

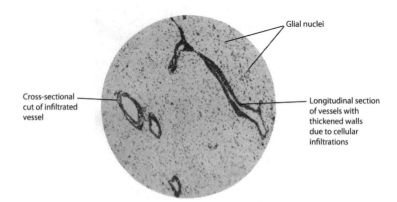

Figure 10.3 Encephalitis lethargica, showing substantia nigra with infiltrated tissues and vessels. (Toluidine blue stain ×110; modified from Bassoe and Hassin [1919].)

Cellular infiltrate surrounding cortical vessel

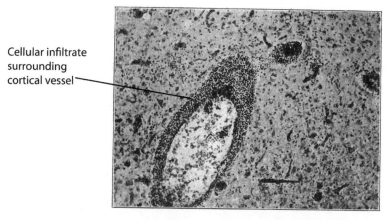

Figure 10.4 A 54-year-old-female victim of encephalitis lethargica; image shows thickly "cuffed" cortical vessel (Zeiss 16 mm objective). (Modified from Buzzard & Greenfield [1920].)

In less damaged cells, the appearance of "inclusion bodies" is apparent as a result of the infection. In EL and rabies, Greenfield stated that the microglial cells (he considered them to be mesoblastic in origin) formed small groups called "nodules inflammatoires." He also indicated that in EL inflammatory cuffing of vessels may be the only evidence of the disease, usually concentrated in the midbrain. Greenfield noted that in EL several different forms of intracytoplasmic granules had been described without any consensus on how to interpret them. He posited that in EL damage to the nerve cell was primary and did not depend on alterations in the vascular supply. Greenfield reported that EL apparently had a selective affinity for certain parts of the nervous system; not only was the greatest destruction seen in those parts, but the virus also lived longer in them. In this regard, he believed it similar to poliomyelitis and louping ill.

In his 1940 textbook, Wilson stated, "Broadly speaking, the lesions of epidemic encephalitis combine interstitial (mesodermal) reactions with parenchymatous changes often independent as regards both position and amount. Meninges and brain are flecked with hemorrhagic effusion of irregular distribution and quantity. Vascular congestion is everywhere apparent, and arterial or venous occlusion may be seen" (p. 133). In contrast to von Economo, Wilson observed that neurons may lose their myelin, although only to a moderate extent. He also reported that mucin or mucin-like bodies had been reported to be lying in neuroglial meshes, without any cytological structure.

In a 1942 review of EL pathology (see Neal, 1942), Stevenson, a New York University neuropathologist, stated that, similarly to von Economo, the most striking microscopic lesion was cell infiltration most marked about small veins. However, in contrast to von Economo, he reported possible perivascular infiltration around the cranial nerves. He reported that the various types of EL do not show correlated pathology that might explain their varying symptomatology.

Thirty years later, Greenfield (1963), in the second edition of his textbook, reported that, in patients dying within the first 2 weeks of symptoms, the cerebral cortex appeared intensely congested and sometimes plum-colored. Congestion was evident in the gray matter of the cortex, basal ganglia, and brainstem. Microscopically, the majority of his cases showed perivascular infiltrations of lymphocytes or plasma cells. Inflammatory cells also infiltrated the cerebral tissue, and this, he reported, was closely related to that of the perivascular infiltration. The infiltration was greatest in the midbrain, both in the tegmentum and SN, but was also evident in the cortex, basal ganglia, and lower brainstem. Lesions of the nerve cells were less obvious, but were present in most cases (this was thus somewhat discrepant from his earlier view).

From these descriptions, inflammatory changes most characterized by venous vessel infiltrations would seem to be the most consistent neuropathology associated in EL. Unfortunately, such inflammatory changes are common to encephalitis and have no diagnostic value relative to the nature of the infecting agent. Furthermore, and again unfortunately, the viral or bacterial EL agent (assuming there is such an agent), appears quite capable of variably affecting almost all areas of the CNS. Thus, it is unclear whether the discrepancies and inconsistencies among the epidemic-period reports are due to different forms of the disease, different phases of the disease, different investigators, different technologies or, in fact, different diseases. This variation suggests that, although neuropathology can rule out non-EL causes of a patient's symptoms (e.g., tumor, tuberculosis, meningitis, etc.), it is not able to *confirm* a diagnosis of EL.

Location of Changes

In his second 1917 article, von Economo reported that the distribution of degenerative changes in the EL brain varied on a case-by-case basis. For those original cases who died, he noted the locations of the lesions as follows:

Case 1. Subthalamus to pons
Case 4. Mainly in midbrain, secondarily in cortex
Case 5. "Posterior parts" most affected with some damage to midbrain
    and diencephalon
Case 10. No damage at all in cortex, basal ganglia, di- and
    mesencephalon. Midbrain and infundibular region severely damaged.

Interestingly, in this article, von Economo makes no conclusions as to those regions of the brain that are most affected.

Bassoe and Hassin (1919) found changes throughout the CNS. They noted that parenchymatous changes involved typically the cortex, peduncles, internal capsule, lower pons, bulb, and cord. Both interstitial and parenchymatous changes were found in the basal ganglia and midbrain.

Buzzard and Greenfield, in their 1919 article, indicated that there are three groups of EL patients with some degree of internal consistency in the anatomical loci of their brain lesions (in contrast to Stevenson; see above):

1. Cases characterized by hemiplegia, hemianesthesia, hemianopia, etc.
2. Cases characterized by symptoms resembling those of paralysis agitans; the basal ganglia group
3. Cases characterized by disturbances in function of the cranial nerves.

Buzzard and Greenfield made it clear that, despite these groups, the disease was always more widespread than might be suspected, especially in the initial stages. Surprisingly, however, they did not use their case data to summarize exactly the topography of the lesions associated with each of the groupings.

In contrast to earlier studies, Hall (1924) reported that the cerebral cortex showed degenerative changes in EL, although he observed most of the changes in the basal ganglia, midbrain, and pons. And, within these regions, maximum damage was found in the mesencephalon, in the region of the crura cerebri, extending toward the subthalamic and thalamic regions down to the pons and bulb. The dorsal region of the gray matter was chiefly affected. He reported that the tegmental region, the SN at the level of the crura and in the pons in the neighborhood of the aqueduct of Sylvius, and the gray matter beneath the floor of the fourth ventricle were the most commonly affected sites.

In contrast to his 1917 article, in his 1929 monograph, von Economo referred to the "constancy of the anatomical picture" pertaining to EL neuropathology. He stated that, "From the very beginning I have directed attention to the fact that, though every gray part of the central nervous system may be attacked, from cortex to sacral cord, it is the brainstem above all which encephalitis lethargica selects as its favorite target; particularly in the region of the aqueduct, the tegmental region, the posterior wall, the floor, and the basal part of the lateral walls of the third ventricle there are the greatest number of encephalitic foci" (p. 87). He further stated that the considerable variation on lesion localization reported by different authors reflected the fact that there were different main sites for different epidemics, with the cerebral cortex showing more frequent lesions in later epidemics. Other authors, however, claimed to have seen increased foci in the corpus striatum and in the SN.

Margulis, in his 1923 Russian monograph on EL, provided a non–Western but generally similar account of EL neuropathology. He reported that, in acute EL, neuropathology was dominated by prominent hyperemia, edema of meninges and brain tissue, and small, punctuate hemorrhages. Microscopy revealed vascular inflammatory processes without sharp borders. The lesions were localized mostly in the gray matter of the brainstem, tegmentum, cerebral peduncle (oculomotor nucleus), SN, striatum, thalamus, and medulla oblongata. Less commonly, the cerebral and cerebellar cortices and the spinal cord could be affected.

In addition to perivascular cuffs, Margulis reported focal perivascular proliferations of adventitial and glial elements (node-like or rosella in shape). In addition, he sometimes found degeneration and lysis of neurons in acute EL. In contrast to Western reports, Margulis also reported that the proliferative-exudative processes consistently affected the meninges.

Wilson, in his 1940 textbook, *Neurology*, stated that the "brunt" of the inflammatory process fell on the brainstem, basal ganglia, and cerebellum, although he also noted that the pathology was as variable as the clinical signs, with the cerebral cortex sometimes the site of profound reaction. However, Wilson also reported some affinity between the invading virus and tissues of the SN because the latter pigmented cells often succumb early, undergoing the usual changes from pallor and swelling to final disappearance. He also noted that a similar affinity was present in rabies. Finally, Wilson believed that a wrong impression was conveyed if the lesions were thought to be so largely located within basal regions as to exclude those at higher levels; thus, some brains may show almost no lower brain pathology whereas the cerebral white matter may show significant abnormalities.

Stevenson (1942), in summarizing previous works and in common with Wilson, noted that the variation in pathology was not as great as might be expected based on clinical signs. He believed that the cranial nerve palsies seen in the typical form of EL were readily explained by infiltration of their nuclei, although little destruction of the neurons might be present.

Finally, in his 1963 textbook, Greenfield stated that both the perivascular and parenchymatous infiltrations were greatest in the midbrain, both in the tegmentum and SN, but were also present in the cortex, basal ganglia, and lower brainstem, and in many cases, in the cervical segments of the spinal cord.

Recent Analysis

To obtain a clearer picture of acute EL neuropathology, both in terms of the nature of the lesions and localizations, in 2009, we (Anderson et al.) reviewed EL neuropathology based on the information in 35 epidemic-period case reports from all over the world that included data on 112 acute EL cases.

The results were generally consistent with reports from the epidemic period in terms of the nature of the lesions, suggesting extensive cortical and meningeal damage along with basal ganglia and SN lesions. However, our review found that cortical damage was the most consistent finding (81% of cases) rather than damage to basal structures (e.g., basal ganglia was lesioned in 40% of cases; Table 10.1). Some of this discrepancy may relate to various definitions of the length of time that was considered consistent with an "acute" versus a "chronic" case, and the fact that our review simply described the frequency of pathology in specific neural regions without regard to its intensity or severity, whereas earlier reviews may

Table 10.1 Frequency of Pathology in Acute Encephalitis Lethargica Cases

Lesions	Number of cases (n = 112)	Percentage
Meninges	67	60
Cortex	81	72
Surface pathology	51	46
Hemorrhage	39	35
Vessel dilation	38	34
Cortex/Meninges	109	97
Perivascular infiltrate	51	45
Glial cell proliferation	25	22
Thrombosis	14	13
Midbrain	47	42
Perivascular infiltrate	27	24
Congestion	12	11
Hemorrhage	10	9
Thrombosis	2	2
Glial cell proliferation	9	8
Pons	41	37
Perivascular infiltrate	26	23
Congestion	20	18
Hemorrhage	19	17
Medulla	53	47
Perivascular infiltrate	35	31
Congestion	19	17
Hemorrhage	15	13
Glial cell proliferation	8	7
Pyramids	4	4
Thrombosis	6	5
Thalamus	28	25
Perivascular infiltrate	24	21
Glial cell proliferation	10	9
Basal ganglia	40	36
Cerebellum	34	30

have been attempting to potentially determine unique lesions associated with EL. One observation not noted by the prior reviews was that, within individuals, cortical damage tended to be confined to a single lobe, implying a somewhat localized infectious process. Our review also attempted to correlate the specific pathology found in each case with the clinical history of the patient before death. In general, poor relationships were found between clinical signs and symptom, and neuropathology (Table 10.2). However, 64% of those with cognitive impairment showed cortical damage and 23% showed thalamic damage. Furthermore, nearly all patients who demonstrated aphasia also had cortical damage upon

Table 10.2 Correlation Percentages Between Pathology and Signs/Symptoms

	Cortex	Meninges	Midbrain	Pons	Medulla	III	VII	XII	SN	BG	Thalamus	Cerebellum
Cognitive impairment	64	52	35	29	37	20	6	10	9	27	23	21
Headache	45	38	17	21	26	11	6	5	4	20	14	19
Lethargy	54	38	21	24	28	12	4	6	6	20	15	16
Vomiting	20	13	5	4	5	1	1	1	2	8	4	4
Incontinence	27	19	15	12	14	6	4	3	3	7	8	8
Autonomic	21	19	13	10	13	5	3	4	4	10	9	8
Ptosis	38	30	17	18	20	11	8	6	4	11	6	13
Ocular palsy	24	20	13	12	12	6	4	4	3	11	7	13
Pupillary abnormalities	16	13	10	12	11	6	2	4	4	8	5	5
Tremor	31	21	14	14	19	10	4	4	4	12	10	10
Hemiparesis/ Hemiplegia	31	23	15	17	14	7	4	5	4	10	7	9
Hyperkinesia	15	13	7	8	8	3	3	2	4	6	9	7
Rigidity	8	9	3	6	5	1	2	1	1	6	4	5
Pains	25	19	13	14	17	7	4	3	2	11	9	12
Speech impairment	21	16	11	12	13	5	5	3	2	6	8	7
Seizure	15	11	4	4	4	4	1	1	0	5	3	3

SN, substantia nigra; BG, basal ganglia.

examination. Similarly, most patients with motor disabilities, lethargy, and visual disturbances also demonstrated cortical damage, as well. On the other hand, little correlation was found between patients exhibiting tongue deviation upon protrusion and cranial nerve (CN) XII damage. Similarly, no correlation was found between facial weakness and CN VII or other cranial nerve damage. This lack of correlation between neuropathology and clinical symptoms is not unusual for degenerative neurologic diseases (Geddes et al., 1993).

In summary, the neuropathology of acute EL based on cases from the epidemic period is very diverse, reflecting in general the neuropathologic correlates of most types of encephalitis. It is often forgotten that, initially, at least some of the investigations found no differences between EL and African sleeping sickness. Certainly, when reviewing reports from the epidemic period, we have problems associated with variability in length of illness and symptomatology, thoroughness of analyses, and also that some of the described neuropathology might have occurred as a result of hypoxia because many of these patients had respiratory problems, and artificial respiration was not then available. Furthermore, many of the analyses were done by those with little or no formal training in neuropathology. Unfortunately, our analysis provided here offers little toward using the available neuropathologic data to facilitate a differential diagnosis of acute EL using modern imaging technologies of the brain.

CHRONIC EL

Introduction

As described in Chapter 2, the exact definition of chronic EL confounds the difficult problem of also determining when chronic EL begins; that is, chronic EL could be considered present in a patient virtually immediately after an acute EL phase, or it could be considered to develop in a patient 30 or more years after an acute EL episode, or in a patient without a defined acute episode (see Chapter 7). Furthermore, possibly because the time frame between the acute and chronic stages could be vast, the number of cases of chronic EL with neuropathologic findings described in the literature is quite large, with perhaps a few hundred available, and in many different languages. Because of this vast quantity of material and the variability in definitions of EL stages, we chose to be selective in our review of available material. We examined many case reports, monographs, and review articles and based the following analysis primarily on those we considered to be the most important; these are summarized in Table 10.3. Prior to that analysis, however, we provide a brief historical review of the early 20th-century questions pertaining to the lesions associated with parkinsonism because those were the underlying questions guiding much of the analysis of chronic EL brains, especially those showing signs of parkinsonism.

Table 10.3 Major Articles/Monographs/Reviews on Chronic Encephalitis Lethargica Pathology

Source	Year/type	Findings
Levy	1922 (monograph on chronic EL)	Described pathological changes in four cases of parkinsonism following EL; stressed the perivascular disintegration of the basal ganglia; the substantia nigra (SN) in all. Also showed depigmentation; cases showed degeneration in the anterolateral columns of the spinal cord. Stated that no conclusions can be made as to the lesions that cause the symptoms of parkinsonism.
Lucksch & Spatz	1923 (article based on 18 PEP cases)	Considered the constancy of changes in the SN as pathognomonic for PEP; fading of dark band and atrophy of cells; no loss of nerve cells in striatum. Did not find similar changes in PD.
Van Boeckel, Bessemans & Nelis	1923 (monograph)	In chronic cases, signs of inflammation disappeared; instead, neuronal loss, most severe in the midbrain, especially the SN, and in the locus ceruleus (LC), and gliosis, which was sometimes very intense. Described microscopic fields with total absence of neurons and intense gliosis; also described amyloid bodies considered to be lipid material being digested and transported to the blood vessels.
Wimmer	1924 (monograph on chronic EL)	Macroscopically, PEP brains were typically virtually normal (no cortical atrophy); microscopically, generally an inflammatory process was evident, showing perivascular, exudative, infiltrative inflammatory phenomenon, aggregations of lymphocytes, and plasma cells. Within these changes are degenerations of neurons; these findings indicate a "constantly active morbid process within the central nervous system" (p. 284). In some cases, inflammatory processes are virtually inapparent, such that only a chronic degeneration of the parenchyma is evident (although not stated, this would seem to have occurred with longer latencies between the acute and chronic stages).
McKinley & Gowan	1926 (article based on three PEP cases)	Reported a decrease in cells in the SN ranging from 58% to 87% compared to normals; no decrease in cell counts was found for the putamen or globus pallidus (GP); concluded that PEP can result without a significant lesion in the GP.
Margulis	1928 (monograph)	Combination of old and new inflammatory changes seen together; degenerative changes in chronic cases concentrate at the same loci as in acute EL: corpus striatum, SN, subthalamic area, thalamus, cortex; sometimes demyelination of nerve fibers similar to multiple sclerosis is seen.

Von Economo	1929 (monograph)	Divided pathology into subchronic and chronic conditions, although does not describe basis of differentiation; typically, some atrophy of convolutions in subchronic EL. Microscopically, for subchronic cases, considered the lesions to be signs of a previous "polio encephalitis" and, in addition, signs of recent inflammatory activity such as perivascular hemorrhage, cuffing of veins, and cell changes of various types; considered the principal sites of both the old and more recent changes to be in corpus striatum (caudate nucleus and putamen), caudal and ventral portions of the thalamus, in the hypothalamic region (but not the subthalamic nucleus), in the posterior wall of the third ventricle, and in the SN. Considered the presence of both old and new lesions to indicate that the virus was still active in the brain; for chronic EL (PEP), indicated that the neuropathology is dominated by loss of neurons and that the inflammatory changes are relegated to the background. Considered the loss of ganglion cells to be a degenerative rather than an inflammatory process.
Stern	1928 (monograph)	Stated that the degree of severity of the amyostatic symptoms and the degree of degeneration within the SN do not correspond.
Fenyes	1932 (article based on one PEP case)	Reported the "odd" fact that a 28-year-old female who showed no signs of dementia had the same type of neurofibrillary tangles (NFTs) that had been described by Alzheimer in 1907 for dementia patients; these NFTs were not found in the SN but were found in many other brainstem nuclei (as per Greenfield & Bosanquet, 1953).
Halloverden	1933, 1935 (articles based on 21 PEP cases)	Consistently found NFTs in the SN and also the pontis tegmentum (as per Greenfield & Bosanquet, 1953).
Hassler	1937 (article based on 11 PEP cases)	SN was more severely damaged than other gray nuclei.

(Continued)

Table 10.3 continued

Source	Year/type	Findings
Neustaedter & Liber	1937 (article based on 13 PEP cases)	Noted that the GP showed marked damage in all cases, with a paucity of cells, and the few remaining cells shrunken or swollen. Red nucleus was also affected in all cases except one. The SN was severely affected in all cases; dentate nucleus was degenerative in 12 of the PEP cases; concluded that "it would be futile to attempt any definite localization for any one symptom or the entire syndrome of the various types of Parkinson's disease" (p. 283).
Wilson	1940 (neurology textbook)	Fatty granules around all vessels; residual ganglion cells in affected zones full of fat (lipoidosis); much glial overgrowth especially in PEP and especially in SN, in which there are few remaining cells, and atrophic sclerosis is common: "But the relationship of this finding to the phenomena of parkinsonism has to be considered with much reserve." Also referred to the presence of NFTs and noted that they may prove to be important.
Klaue	1940	Could not identify neurofibrillary changes and concluded that, although there may be quantitative differences in degeneration between PD and PEP, the two had identical topographic lesion patterns (no qualitative differences) (as per Greenfield & Bosanquet, 1953).
von Braunmuhl	1949 (review)	Confirmed NFTs in PEPs; found them in order of frequency in SN, locus ceruleus, tegmentum pontis, corpora quadrigemina, hypothalamus, nuclei around the third ventricle, subthalamic nucleus, red nucleus, GP, corpus striatum, dentate nucleus, cornu ammonis, insula, and last, the remainder of the cerebral cortex (as per Greenfield & Bosanquet, 1953).
Greenfield & Bosanquet	1953 (article based on ten PEP cases)	Could not make qualitative division between PD and PEP: "Our observations do not allow us to place all cases with Lewy bodies in the idiopathic group and all those with neurofibrillary tangles in the postencephalitic group, although for the great majority of our cases this distinction holds" (p. 225).
Torvik & Meen	1966 (article based on three PEP cases)	Results similar to prior findings in that the lesions involved not only the SN but also LC and substantia innominata, reticular formation, and periaqueductal mesencephalic gray; also noted no good correlation between the number of cells with neurofibrillary changes and the severity of damage.

Alvord	1971 (article)	The loss of neurons in the SN of PEP is much greater than in PD, and the foci are less systemized (medial as well as lateral cell groups tend to be destroyed in PEP).
1981 (article based on four PEP cases)	Ultrastructurally, the NFTs in PEP consisted almost exclusively of twisted tubules (TT) that were the same as those found in patients with parkinsonian dementia complex of Guam and Alzheimer disease, whereas patients with progressive supranuclear palsy (PSP) have predominantly straight tubules (ST); NFTs were primarily found in the SN, periaqueductal gray matter, raphe nuclei, reticular formation, LC, hypothalamus, and part of Ammon horn. Except for a rare NFT in the striatum, none was found in the cerebral or cerebellar cortices, or basal ganglia.
Geddes et al.	1993 (article based on eight PEP cases)	No correlation between the severity of disease and severity of pathology; most affected structure in 6/8 cases was the SN, other two cases only had moderate damage in the SN. Additional structures containing NFTs were LC, hippocampus, amygdala, striatum, pallidum, thalamus, subthalamus, hypothalamus, nuclei of the reticular formation, pons, and medulla. In seven cases, and in contrast to prior reports, NFTs were found in the neocortex, with the insular, frontal, and temporal lobes being the most involved. In a minority of cases, NFTs were also seen in the spinal cord; concluded that in PEP no anatomical site is exempt from NFTs, although there is a tendency for the principal oculomotor nucleus, IV nerve nucleus, and the inferior olivary complex to be spared.
Ikeda et al.	1993 (article based on four PEP cases)	Reported the presence of NFTs in glial cells, which are referred to as glial fibrillary tangles (GFTs); indicated that they were found in PEP, not in the cortex, but in the areas "heavily affected by encephalitis," specifically in the walls of the third ventricle and cerebral aqueduct, and in the marginal region of the midbrain.
Buée-Scherrer et al.	1997 (article based on three PEP cases)	NFTs in variable densities in the hippocampus and entorhinal cortex, areas 4, 9, and 20, and in subcortical regions such as the GP and putamen. NFTs were denser in the hippocampal formation and area 20, compared with areas 4 and 9, and the putamen, suggesting that some regions were preferentially affected by the disease. Furthermore, NFTs were more plentiful in supragranular than in infragranular cortical layers. First study to determine that the τ pathology in PEP is primarily composed of 3R τ isoforms.

(Continued)

Table 10.3 continued

Source	Year/type	Findings
Josephs et al.	2002 (article based on three PEP cases)	Reported absence of α-synuclein (a protein found in the nucleus of neurons and that are inherent in the Lewy bodies of PD) pathology in PEP, which is similar to what was found previously in progressive supranuclear palsy; was unable to differentiate between the two conditions using routine stains. Also found that glia cells have τ pathology in PEP.
Jellinger	2003 (review)	Marked neuronal loss and gliosis throughout brainstem, particularly in SN (all of pars compacta with no preference for ventral tier as in PD) and to a lesser extent in LC; no Lewy bodies but globose NFTs in residual neurons in SN, LC, and other nonpigmented brainstem nuclei; severe involvement of various nuclei, including the oculomotor nuclear complex, colliculi, midbrain raphe, pontine tegmentum, reticular formation, subthalamic nucleus, amygdaloid complex, and the basal nucleus of Meynert.
Jellinger	2009 (article based on ten PEP cases)	Confirmed previous findings on PEP; found PEP is a tauopathy characterized by widespread neurofibrillary lesions composed of both 3- and 4-repeat τ isoforms; further confirmed the absence of Lewy body and other α-synuclein pathology, thus rendering PEP as a pure τ pathology.

During the first few decades of the 20th century, there was an active debate as to whether the primary lesion associated with parkinsonism (of any type) was in the globus pallidus (GP) or SN. The renowned American neurologist, J. Ramsay Hunt, as well as German-Danish and French neurologists, Oskar and Cecile Vogt, and French neurologist, Jean Lhermitte, all supported the GP school, whereas Russian neurologist Konstantin Trétiakoff was the initial and main supporter of the SN school, which proved eventually to be correct (although the GP is often also affected in parkinsonism). For a period during these decades, it was believed that both schools were correct in that PD was considered to have a primary lesion in the corpus striatum, whereas for PEP the SN was thought to be principally involved (Hassin, 1933); even as late as 1940, Wilson, in his textbook, was unwilling to firmly establish the primary relationship between degeneration in the SN and parkinsonism (see Table 10.3; Fig. 10.5 top, middle).

Trétiakoff's 1919 doctoral thesis, *Contribution a l'etude de L'anatomie pathologique du locus niger de Soemmering avce quelques deductions relatives á la pathologénie des troubles du tonus musculaire et de la maladie de Parkinson* (A Study of the Pathological Anatomy of the Locus Niger [SN] of Somemerring and Its Relevance to the Pathogenesis of Changes in Muscular Tone in Parkinson's Disease), involved the analysis of the locus niger (SN) in 11 PD cases (two were cases of "atypical" parkinsonism) and three patients with the parkinsonian type of EL. Unfortunately, Tretiakoff provided very little clinical information about these patients. He concluded that the SN is mainly involved in parkinsonism, meaning both the idiopathic disease and the parkinsonism type of EL (it should be mentioned that, at this time, postencephalitic parkinsonism as a chronic condition had not yet been recognized; see Chapter 7). It was not until much later (1962), with the development of the histofluorescence technique for tracing neuronal pathways, that it was discovered that the SN produces dopamine that flows to the striatum and that dopamine deficiency in this pathway is associated with the development of parkinsonism signs. However, parkinsonism can also be produced without SN lesions (Duychaerts, 2005). Furthermore, whereas PEP is associated with the development of a tau (τ) protein pathology and the development of neurofibrillary tangles (NFTs) (Table 10.3 and below), PD is associated with α-synuclein pathology (i.e., the development of Lewy bodies in many brain structures) (Duychaerts, 2005).

Case Analyses

As time passed between the EL epidemic period and the present, the chronic phase of EL became more and more synonymous with PEP. We could only find two reports during the epidemic period that specifically described the pathology of non-PEP cases of chronic EL (although the large monographs on EL included some cases; see Table 10.3). In 1920, Schaller and Oliver described one case in which the SN was found to be normal, as was the cortex, but the cranial nerve

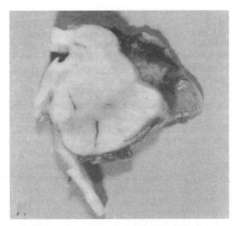

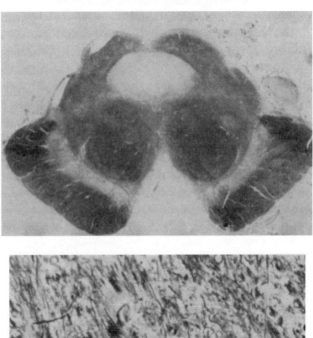

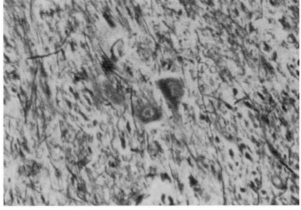

Figure 10.5 Top: A macroscopic cross-section of the substantia nigra in a case of postencephalitic parkinsonism (PEP). Note the great loss of pigmentation in the substantia nigra (*arrow*; from Geddes et al., 1993). **Middle:** A stained section from a PEP patient, again showing pallor in the substantia nigra, which has been depleted of neurons (from Rail et al., 1981). **Bottom:** Neurofibrillary tangles in the substantia nigra of a PEP patient (from Rail et al., 1981).

nuclei were generally severely affected, as were most of the medullary nuclei. The patient's symptoms included dysarthria and dysphagia, headache, generalized burning pains, and nervousness. Based on a case of chronic EL characterized by decerebrate rigidity, Weisenburg and Alpers (1927) found damage primarily in the SN and red nucleus. They attributed the decerebrate rigidity to changes in the red nucleus.

The summaries presented in Table 10.3 reveal that during the epidemic period some "chronic" (or subchronic) cases were found to show inflammatory changes similar to those reported for acute cases but that, as the time frame between the period and death increased (i.e., the time elapsed between the acute and chronic phases increased), there were fewer descriptions of inflammatory lesions in chronic EL patients (virtually all the patients in these studies were believed to have had their acute EL phase during the epidemic period, even if no identifiable acute EL phase existed in their histories).

Although the summaries in the Table 10.3 consistently indicate the involvement of the SN (and also the basal ganglia and locus ceruleus) in chronic EL, the involvement of other structures is quite variable and to some extent inconsistent. For example, von Economo (1929) and von Braunmuhl (1949) reported degenerative changes in the cerebral cortex, whereas most reports did not; but it is not clear how many of the reports actually examined the cerebral cortex. Intuitively, it would seem that the degenerative changes reported for each case should correlate to some extent with the clinical signs exhibited by the patient; however, as is apparent in the table and as was found for the acute lesions, many of the reports commented on the apparent lack of correlation between the lesions (generally the extent of the damage) and the clinical signs.

In contrast to the view that the SN was the primary lesion in EL and its chronic states, as late as 1949, Bucy and Brinker stated in their textbook that, "The cerebral cortex is often severely damaged both in the acute and chronic forms of the disease. Therefore, the mental symptoms are not psychomotor disturbances from disease of the basal ganglia" (p. 656). Thus, much confusion of about EL/PEP neuropathology persisted until at least the mid-20th century.

Neurofibrillary Tangles

The neuropathology and probably the clinical manifestations of chronic EL (presumably just PEP) cannot be understood without a discussion of neurofibrillary tangles (NFTs). These pathological protein (τ) aggregates result from hyperphosphorylation of τ, causing it to aggregate in an insoluble form in various shapes, depending on the condition. They are found in a variety of neurodegenerative diseases besides PEP, including Alzheimer disease, progressive supranuclear palsy, corticobasal degeneration, argyrophilic grain disease, Pick disease, and parkinsonism-dementia complex of Guam (Duyckaerts, 2005). It is unknown whether the tangles are primary or secondary to the disease process.

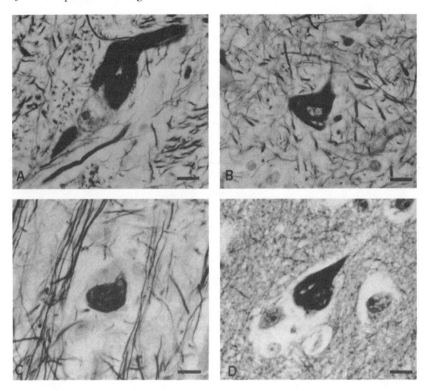

Figure 10.6 Neurofibrillary tangles of different shapes in the red nucleus (*A*), subthalamus (*B*), putamen (*C*), and cortex (*D*). (From Geddes et al. [1993].)

Alois Alzheimer first provided a description of these tangles in a demented patient in a 1907 article. István Fényes, after an article published in 1932, is typically given credit for first describing the identical tangles in the brainstem of a PEP patient who was not demented (Fig. 10.5 bottom; Fig. 10.6). However, considering the large number of careful studies devoted to describing the histopathology of chronic EL (especially PEP) during the 1920s, it is quite surprising that NFTs were not reported earlier for PEP cases. So, either NFTs take a very long time to develop after the initial insult (presumably acute EL), or PEP that developed quickly after the acute phase was different from that condition that developed after a delay. Interestingly, as far as we can determine, there has never been a specific (recent) search for NFTs in PEP tissue from patients who died during the 1920s. On the other hand, and in accord with the first view, Chavany et al. (1951) stressed that encephalitis may change the normal metabolism of a nerve cell in such a way as to cause the development of a degenerative process that might become apparent only after a long period. Similarly, Steele et al. (1964)

emphasized that viral infections do not necessarily result in florid inflammatory reactions. Rather, they may cause either destructive or proliferative lesions that linger in cells for years without causing any apparent change, and they may produce chronic lesions in which the inflammatory component is very slight.

It is evident from Table 10.3 that, as time passed, more and more neural structures were identified as containing NFTs in PEP patients, eventually reaching the condition noted by Geddes et al., in 1993, that no anatomical site can be said not to contain them. This again raises a question: Why weren't NFTs in some of these sites (e.g., cerebral cortex) found earlier? Part of the explanation may be that, for many of the pathologic studies, the brainstem was the primary region analyzed (e.g., Greenfield & Bosquanet, 1953). However, this may also reflect that NFTs develop in these sites only with very long-term disease progression.

As is also apparent from Table 10.3, the issue of NFTs as a means to distinguish various degenerative neurologic conditions has been a recurrent topic of interest. In their initial 1964 description of PSP, Steele et al. noted that PEP and PSP are very similar in histopathology, both in locations of lesions and presence of NFTs. Almost 40 years later, following a detailed study, one of us (KJ) also found that, despite the very different clinical features between PEP and PSP, the two are almost identical histopathologically (Josephs et al., 2002). Both are characterized by primary pigmentary incontinence in the SN and the presence of globose NFTs in subcortical and brainstem nuclei. Similarly, both lack the α-synuclein (Lewy body) pathology found in PD. However, PSP and PEP do differ in their biochemical signature. In PEP, the NFTs are composed of hyperphosphorylated τ protein that is immunoreactive for both 3 and 4 repeat (3R and 4R) τ isoforms (as in Alzheimer diseases), whereas PSP predominantly contains 4R τ isoforms (Jellinger, 2009). The significance of these tangles in general and the difference in their compositions remain to be determined.

CONCLUSION

As with most degenerative conditions, the neuropathology of EL and PEP is intriguing and puzzling. It would seem that structural lesions should correlate with symptomatology, but beyond broad generalities (e.g., SN lesions) they don't, presumably because the lesions only indirectly reflect functional damage. Furthermore, although we do know that PEP brains show 3R and 4R τ isoforms, we have no idea exactly what this means functionally, and if these coagulated proteins result from the cause or the effect of the underlying disease. Nevertheless, a large amount of case pathology data is available for PEP, and as yet no one has performed a thorough analysis of all of it. Such a meta-analysis may reveal heretofore unknown insights into the cause and manifestations of EL/PEP.

REFERENCES CITED

Alexander, M. (1921). Epidemic encephalitis; clinical and pathological study of twenty-five cases. *Archives of Neurology and Psychiatry, 6,* 44–60.

Alvord, E. C., Jr. (1971). The pathology of Parkinsonism. Part II. An interpretation with special reference to other changes in the aging brain. *Contemporary Neurology Series, 8,* 131–161.

Anderson L., Vilensky J., & Duvoisin R. (2009). Neuropathology of acute phase encephalitis lethargic: a review of cases from the epidemic period. *Neuropathology and Applied Neurobiology 35,* 462–472.

Bassoe, P., & Hassin, G. B. (1919). A contribution to the histopathology of epidemic ("lethargic") encephalitis. *Archives of Neurology and Psychiatry, 2,* 24–40.

Booss, J., & Esiri, M. M. (2003). *Viral Encephalitis in Humans.* Washington DC: American Society for Microbiology Press.

Brinker, R., & Bucy, P. (1949). *Neurology.* Springfield, IL: Charles C. Thomas.

Braunmuhl, A. V. (1949). Encephalitis epidemica und Synaresislehre. *Grundsatzliches zur Anatomie und Pathogenese des postencephalitischen Parkinsonismus. Bd. 181*(Suppl), 543–576.

Buzzard, E. F., & Greenfield, J. P. (1920). Lethargica encephalitis; Its Sequelae and morbid anatomy. *Brain, 42,* 305–338.

Buee-Scherrer, V., Buee, L., Leveugle, B., Perl, D. P., Vermersch, P., Hof, P.R., & Delacourte, A. (1997). Pathological tau proteins in postencephalitic parkinsonism: Comparison with Alzheimer's Disease and other neurodegenerative disorders. *Annals of Neurology, 42,* 356–359.

Chavany, J. A., van Bogaert, L., & Godlewski, S. (1951). Sur un syndrome de rigidité a predominance axiale, avec perturbation des automatisms oculo-palpébraux d'origine encéphalitique. *La Presse Médicale, 59,* 958–962.

Chavany, J., Bogaert, L., & Godlewski, S. (1951). Syndrome of rigidity with axial predominance with perturbation des automatismes ocul-palpebraux d'origine encephalitique. *La Presse Medicale, 59,* 958–962.

Duychaerts, C. (2005). Neuropathology and Nosology. In: Litvan I (Ed). *Atypical Parkinsonian Disorders Clinical and Research Aspects* (pp. 111–138). Totowa, NJ: Humana Press.

Fenyes, I. (1932). Alzheimersche Fibrillenveranderung im Hirnstamm einer 28 jahrigen Postencepalitikerin. *Archiv für Psychiatrie (Berlin), 96,* 700–717.

Geddes, J. F., Hughes, A. J., Lees, A. J., & Daniel, S. E. (1993). Pathological overlap in cases of parkinsonism associated with neurofibrillary tangles. *Brain, 116,* 281–302.

Greenfield, J. G. (1933). Some recent advances in the pathology of encephalitis. *The Medical Forum, 1,* 334–348.

Greenfield, J.G. (1963). *Greenfield's Neuropathology.* London: Edward Arnold Publishers, Ltd.

Greenfield, J.G., Bosanquet, F. D. (1953). The brain-stem lesions in parkinsonism. *Journal of Neurology, Neurosurgery, and Psychiatry, 16,* 213–226.

Greenfield, J. G., Blackwood, W., McMenemey, W. H., Meyer, A., & Norman, R. M. (1963). "Encephalitis Lethargica." *Neuropathology.* London: Edward Arnold Publishers, Ltd.

Hall, A. J. (1924). *Epidemic encephalitis (encephalitis lethargica).* Bristol: John Wright & Sons.

Halloverden, J. (1933). Zur patogenese postencephalitischen parkinsonismus. *Klinische Wochenschrift, 12,* 692–695.

Halloverden, J. (1935). Anatomische untersuchungen zur pathogenese des ponstencephalitischen parkinsonisumus. *Deutsche Zeitschrift für Nervenheilkunde, 136,* 68–77.

Hassin, G. B. (1933). *Histopathology of the Peripheral and Central Nervous Systems.* Baltimore, MD: Williams & Wilkins.

Hassler, R. (1938). Zur Pathologie der Paralysis agitans und des postenzephalitischen parkinsonismus. *Journal für Psychologie und Neurologie, 48,* 387–476.

Ishii, T., & Nakamura, Y. (1981). Distribution and Ultrastructure of Alzheimer's neurofibrillary tangles in postencephalitic parkinsonism of Economo type. *Acta Neuropathologica, 55,* 59–62.

Jellinger, K. A. (2009). Absence of α-synuclein pathology in postencephalitic parkinsonism. *Acta Neuropathologica, 118, 371–379.*

Josephs, K. A., Parisi, J. E., & Dickson, D. W. (2002). Alpha-synuclein studies are negative in postencephalitic parkinsonism of von Economo. *Neurology, 59,* 645–646.

Levy, G. (1922). *Contribution A L'Etude des Manifestations Tardives de L'Encephalite Epidemique.* M.D. Thesis. Faculte De Medecine De Paris.

Lucksch, F., & Spatz, H. (1923). Die Veranderungen im Zentralnervensystem bei Parkinsonismus in den Spatstadien der Encephalitis epidemica. *Munchener Medizinische Wochenschrift, 70,* 1245.

Margulis, M. S. (1923). *Acute Encephalitis: Epidemic and Sporadic.* Moscow: Government Publishers.

McKinley, J. C. (1926). Neuron destruction in postencephalitic paralysis agitans: a micrometric study of the lenticular region and substantia nigra. *Archives of Neurology and Psychiatry, 15,* 1–27.

Neal, J. (1942). *Encephalitis: A Clinical Study.* New York: Grune & Stratton.

Newsholme, A., James, S. P., MacNalty, A. S., Marinesco, G., McIntosh, J., & Draper, G. (1918). *Report of an Enquiry into an Obscure Disease, Encephalitis Lethargica.* Reports to the Local Government Board on public health and medical subjects, new ser., no. 121. London: Printed under the authority of His Majesty's Stationery Office by Jas. Truscott and Son.

Neustaedter, M., & Liber, A. F. (1937). Concerning the pathology of parkinsonism (idiopathic, arteriosclerotic, and post-encephalitic). *Journal of Nervous and Mental Disease, 86,* 264–283.

Rail, D., Scholtz, C., & Swash, M. (1981). Post-encephalitic Parkinsonism: current experience. *Journal of Neurology, Neurosurgery, & Psychiatry, 44*(8), 670–676.

Schaller, W. F., & Oliver, J. (1922). Chronic epidemic encephalitis; report of a case; clinical record, complete necropsy and detailed histologic study of the central nervous system. *Archives of Neurology and Psychiatry, 8,* 1–14.

Steele, J. C., Richardson, J. C., & Olszewski, J. (1964). Progressive supranuclear palsy: A heterogeneous degeneration involving the brain stem, basal ganglia and cerebellum with vertical gaze and pseudobulbar palsy, nuchal dystonia and dementia. *Archives of Neurology, 10,* 333–359.

Stern, F. (1928). *Die Epidemische Encephalitis.* Berlin: Springer.

Torvik A., & Meen, D. (1966). Distribution of the brain stem lesions in postencephalitic parkinsonism. *Acta Neurologica Scandinavica, 42,* 415–425.

Tretiakoff, C. (1919). L'Anatomie pathologique du locus niger, avec queleques déductions relatives à la pathogénie des troubles du tonus musculaire, et de la maladie de Parkinson. (Thesis for the doctorate of medicine.) Paris: Imprimerie de la faculté de Médecine, Jouve & Co., Editors.

van Bogaert, L., & Théodoridès, J. (1979). *Constantin von Economo (1876–1931): The Man and the Scientist.* Wien: Ernst Becvar.

Van Boeckel, L., Bessemans, A., & Nelis, C. (1923). *L'Encephalite Lethargique.* Bruxelles: Imprimerie Ch. Nossent.

von Economo, C. (1917a). Encephalitis lethargica. *Wiener Klinische Wochenschrift, 30,* 581–585.

von Economo, C. (1917b). Neue Beitrage zur Encephalitis lethargica. *Neurologisches Centralblatt*, 5, 866–878.

von Economo, C. (1929). *Die Encephalitis lethargica, ihre Nachkrankheiten und ihre Behardlung.* Berlin: Urban & Schwarzenberg. (Published in English in 1931: Translated by K. O. Newman; London: Oxford University Press.)

Weisenburg, T. H., & Alpers, B. J. (1927). Decerebrate rigidity following encephalitis: Report of a case with necropsy. *Archives of Neurology and Psychiatry, 18*, 1–15.

Wilson, S. A. K. (1940). *Neurology.* Baltimore: The Williams & Wilkins Company.

11

SELF-REPORTS OF ENCEPHALITIS LETHARGICA

Joel A. Vilensky, Judith Cameron, and Roger C. Duvoisin

To the doctor, with our best wishes for rapid improvement, a devoted patient.

Duff Gilfond

The encephalitis lethargica (EL) literature includes thousands of case reports, some very detailed, many not. But, considering the epidemic nature and apparent prevalence of the disease, there is a surprising dearth of personal descriptions of the disease, especially in the popular media. In this chapter, we present the only compilation of such personal insights (i.e., self-reports, from both the popular and professional media) into this enigmatic disease, including some translated from French and German. We have included nine reports, from eight patients. The majority of these nine self-reports were written (or based on records) by physicians recording their own condition, and thus may provide greater clinical insights than most of the available case studies. In one case, two separate articles were published in *Paris Medical* by a physician who first described his experience with EL in 1920 and then reported on the sequelae almost 30 years later, in 1948, in the same journal. We also provide one self-report of a patient with putative postencephalitic parkinsonism (PEP), who may initially have had EL in 1924. After each account, we provide brief comments/analysis, with an overall perspective at the end of the chapter. The cases are presented in presumed (approximate) chronological order of EL onset.

Case 1. Early description by an anonymous physician

In 1922, the British Ministry of Health published *Reports on Public Health and Medical Subjects. No.11: Report on Encephalitis Lethargica.* "Being an account of further enquiries into the epidemiology and clinical features of the disease; including an analysis of over 1,250 reports on cases notified in England and Wales during 1919 and 1920, together with a comprehensive bibliography of the subject" (p. i). Appendix L of that report provides ten case histories (cases A–J), of which two are self-reports. One of them, reproduced below, was compiled from a physician's own notes on his condition. The entire volume was authored by A.C. Parson, A.S. MacNalty, and J.R. Perdrau.

History of a non-fatal attack of encephalitis lethargica in the case of a medical practitioner, complied mainly from notes supplied by the patient himself.

"X," a medical practitioner of 49, was attacked on 25th December 1918, with vomiting and diarrhea, which incapacitated him for 5 days; this gastrointestinal illness could not be associated with any dietetic indiscretions, against which, at this time, the patient was particularly on his guard.

From now onwards he was never quite well; he continued at work, however, despite languor, pains in the back and limbs, as well as headache and earache. There was also a feeling of contraction down the anterior aspect of the body associated with a flexure of the head downwards and forwards.

Meanwhile his patients and members of his household had been noticing his expression was altering, and that he had evidently some difficulty of vision. Early in January 1919, there was definite diplopia.

Dr. "X" carried on, however, until 11th February, when the disease unmistakably declared itself, and the patient retired to bed with a temperature of [38°C]. The fever, which averaged about 38°C remained for 8 weeks, and the highest temperature recorded was 40°C [104°F]. There was a much quickened pulse, the rate of which varied between 120 and 150; profuse and continuous sweating, and troublesome constipation. The urine was normal in every respect, and there was nothing abnormal found in the lungs or abdominal viscera. No rash.

These general symptoms were accompanied by various manifestations of mental disturbance and neuromuscular disability.

There was marked lethargy; patient lay like a log, in the supine position, with arms folded across the chest, legs fully extended, and face devoid of all expression. For weeks the voice was not raised above a whisper, but all questions and answers were quite normal as regards articulation. Dull and apathetic notwithstanding, the patient's condition never approached unconsciousness, and he spontaneously discussed the symptoms and treatment of his case, but during this time there was considerable confusion of ideas as remembered by the patient during his convalescence. Neither during the few outbursts of nocturnal delirium nor in his irrational thoughts and remarks did the patient "give himself away" or "live over again" in scenes of his professional occupation. Among the delusions recalled by the patient were the following: "Thought he was in an institution and was being changed from room to room"; "spending the night in a dock unloading vessels"; "with a dog in a country lane, where he was expected to curl up and sleep under a tree."

There were curious delusions concerning his anatomical configuration. Thus, under the impression that he possessed more than one entrance to the pharynx, he would poke various parts of his face with the tooth brush in an attempt to find other mouths and attend to other sets of teeth; he imagined that he had several rows of eyes and a double set of finger nails. He associated his legs with those of a grand piano, so that he pointed out to the nurse who was attending to the toilet [washing] of his limbs the apparent absurdity of the proceeding.

During the latter part of the patient's 3 months' confinement to bed, insomnia was a troublesome feature.

> a. *Ocular Affections.* Diplopia was a very early symptom, but no sign of strabismus was recorded. There was a double ptosis early in the course of the disease and this was preceded by conjunctivitis. The right pupil was dilated and twice the size of the left. Nystagmus was a later sign.
>
> b. *Other Paralyses.* Weakness of muscles of right face, paralysis of right alae nasi [small muscle of face]. Paralysis of intercostals on both sides and partial paralysis of diaphragm. Retention of urine for 5 days. Dysphagia. Slight general tremors.

Progress. Dr. "X" came downstairs on 21st May 1919, and on 13th June he went to Margate, where he was wheeled about in a bath chair for 3 weeks. He resumed general practice in September 1919.

Present Condition, December 1920. The face has resumed its normal symmetry. Breathing is easy and regular. The sphincters function properly and there are no obvious tremors. Weight has recovered and capacity for physical and mental work largely regained. Memory appears good and questions are answered intelligently and promptly. There is, perhaps, a certain deliberateness of manner and action, and a far-away expression at times; patient gives the impression of having passed through a severe illness. Dr. "X" himself finds that he is much more inclined to nervousness, and easily gets upset, while his emotions are much less under control. He "nearly always falls asleep at a concert or while in the theatre or church." Sexual desire is practically lost. In addition, Dr. "X" is subject to what he calls "paretic crises," in which there may be very troublesome dysphagia or stiffness and weakness of the right arm; at such times, too, and at others, there is excessive salivation and tremors. The power of writing has been greatly impaired, so that the hands need re-educating in this respect; walking, too, is not quite the automatic action it should be, and there is tendency to drag the feet.

June 1922. There is still some inequality of pupils, and diplopia often occurs.

COMMENT: The initiation of the disease by gastrointestinal problems (e.g., diarrhea) seems to be common in some epidemics, but not others (see Chapter 2). Hallucinations were not often reported during EL. Generally, however, this patient exhibits a very typical, somewhat prolonged course of EL. He showed lethargy, pseudosomnolence, diplopia, and ptosis. Subsequently, he developed "crises" of parkinsonian signs, such as stiffness, walking difficulties, and dysphagia (but apparently these were not consistently present). An especially valuable aspect of this description is that it is relatively detailed over a 3.5-year period. It is noteworthy that diplopia remained a persistent symptom, as did a proneness for nervousness and dysphagia.

Case 2. Early description by an anonymous attorney

This case is another taken from the British Ministry of Health's *Reports on Public Health and Medical Subjects. No.11: Report on Encephalitis Lethargica*, published in 1922. The patient was an attorney ("solicitor"), who wrote of his experience in diary form.

Case 2. Autobiographical notes by a solicitor who suffered severely from encephalitis lethargica and continued at work during the early stages of his illness (ambulatory case).

April 9–29. Bad attack of influenza.

December 4. Feeling fit, but had a busy day in London and a rush to catch 6 o'clock train. Had dinner on arrival home and went out after to a lecture. In bed about eleven. Woke up about 1 o'clock with temperature, headache. Did not sleep again that night.

December 5. My sight began to go wrong. Everything I looked at seemed duplicated. I put it down to a liver attack. Went to bed early, but only slept a short time, and then woke up with headache and had no further sleep.

December 6. Did not go to work. Sight getting worse. Rested most of day, but only had a short sleep, and lay awake rest of the night with the headache the same as before.

December 7. The double vision seemed less accentuated and had more sleep at night, but lay awake from about 2 to 6 a.m.

December 8. Went to London. Sight very bad. Could not read either with or without glasses unless I closed one eye. Came home and went to bed early. Slept very heavily and could hardly rouse myself in the morning to get up.

December 9. Slept at every available opportunity in the train and in office. Eyes practically useless; had to get clerk to read letters to me. Went to bed early and slept heavily, and had the same difficulty in waking up in morning.

December 10. Practically a repetition of the previous day. My clerk rang up my oculist and explained the trouble with my eyes, and he appointed to see me the next day.

December 11. Could scarcely keep awake all day. Went to see G. He tested my sight and said he could do nothing, and advised me to see nerve specialist at once. He said he thought I had a nerve infection, which was very rare. I was too tired to go to see doctor that night, so asked him if he would write to my own doctor and I would see him the next day. My sight was now very bad, and it was only with difficulty I could keep awake.

December 12. I went to bed in the course of the day and the doctor came to see me. I was now in a kind of stupor and practically unconscious. A London specialist and my brother came to see me and a nurse was put in charge. Relations also came to see me; but I knew nothing and lay practically in a stupor until, I think, December 26.

December 26. From this date I gradually became less drowsy, and my vision by degrees ceased to duplicate the object. While in the stupor I felt nothing; no pain or any sensation. It was absolutely dreamless, heavy sleep. I believe my temperature was generally below normal and pulse erratic, but this I cannot speak of with certainty. The chief medicine I had was Hexamine. When I stopped taking it the first and second times, my vision was again slightly affected. I had no paralysis.

January 27. I dressed for first time and went down for a few hours. I was very weak.

February 6. Went down to Budleigh Salterton and Wiltshire for a month. Much better on return, but have since developed a slight difficulty in speaking. Capacity for work just as good, but tire more quickly.

COMMENT: In this patient, the lethargy became stuporous. He also had diplopia. He does not mention pseudosomnolence, which was clearly apparent in the first patient. He does not show any hallucinations, intestinal problems, or parkinsonian signs, and his sequelae seem to be dysarthria and a tendency to tire easily. Note also that he calls his sleep "dreamless."

Case 3. (1) Initial report by the French physician, G.A. Delater: *Auto observation d'encephalite lethargique* (Self-observation of encephalitis lethargica)

The following 1920 self-report is by a French physician, Dr. G.A. Delater, who describes his experience during the acute phase of EL and subsequent convalescence. Remarkably, he also wrote a 30-year follow-up article, describing the chronic condition, which is included following this initial report.

Perhaps it is not unimportant that a doctor, who developed a severe form of this very polymorphic disease, relates his experience. The psychological effects have not often been reported previously.

The first symptoms arose 3 weeks after my return from Morocco. I had been summoned there to attend to a Jewish woman who "slept": I could not understand it and could not give a diagnosis. One could only say that it was a very rare condition in this country.

The 3 weeks in France were very active, and I had entered into my new service without having taken any vacation. On the 30th of November in 1919, I noticed a certain irritation; waiting tormented me, talking caused tension, the fear of being late caused me (to be) agitated and impatient. Then, as soon as I boarded the train that was to take me to Paris, I felt an irresistible need to sleep. It seems that I did find myself in sleep and that I slid vertiginously there. I managed, however, by reading a little; but upon my arrival to Paris, I was light-headed (in a similar state to vertigo) and a little nauseous, and nearly asked a friend to accompany me to my house. For 3 days, I struggled in my service and succeeded in not falling asleep while working. I was drowsy in the metro, but got to the station where I had to get off. Upon my arrival in Épernay I had a fever, muscle aching, and finally became exhausted and bedridden.

Here, for 10 days, I slept all the time, without any agitation, and was awakened from my sleep only by the person who took care of me and forced me to eat, which I readily accepted. The fever stayed at 39°C [102.2°F] for the first 2 days, then dropped only to 38°C [100.4°F]. The physician who saw me suspected fatigue caused by a brief, unspecified infectious illness. On the sixth day, he believed that it was meningitis after seeing that my speech was becoming increasingly poor, that my lower lip and tongue were drooping, and that saliva flowed as soon as I lay my head back. (In this position, saliva filled my mouth up; hence, I swallowed it intermittently.) Then, after a colleague of his saw that I had normal reflexes, muscular strength in my limbs, and had my sensibility intact, they both decided to send me to Val-de-Grâce [a Paris hospital]. I was aware of what was happening, of its awkwardness, of my progressive weakening (for I could rise only with difficulty), of the dulling of my faculties that left me only with a heightened, clear sense of awareness, but this was accompanied with a sort of smug indifference, so I did not suffer in any way.

Upon my return to Paris on December 14, I could get dressed and board the train without assistance; I only wanted a handkerchief to collect the saliva that flowed abundantly from my mouth. (Remember that when I arrived at Val-de-Grâce I could not even articulate my name distinctly enough to be understood.) I quickly became frail but stayed awake long enough to see, shortly after my arrival, the presence of senior professors meeting around my bed. It gave me joy to see that they finally had a diagnosis and to hear that Monsieur Netter was arriving the following day. And it was here that I remembered, while repeatedly feeling delirious, an article by Sainton about encephalitis that I read a few months ago, and articles by Netter. [A. Netter originally diagnosed EL in France; see Chapter 2].

The night weighed heavy, and the following morning I could for the last time eat breakfast by myself. Professor Dopter [see Chapter 6 for his views on transmissibility of EL], who took care of me, made a gentle lumbar puncture that revealed normal lymphocytosis, a normal quantity of albumin, and an excessive amount of sugar, and a test for syphilis that was negative.

From this moment, I was in my bed and only capable of sluggish movement—with great difficulty—not only in using my wrists to sit up or to move a leg, but also in being unable to turn to my side, in spite of the persistent fear of a sacral ulceration. I had a profound weakness in all of the muscles. This was reflected by the slowness with which I raised or withdrew my hand when anyone came to see me, but I did not have paralysis. The face, which was fixed, but could limply move when I tried, presented signs more reminiscent of pseudobulbar syndrome, with the muscular system of the eyes almost intact. I gazed only at the ceiling with the same obstination as sitting down, but I took the liberty of conserving the energy used in extreme movements. I did not have diplopia, but a certain degree of discomfort and pain when viewing things up close. I could bring my lips close together, though poorly, for drinking, but I could not whistle. I could move my jaw, but could not masticate, nor even roll solid food between the tongue and the palate. And when someone "swabbed"(so as to clean) my mouth, one could not, so to speak, pass over my tongue. I nourished myself with only liquids: milk, beaten egg yolks, boiled and finely puréed meat. I could not, particularly, swallow bread because the palate always remained hard. When one asked me to, I could slowly and with difficulty stick my tongue out, but for the most part experienced paresis, i.e., the tongue musculature would not contract.

A little later on, I noticed that I could not blow my nose. The tongue and the lips were unable to prevent the air from leaving my mouth. A marked dysarthria [difficulty in speaking] was often present. To be understood, I attempted to write down things that I desired. Even so, I was not often successful because I could barely detach my gaze from the ceiling, and my hand was too weak and clumsy to form letters.

I never had reflex abnormalities. My sensations were normal. I only experienced a continual soreness along the mastoid branch of the superficial cervical plexus, along with continual itching, even to the slightest touch, of the scalp over the vertex to the mastoid process. It is the only true pain that I experienced, although it was always minor and bothered me very little. However, I have not considered the painful bed sores of the sacral region, which were virtually torture all of the time, exaggerated by a little delirium due to the weight of my blankets that distorted my feet and "crushed" my heels.

Although hardly able to move my legs, I imagined how agonizing travel would be. When I was able to be understood, I requested that my blankets be lightened, and that a cotton padding to be placed under my heels. I also asked for a round, inflatable, rubber "bag" to be placed under my sacrum.

A light sweat would appear with the slightest effort, even when I did not have a fever. I feared the heat, and my hands were constantly looking for a cool place that I finally found under the mattress or on the rungs of my headboard. The salivary secretion was overabundant. To avoid the wetting of the front of my shirt, I had to accept the wearing of a type of bib.

I clearly had polyuria [excessive urination], which succeeded 3 or 4 days of oliguria [a decrease in urination], and was obligated to wake up several times a night. Also, I had a rather strong constipation, which necessitated some laxatives and an enema every 2 days.

I remember, of this period, certain episodes of awareness/consciousness when I did not sleep. I have to emphasize a "dissociation" in my psyche. I noticed a hastening of those who treated me and was surprised at their concern, and sometimes, despite their concealment, I saw their grief. I was not shocked or alarmed by this, though I felt myself imperceptibly slipping toward total exhaustion. All of my perception was preserved but I never experienced an associated emotion. I was basically a spectator. I thought of my children, who would be deprived of their father, as if I was not involved and I did not think that this absence of emotion was due to a lack of cortical functioning, but rather due to a numbness. All of my faculties disappeared, just like my muscle strength. The only thing that persisted was my higher thinking when I was awake, such as promotion to a higher rank, winning a million in the lottery, and desiring to be autopsied if I died.

Despite the rapid worsening of my symptoms and "general state," my temperature returned almost to normal, seldom reaching 38°C [100.4°F].

It was at this moment, 19th December, the 20th day of my disease, 5 days after my entry into the hospital, that, in order to attempt to prevent the peduncular syndrome, Professor Vincent attempted for the first time "an abscess of fixation" by injecting me with turpentine.

On the 30th day, my temperature rose again to around 40°C [104°F]. I felt more exhausted and more impatient for the end of this illness. All the symptoms persevered, but the salivation diminished, and at this moment I noted a clearer awareness of things. After the initiation of the abscess [from the turpentine injection], my temperature increased again for 3 days to above 39°C [102.2°F]; I dreaded my death. Then, three quick declines in temperature occurred. Furthermore, my physical exhaustion was gone, my smile returned, and I experienced rapid euphoria because I could roll over in my bed. This was quite a transformation for my visitors. Ten days after the absence of any fever, I arose and walked to the chair for the first time. My excess salivation was gone, my everyday speech was becoming comprehensible; however, it remained laggard, monotonous, and had mumbled pronunciations of s, of j, and of ch, as if the paresis of the tongue would not lead the air to its point and allow it to escape. Later, I had an immense, childish joy upon discovering that I could now masticate. And when I was able to whistle, I did, though sometimes awkwardly, numerous times.

With regard to my legs, relaxed walking was very slow to return. My legs could now bend, and I could support myself so that I would not fall. However, for most of the 3 weeks, I maintained a certain stiffness in my walking posture. My head was kept stiff as that of someone with Parkinson's, and the muscles of both legs flexed with difficulty and with terrible pain in their full extent.

The abscess, after an infectious burning that accompanied it, seemed to have rapidly diminished the acute phenomena of the disease which, having been grave, dragged on before ending. This persistence, despite the maintenance of my temperature around 37.5°C [99.5°F], troubled for a moment even Professor Dopter, because it added a severe form of deep venous thrombosis, which led to the idea that my legs and feet were cachectic. This period lasted only 4 to 5 days.

During the beginning of my recovery, my emotional reactions were exaggerated. I laughed easily and often, and in response to the slightest emotion, whether happy or sad, I wept convulsively to the point of not being able to speak. Any expectation was met with impatience. For example, I wanted Band-Aids or meals that someone had promised me "right away." These episodes showed my strenuous and potential nervousness and slowly diminished or otherwise transformed themselves.

Two months after entering the hospital, two and a half months after the debut of the disease, I was able to leave in convalescence, having gained back more than the 8 kg I had lost.

I was in a perfect general state; just tired. There was, however, no reduction of the pain of the mastoid branch of the superficial cervical plexus. It did not even yield to the helpful massages of the "hot air" showers.

In the mountains, my strength came back quickly. Later, 15 to 18 days after my departure from the hospital, I noticed multiple resurgences of a very light and rapid twitching in the bending of the fourth and fifth fingers of my left hand when I skimmed my moustache. Ten days after this appearance, I had the same trouble in the fourth and fifth toes of my left foot while I walked, with quick "movements" in the arch of my foot.

Successively these spasms appeared in the right foot, but attenuated more frequently. These contractions appeared in the quadriceps muscle group above the left knee-cap, and the elusive, muscular jolts barely affected my speech. Also, the twitching in my hands did not progress.

Today, 8 months after the start of the disease, 5 months after the start of the myoclonic jolts, all of the manifestations persist without change, except that the contractions are perhaps stronger and sometimes longer, primarily localized in the quadriceps. In the lower limbs, they hardly occur while standing, but rather during walking, which makes me tired. They appear very irregularly, every 30 seconds or more rarely. They are separated more when I am distracted and are almost completely beyond my control. If I conduct an act in which my movements are repeated frequently all the time (as, for example, in brushing my teeth), I sense that the twitchings are increasing in number, to the point of almost being continuous. They appear to me as a type of "trigger," which is foreign to my control, an intermittent excitation. They vary little in intensity, and are accompanied at times with a twitching in the left side of my lips, which then lowers the corners of my mouth. It was at this time that I initially experienced very minor vertigo, like a cerebral cloudiness without an inclination to fall, and a kind of tightening beneath the diaphragm or behind the sternum, which had, consequently, a deep, inspiratory movement. At the same time, I sensed myself tensing my limbs and my face. There was not, however, a modification in walking or a significant displacement of the parts of my limbs. Seated, I did not have more than a few, small, bending movements of the toes, mostly on the left side, and inconsistent, adductive movements of my thigh. Lying down, I felt, in general, nothing. The untimely muscle contractions of the oral pharynx and the constrictions of the jaw or the lips sometimes distorted my speech, as if it passed through a vent too narrowly. The syllables squished themselves together and the consonants disappeared. I rarely felt a muscular contraction. I felt only the modification of my speech that the people with whom I spoke did not always notice. By the way, I was able to correct those words that I pronounced poorly an instant after I spoke them.

I frequently experience a difficulty when using the same phrase; a "stop" that is like a spasmodic rippling particularly in the tongue occurs, so that the thought remains linked to its associated muscular movements.

My sensations are normal, but I experience constantly in the upper part of my cervical plexus the same sharp pain that existed throughout my disease, although it has decreased, and occurs mainly in the night when I lie down. I have no shaking, clumsiness, or modification of reflexes; only, in total, muscle spasms that are manifested again by cramping in the limbs in the morning when I get out of bed and stretch.

This is indeed the peripheral translation of a state of nervousness that make me feel as if I was under pressure with the slightest solicitation of my emotions. My throat tenses, I am a little fearful, and I burst toward the end of that which I have started. My speech is very loud, bursting forth, and is often distorted. I talk so fast that sometimes I use one word for another. I have no control over the words used "in the moment" from the ones already used. This straining, nervous potential exists without any modification of other faculties: ideation, memory, affectivity. My character appears normal, but I feel my personality diminish in this struggle.

To complete the clinical picture, I will discuss a little of the edema of my limbs, noticeable mainly in the left, which has reappeared since the start of my recovery. It shows up in the evening and departs in the morning and is more or less noticeable during the day. I do not have albuminuria, and all of my vegetative functions are otherwise perfect, but I perspire easily when I walk.

These observations offer a little more complete picture of the encephalitis known as lethargic. It involves paresis, modification to hyperexcitability, hypersecretive salivation, intact psychological functions with torpor but without infringement on the conscience, a little dreamlike delirium, prolonging of the disease under an unstable, emotional and motor state, relapses or slow progress, and a prognosis that is still perhaps mysterious. These facts, which a physician has experienced himself, perhaps offer a reasonable justification for this publication.

COMMENT: The hyperexcitability caused by EL is emphasized in this case, both physically and mentally. There is a slight indication of pseudosomnolence during the lethargic phase, and Dr. Delater highlighted that he did not have diplopia, but noted that he stared at the ceiling, and he also had vertigo. He had consistent pain along his chin and neck, and also had dysphagia and dysarthria. He also discussed severe sacral ulcers and itches, the latter being not commonly reported in EL. His EL could have been transmitted from the Jewish woman he treated in Morocco; this would be consistent with the idea that EL was sometimes transmissible from person to person (see Chapter 6). His treatment included the creation of an abscess by injection of turpentine. Dr. Delater had clear parkinsonian bradykinesia, sialorrhea, and rigidity, but there is no indication that it persisted during recovery, although he did have twitchings, which seem more like myoclonus than tremor (see below). His persisting symptoms also included a state of nervousness and daily limb edema, which seems very difficult to explain. His speech was also very fast, perhaps analogous to festination.

Case 3. (2) Follow-up report by the French physician, G.A. Delater: *Suite sur trent ans et fin d'une auto-observation d'encephalite lethargica (Follow-up during 30 years and completion of a self-observation of encephalitis lethargica)*

Nearly 30 years after his initial self-report, Dr. Delater wrote a follow-up report describing the chronic condition, which was published in the same journal, *Paris Medical*, as his initial report. This is one of only two detailed self-descriptions of chronic EL that we could locate (the other is presented here as case 6).

Some will perhaps remember the published account of a young medical officer's own experience with encephalitis lethargica printed in Paris Medical on October 30, 1920, in which he described in detail the specific psychological changes that occurred during the serious, acute phase of the illness; the contraction of the illness as he examined a sleeping woman in the Jewish quarter of Marrakech in September 1919; a certain panic attack that was followed by dizzying sleep during the day of November 30, 1919; two months of total paralysis with pseudobulbar syndrome spent at the Val-de-Grace, while he restfully remained under the enlightened and affectionate care of Prof. Dopter, his wife, and his devoted nurse, Miss Baudriot; then a rapid recovery that left him at the end of 8 months with only spasticity, discreet myoclonic jerks in the limbs of the left side when standing in an upright position, spasms in the lips, and adiadochokinesis [inability to perform rapid alternating movements, typically associated with cerebellar damage], ultimately leaving him with a certain nervous irritability that led him to compare himself to a boiler under pressure, always on the point of bursting the closed valves.

It is the continuation of this self-observation over the past 30 years that I would like to present to you now.

I can thus resume [1948] the notes that I have taken irregularly since 1920:

Since 1922, I have had excessive pain (in the sciatic nerve initially, then in 1924 exclusively in the lumbosacral region, accompanied by atrophy of the calf muscles and the right thigh). Since 1936–1937, and above all since the campaign of 1940 in which I served in the armored division, the 3rd D.L.M., this pain has prevented me from walking for more than 300 meters or even standing upright for more than 15 minutes. All of these manifestations were ascribable to spondylolisthesis, located by X-rays in 1932, with subluxation and compression of the 4th lumbar vertebra and reactional osteophytes with abnormal tearing. The radicular compressions, as a result of these deformations, had similar consequences, and as long as I persisted in walking, from this date until 1940, the paresthesia phenomena (tingling sensations, then heat, then hypoesthesia in the two lower limbs, the buttocks, and the perineum) and paresis of the right knee occurred at the end of 10–15 minutes of walking.

Approximately 20 days after the beginning of my recuperation, I started to experience very light myoclonic jerks in the upper left and lower left limbs while walking (occurring irregularly every 30 seconds, or even less frequently, and becoming more spaced apart when I was inattentive). With the spasticity, the stiffness, and the adiadochokinesis, the myoclonus slowly bilateralized, eventually disappearing from the left side, but since 1943 has persisted only in the right upper limb when I am lying down, particularly when I have smoked two cigarettes at the end of the day and especially when I want to go to sleep between 2 and 3 o'clock in the morning.

This myoclonus must be related to the bizarre sensations that I have experienced since 1943 when trying to fall asleep, and which seem to be connected to the onset of agonizingly painful contractions, such as the beginning of a cramp in my right quadriceps, where the movements of my muscles were at first slow, then completely diminished upon execution.

Also in 1943, after the strains suffered during the Resistance in which I served beside Lt. Yves Le Henaff, who was killed at Dachau, I again observed vasomotor problems in the lower right limb, the location of muscular atrophy since 1925, and observed that my right leg dragged more and more. Then I observed that my right arm dangled and hung limp more and more and included scapular pain and atrophy of the shoulder, upper arm, and forearm. I also had vasomotor problems (severe coldness and cyanosis) in the right hand, fingers, and wrist, accompanied by paresis in the extensor and interosseous muscles, especially in the cold weather. It was at this point that I stopped writing completely.

I had already mentioned in 1920, a kind of "inexpressible malaise," as noted by Sicard in his article in Presse Medicale, *March 21, 1923, which still occurs today "every time my emotions are stirred," and which I find to be exactly the same as in my notes taken in 1925:*

Emotivity*: I am so clumsy in the laboratory, and in danger in the street because of stumbling, that I get seized by a sudden, severe anxiety attack,* *while at the same time noticing the tensing of the lips and immobilization of the arms and legs.*

Nervous Instability*: I am no longer the master of myself, and I operate as if I am a machine without brakes. It is as if I am under pressure and about to burst, especially when I am explaining something that interests or agitates me. Then I talk volubly, and without taking time to think, I hurl myself feverishly into finishing that which I've started, to some uncertain end, and I feel anxious, as if my resources are suddenly going to fail me. Words do not come at all or I use the wrong words, and I sometimes get led astray by a simple relationship that has no connection to their meaning. Or, I tense and distort words, turning my head—I have to watch myself carefully and try to talk very slowly.*

These problems are nothing compared with the bradykinesia and bradyphrenia noted by Cruchet and Verger in Presse Medicale, *November 15, 1922, and by Lhermitte in the prolonged form of epidemic encephalitis in the* Journal of Medicine, France, *April 1923. They were in fact, for me, accompanied by tachyphrenia and tachythymia, against which bradykinesia and ideative bradyphrenia were, in my opinion, simply functional reactions and nothing more. Just as I have my involuntary movements caused by myoclonus, I have this inexactness in my words and ideas that outrun my thinking. My psychological state runs ahead of its center of gravity!*

Consequences*: I worry constantly about these problems, subjectively and objectively. They include loss of confidence in myself and worries about social demotion, e.g., criticism from my supervisors, remarks by other people, their mistrust of my qualifications, etc. Is it possible to ascribe to these excessive problems, this "speeding up," the basis of my scientific and literary hyperproduction since 1924? (Two hundred medical articles and eight technical works or novels, of which two were awarded prizes by the Association of Doctors and Pharmacists.) In any case, this achievement provides an argument in favor of the hypothesis "neurosis produces genius" put forward by Grasset, and against the converse proposition (presumably, "genius makes one neurotic"), and strengthens the Christian reservations about the expedient claims of modern eugenics.*

I don't think that one can put this group of pathologies under the label of postencephalitic parkinsonism. Obviously, I take a firm position on this because I have taken more than a few steps on this road. I am forced to confront that which accompanies me: the impaired mobility in my right arm that inhibits my writing and also, quite often, constrains my ability to help with meals and to dress myself. However, if I am not under pressure, I can write very slowly and legibly for quite a long time. It was in this way that it took five entire afternoons to write the rough draft of this article. However, I do not have the walk of old Parkinson's sufferers, i.e., with small steps, close together, and I don't "cogwheel" like them.

Obviously, I also lack any get-up-and-go, any dynamism. I have very little energy except when I have taken one or two tablets of Phenedrine or Ortedrine. I am in slow motion, always quiet. But I have had very little of the frozen visage since my journey began, and the myoclonus that I've experienced cannot be called a tremor. Moreover, the latter has disappeared completely and the former has ameliorated considerably to the point of only appearing when I smoke, thanks to the vitamin B made available to me at the end of 1946, per the suggestion of my friend Dr. Hillerate in Vichy.

I will allow myself to note on this subject, a method of absorption that experience has shown me to be especially effective. It is derived from oral absorption. Because of the proximity of the nasopharynx to the substantia nigra of the mesencephalon, using an atomizer, I sprayed the vitamin in liquid form through the choanae into the nasopharynx. However, the liquid produced disagreeable reactions. Then the idea came to me to hold the 3–4 tablets of vitamin B, which I was taking 3–4 times a day, in my mouth for 3–5 minutes. Administered this way, it seemed to me that the product had certain restorative properties. (It is easy to hold the tablets for 20 minutes in the vestibule of the mouth—often there follows the satisfaction of feeling a rapid strengthening of a tooth weakened by the slow process of gingivitis.)

Thus it was, that from the outset of this treatment, I began to write again and stopped having the various auditory problems, the whistling, buzzing, vertigo, deafness, which, after 1937, were the result of congestive processes associated with the eighth cranial nerve. And I do not despair, God willing, of achieving a relative recovery. And now I hope you will excuse me for voicing a wish that I have, which this publication conveys with a sort of solemnity: I desire that my brain will end up under the microtome of my old friend and colleague from St. Luc, Professor Lhermitte. In that way, up to the end, I will have been able to contribute to medical science.

And, there is a further follow-up of self-observation:

October 1947. On my return from vacation after a drop in temperature and a forced walk of 300 meters, I was stricken with a syndrome of spasmodic arterial blockage in the right leg and foot, a worsening of numbness, hypoesthesia, and paresis in the right-side extremities, which I interpreted as an extension of the mesencephalic lesions to the vasomotor nerves. These problems responded to antispasmodic medication.

COMMENT: Dr. Delater was indeed very productive during his lifetime, writing many articles and books despite his illness. His first statement about his chronic EL refers to the pain and muscle atrophy, which nevertheless did not prevent him from serving during the early part of World War II. These symptoms may be more associated with his vertebral pathologies than with EL. He also seemed to have been more affected by paresis in cold weather, which is suggestive of Raynaud disease. He continues to be nervous, and he mentions a speeding up of his thought processes and speech, which could be considered analogous to festination. Myoclonus was present throughout much of his illness—he indicated that it could not be considered tremor and that vitamin B treatments appeared to eliminate the movements. In Dr. Delater's description, he associated his condition with pseudobulbar syndrome and is quite emphatic that he does not have PEP. Dr. Delater indicated that EL affected the function of some of his cranial (e.g., the eighth) and peripheral nerves.

The most valuable aspect of Dr. Delater's contribution is that it spans more than 30 years and thereby exemplifies how, despite EL and its sequelae, some patients continued to lead productive lives.

Case 4. Self-report by an anonymous American physician

This self-report, by an anonymous American physician, was published in the *Journal of the American Medical Association* in 1922.

With the hope that my experience may be of assistance to others in the diagnosis, prognosis, and convalescent care of persons suffering from epidemic (lethargic) encephalitis, I will record my symptoms, with special reference to the subjective symptoms, as they occurred, without attempting to make any deductions or any reference to literature, which is not available to me at this time.

Personal History. *At the time of the illness here recorded I was 34 years of age, married, and had one child, aged 7 years. For the 20 years preceding I had enjoyed excellent health. After returning from France and receiving my discharge from the army in August, 1919, I traveled throughout the eastern half of the United States until January 2, when I arrived in Baltimore, where I remained until the end of February. During this period of moving from place to place I had had no illness of any sort except a severe coryza at Christmas time (1919); and I had knowingly come in contact with but two persons who had been ill: my son, who had a gastric disturbance following a long ride on a train during the second week in February, and a man who had recently been ill with influenza.*

Prodromal Period. *During the latter part of January and the month of February I was exceedingly nervous, and during February there was present an extraordinary sexual excitement, but there were no other signs of illness, and I attributed these symptoms to the strenuous life I had been living for a few months. When my wife met me about the middle of February, she said that she had never known me to be in such a disturbed mental condition.*

Onset. *In New York on the evening of February 27, after an unappetizing meal, I suddenly became nauseated and vomited. Vomiting continued throughout the night. The next day everything eaten was immediately vomited, and I was feverish and chilly by turns, as if I were experiencing the onset of some acute illness. It was but a week since I had been talking with the man convalescing from influenza, and I thought that I was experiencing the onset of that disease. That night I was unable to sleep; on the contrary, my mental processes were exceedingly active. My mind "raced" with thoughts coming and being carried to their conclusion with such speed that the experience was extremely pleasant. These thoughts have stayed with me almost as clearly as though it was* *last night. During that night I had a most unusual experience, in view of the symptoms mentioned under the heading of prodromes, the complete loss of sexual power. This was so startling that I thought that my illness was more severe than I had previously supposed.*

The next day found the symptoms much abated, and though my head ached and I felt weak, I was well enough to go out for a little walk with my family. This night the symptoms of the preceding night returned, but with diminished force, and my thoughts were not nearly so clear.

On the third day, March 1, I lounged around my room all day. This night, the fourth from the onset, I slept.

The following day I went to the office as usual and made final arrangements to leave for Panama on the next day. I still felt as though recovering from a mild attack of influenza.

Apparent Intermission. *During the trip, which lasted 7 days, I had a bilateral earache. Never before that I can remember had I had the slightest trouble with my ears. Herpes labialis developed about the middle of the week. A trip on the ocean would ordinarily have been a pleasure to me, but this time it became tiresome, and I was very nervous and irritable. I attributed these symptoms to the fact that for several months, I had been working very hard and to the illness in New York. Although sexual power had returned as the early symptoms disappeared, I no longer had the excitement mentioned previously. I landed at Christobal, Canal Zone, March 10, 1920, apparently quite well.*

The Attack. *Period of excitement, conscious: No other symptoms occurred until March 13, when I was again unable to sleep. Once more I had the pleasant sensation of my mind racing joyously and clearly, and again I experienced that "mysterious" loss of sexual power. From this time on there was a loss of sexual desire as well as of sexual power.*

March 14: I was happy, bright, and talkative (not my usual habit). Both thoughts and speech were rapid. I discussed the work with my predecessor, and with a lively imagination, I told story after story to my son, speaking so rapidly that he said he had difficulty in understanding me. Again I could not sleep.

March 15: I went to the office. I was still unusually talkative, but spoke through set teeth. The night brought no sleep.

March 16: On arising in the morning, I found that I could not keep from humming or repeating odd, meaningless sounds. The "control" had ceased to function. I noticed that, without any exertion, my respiration became panting in character, and men whom I met asked me if I had been running. I felt as if I were under the influence of alcohol, and talked as if I were. I was so intent on becoming thoroughly acquainted with the various phases of my new work, as my predecessor was to leave in a few days, that I did not realize that I was ill and I felt somewhat ashamed because, as I thought, my nerves were getting beyond my control. Throughout the day my mind was active, but I was becoming more and more irritable. There was no sleep that night.

March 17: The humming had disappeared, my mind was not so clear, and my thoughts were much less rapid. The panting respiration was present in an aggravated form. At night, when I tried to sleep, I found myself setting my teeth, and in breathing I made such "awful noises" that I almost drove my wife to distraction. To me it seemed that I would get almost to sleep and then some interference or irregularity of my breathing would again awaken me. Sleep was impossible. I felt somewhat feverish.

March 18: I left the office early to try to tire myself out by exercise so that I might sleep. I was unsuccessful.

March 19: Repetition of the preceding day.

The Lethargic Period–March 20: *I went to the office as usual, but soon returned to my room at the hotel, where I tried to tire myself out, feeling certain that I had merely lost control of my nerves in a new situation and in the tropics. That afternoon I fell asleep for a few hours and on awakening found that I had a marked diplopia. However, I did not yet feel sufficiently ill to stay in bed, and in the evening I went out on a business errand.*

From March 21 until my temperature became normal about 12 days later, my memory of all that occurred is lacking or extremely hazy. My wife states that while still at the hotel I talked incessantly and that my hands and arms were never still. I gave numerous short connected discourses on subjects related to my work or problems in which I was interested. Most of the time I lay with my eyes closed, mumbling or talking, picking at the bedclothes or groping as if hunting for something to eat. When I found I had nothing I would open my eyes, and a queer, disappointed expression would spread over my face. This happened so often as to be characteristic. As long as my attention could be held, which was for only a few moments at a time, I answered clearly and intelligently. March 24, when two physicians were called in consultation, I evidently made a great effort at self-control for some time. One of the physicians remarked that my case resembled typhoid.

On entering the Ancon Hospital, March 24, I had a temperature of 102.3°F [39°C]. (I had probably had that much elevation of temperature for several days previous to my admission.) My attention could be held only by speaking to me in a loud voice or by calling my name repeatedly. When I did answer, I replied intelligently, but I would immediately pass off into a stupor with delirious muttering.

For the first week in the hospital the nurses' entry on my chart was "irrational." My wife, who visited me every day, states that for 3 or 4 days I was in the same condition as at the hotel. My attention could be held for only a few seconds. My eyes would close and I would begin to grope and to talk about something else or mutter an utterly meaningless jumble of words.

March 28: My wife noticed that she could command my attention for a longer period of time and that I seemed to pass into a more quiet sleep. Of all the tests that were made on me, I remember but one, the spinal puncture, made that afternoon. Before going to the hospital I knew that almost the first thing that would happen would be the spinal puncture, and in the condition I was in

I became very much opposed to the performance of this test. However, my memory of this operation is not of the pain, but of the skill of the physician who did it. I can remember a sensation of "if that is all, it is nothing." From various sources I find that I must have put up rather strong opposition to having the puncture made, but when the physician at last came to do it, I offered no resistance, and as he reports, I was asleep before he was through.

Convalescence. The long and tedious period of convalescence was characterized by marked weakness, an insatiable desire to lie down and sleep, and various nervous manifestations. The most pronounced symptoms disappeared within 6 months, but some of the first to appear, impotence and loss of sexual desire, were more tenacious, and at the present time, 20 months after the onset of the disease, I cannot confidently say that normal sexual life has returned.

Before leaving the hospital, I was conscious of an almost constant desire to urinate, but the flow was very slow in starting and then it was little more than a dribble. At this time I was also very constipated. These symptoms lasted for 1 month after I had left the hospital.

For several months, perspiration was very marked, especially about my mouth.

For months I involuntarily set my teeth when trying to go to sleep or on the slightest excitement.

Often I felt in my throat what I diagnosed as a hysterical bolus.

For about a month my memory was an almost absolute blank, and my past was so hazy that it was impossible for me even to understand why I was living with my family. Why I should not take one of the ships that passed and go to some other place was a question that often arose. It seemed to me as though a dense fog surrounded my whole past; nothing was certain. Any attempt to remember was usually an impossible struggle.

Before these symptoms left (3 weeks after leaving the hospital) I resumed the duties of my office. The walk of two short blocks from my home to the car was almost too much for me, and when I arrived at the office, I could scarcely wait, until I reached a chair to sit down. In spite of the most strenuous efforts I frequently went to sleep. Sleep overwhelmed me during the short street car rides to and from the office. At home it was impossible for me to sit at the table until the meal was finished. I must lie down.

At night I could not overcome a fear of I know not what. I made endless rounds to see that the windows and doors were locked, and at every noise, imaginary or real, I was out of bed prowling around the house to find the cause of it. The nights were terrors for me, and I was glad when daylight returned.

After the other symptoms had disappeared, a weakness remained for at least 6 months, so great that after any special effort I came to expect 2 or 3 days of headache and of neuralgia-like pains in the chest.

After a horseback ride of 4 hours I was obliged to remain in bed for a day and a half, unable to do aught but sleep. The neuralgia-like pains would often prevent me from sleeping. They usually began at night soon after retiring, and *would disappear a few hours after arising in the morning. An attack of these pains would usually last 2 or 3 days.*

*   **Conclusion**. *After 6 months all symptoms had so far disappeared that no one would have thought, to look at me, that I had been ill. (In fact, throughout my illness people remarked about my apparently good condition.) I lacked energy and endurance for walking or taking any other form of exercise, and whether owing wholly to the lack of exercise or to the disease, I have gradually increased in weight 25 pounds [11.3 kg] more than I ever did before. At the present time, 20 months after my illness, I feel as well as I ever did in my life, except for a very rare recurrence of the neuralgic pains previously mentioned. Neither my wife nor my child ever showed any symptoms of lethargic encephalitis.*

COMMENT: There are many interesting features of this physician's signs and symptoms, which share some similarities with those of Dr. Delater—racing thoughts, pain, and weakness. This physician also experienced the extreme lethargy, pseudosomnolence, and diplopia that are the most consistent features of EL. Furthermore, as was often the case, he initially believed he had influenza. He also describes respiratory symptoms probably representing the respiratory tics that were a fairly common manifestation of EL/PEP. These may account, at least in part, for his sleep difficulties. He showed vomiting as an early sign, which also was evident in case 1 above. As well, he had what today would be called loss of libido and erectile dysfunction, from which he gradually and eventually recovered. The author does not mention any parkinsonian signs. Interestingly, considering the possible relationship between EL and herpes (see Chapter 9), he developed a case of herpes labialis during the disease process. Twenty months after the acute episode, he claims a "virtually" complete recovery. However, as with the previous self-reports, it was not a complete recovery, because he still had occasional associated pain. One wonders how this physician fared over the ensuing years. Finally, it is interesting, in contrast to many of the other self-reports, that friends did not identify him as being ill—this would be consistent with the absence of reported parkinsonian signs (rigidity, masked face, stooped posture, etc.).

Case 5. Self-report by a German patient: *Encephalitis lethargica in der Selbstbeobachtung (Self-observation of encephalitis lethargica)*

The following self-report was written by a German patient of Drs. W. Mayer-Gross and G. Steiner in 1921.

*   *I became ill with encephalitis lethargica in the middle of February 1920. Initially, I lay awake for 2 nights but remained remarkably fresh. On the following morning, I felt nauseous with pressure in my head. I then had a sudden feeling, like a current running through my head, and felt certain I was*

going crazy. I took a planned visit to a friend in the country, but instead of looking forward to it, I felt afraid about seeing him. When I returned home in the
evening I felt better, but it was as if I was a little drunk, as well as having pressure in my head. I knew what I was doing, but it was if the "me" in my mind
was not there, and I believed I would never be able to study or enjoy fencing
again.

That night, I didn't sleep again. It was as if the back of my head, where tired-
ness comes from, was a void. My eyes wouldn't close without a conscious effort
and a strong headache set in. I couldn't think properly and was aware of my
heart cramping up. I was short of breath and needed to whistle to ensure
deeper breathing. Then the whistling became compulsive and I seemed unable
to stop. I finally fell asleep towards the morning, but when I woke, discovered
that my body had effectively fallen asleep, with a prickly feeling in my limbs.

The doctor was called and diagnosed a neurasthenic attack, prescribing a
tranquilizer. My headache improved during the day, but I remained unable to
think productively and was still missing the internal "me." I worried that I was
coming down with the flu. The following night, I slept restlessly with a pain
along the left side of my jaw, although it improved the next day and the dentist
found no cause. Since then, I have developed the habit of clenching the inside
of my left cheek between my teeth before releasing it again as at the time it
seemed to lessen the pain, but has now become a compulsion—I can stop
doing it only with a conscious effort.

On the following day, I got out of bed suffering a tortured, almost physical
sensation of fear. Any slightly negative feeling was magnified, to the degree that
attempting any positive act failed due to the paralyzing doubts. For example,
I wanted to visit a friend but felt he would not wish to see me. Doubt came with
every impulse. However, I could play the guitar and did so without interruption.
Music played a beneficial role for me throughout my illness—particularly the
melody and harmony. I particularly liked music that evoked memories.

The following day, I woke with a slight fever and double vision that disappeared during the course of the day but returned in the evening. This problem
has recurred throughout the illness, particularly when I am tired. From this time
until shortly after the spinal tap, my memories are vague. Apparently, I had a
high temperature up to 40.2°C [104.4°F] that dropped after the lumbar puncture but rose again due to a throat infection. There was then a period of hypo-
thermia until, gradually, my temperature returned to normal.

Although I no longer remember them, I also hallucinated day and night, predominantly about the war. I suffered acute headaches in two specific areas—
one where I had a fencing injury, but the other where I had no previous injury.
Following the spinal tap, I slept almost continually for several weeks and was
woken for meals and ate well despite difficulties in chewing and swallowing.
I also started to have problems urinating; it improved at the beginning of April,
although I still do have problems occasionally, albeit of a different nature. Then,
the problem was being able to urinate, whereas now I sometimes cannot hold
my water.

On April 4th my left thigh, which had been badly wounded in the war, started to shake. The shaking consisted of an alternating tightening and loosening of the muscles. The shaking was initially continuous, but by mid-May, I was able to control it if I flexed my leg. However, the shaking started up again soon after and this has been an ongoing problem since.

In mid-April I got up and did not initially notice many movement restrictions. However, I did know that certain movements in my arms were no long possible and when walking I held a stiff posture, needing a goal to aim for to retain my balance. If my head turned, I worried about falling. I also held my arms with elbows flexed. These issues continue to today.

Around this time we moved our family home away from Berlin and I over-reacted with bouts of weeping—my negative feelings were disproportionate, and it took weeks for me to calm down. Even today, I worry unnecessarily about unlikely events happening. In my new home I felt I would never get better and was treated with solar therapy and pine needle baths in addition to Elarson [arsenic] tablets.

That September, I visited a friend in Berlin, and although my movement problems were no worse than earlier in the year, my mental state was poor and my continuous feelings of doubt ruined the trip. I could no longer feel happy or angry about anything; I just thought "What's the point?" about pretty much everything—even music. I also became aware that I was unaffected by other people's moods or emotions. In mid-December, I was able to feel angry again, which actually made me happy. Around this time, I again feared insanity; this problem worsened as the day progressed and my thoughts became more confused. I was no longer able to concentrate on anything.

However, in the middle of October, I returned to my studies in Freiburg and my movement disturbances gradually worsened. On being prescribed scopolamine, they improved but 2 weeks later they returned even worse than before. They are still a problem despite the continued use of scopolamine.

This was when I felt most depressed and I considered suicide. Strangely, these thoughts were at their most intense before a bowel movement. I would prevaricate over everything and question any and every small decision. It was as if I was looking at myself under a microscope. Also, I examined every physical reaction with curiosity, such as sneezing and coughing or urinating. I became obsessive about everything, which then created chains of thought. For example, seeing a person in any occupation (servant, train engineer) would make me wonder what would become of me, and I wondered if I would achieve nothing in life. Or picking up a pen would make me consider its holder and how precious or fragile it could be. At this time I also became hypersensitive to other people's moods—I didn't have any empathy about their feelings, but simply registered them to an unnaturally high degree. I also lacked any natural impulse for insignificant tasks—I would have to think before cleaning my pipe or putting wood on the fire. And although I always had the energy and ability to carry out these tasks, I was fearful that, mid-movement, I would become frozen and unable to finish the chore. To a degree, I thought the problems were all in my mind and that if I could forget that I was sick, the problems would disappear. This was partly because once I spent a whole evening thinking normally and my movement problems disappeared.

During my lectures, I was able to follow the discussion but could not read for very long or do anything that required concentration. If I tried, I couldn't make sense even of individual words, let alone their connection to one another and subsequently, my movement problems worsened which in turn worsened my mental condition.

After Christmas and treatment by hypnosis that had no effect, I had massage, potassium iodide, sweating, and injections of strychnine, as well as a dose of electric shock therapy that was initially successful. However, after a throat infection that, in hindsight may have been a relapse of the illness, I started to have problems sleeping. While hallucinating one night, I was only half aware of where I was and who I was. It was like looking into the room from the outside; I was throwing myself around the bed and my leg shook uncontrollably. I slept eventually and in the morning got up and dressed. That afternoon, I had another electric shock treatment and when I tried to get dressed, the movement problems had become as bad as they are now, although by the middle of February, on the anniversary of the illness, I was suddenly able to move freely again, almost like before. However, as I feared, my mobility decreased and by the end of the third day, I was again requiring hours to get dressed. At the beginning of March, I left the clinic and returned to my parents' home in much the state in which I find myself today.

Present Self-Observation. *With regard to my physical state, the strength in my arms is good but the left one simply doesn't do what it's told. For example, pulling up my pants or holding them while getting dressed, is extremely difficult. If I force the movement, the arm simply shakes violently. It is also difficult to use either arm to wipe my mouth.*

Rotating movements with my hand on my face are very difficult and easier if I hold one hand with the other. Wiping or washing my face is almost impossible with my left hand and difficult with the right. Through practice though, this movement does appear to have improved. Holding my arm vertically and twisting my hand was very difficult when I was in the clinic, but is now almost normal again. However, doing up buttons or my tie is difficult and dusting my suit or washing myself with my left hand remains very difficult.

Playing the piano with two hands is hard—as soon as the right hand starts, the left stops. Eating with my left hand is almost impossible, but executing a similar movement with both hands simultaneously is easier and simple commands such as "stretch arms upwards, sideways, forwards" are easily executed.

Nevertheless, everything is slow and I often need minutes to complete a movement, having stopped halfway through. For example I may hold the napkin to my mouth without wiping or putting it down. I want to finish but am unable to. If I get angry about it, I can usually complete the movement. Or perhaps, I will hear a clock strike, and when it has finished striking, I can finish the movement.

Sometimes I do enjoy free movement for a short while and, with the exception of the rotating movement on my face, my arms obey. There is a change in my mental state, not something I can control, but a feeling of concentration and I suddenly notice that I have free movement. I still need to want to execute the movement and do it without thinking of anything else. And as soon as I do think of something else or of my movement problems, the ability has disappeared. These free moments appear to have become more frequent recently, but I know that even then, my posture remains strongly bent forward.

During dreams it is different, and I am able to execute movements like getting dressed quickly. I can then easily waken and immediately try to move, but am disabled—my thoughts digress and I can do nothing. No matter how hard I concentrate, my arm shakes uncontrollably and with longer-lasting movements, my leg shakes too. However, if it were a life-and-death situation, I feel sure I would be able to move appropriately.

With regard to other physical disturbances, I walk relatively well, but can feel unsure on my legs when dancing or being helped on with my coat when I sway backwards and forwards. But my balance, on the edge or a pavement or rail for example, is good.

My posture is poor and I hold myself strongly bent forward with my head stiffly forward again so that I am conspicuous to others, even when eating. Food remains in my mouth until I consciously remove it with my tongue. I am no longer able to whistle easily and if I hold my pipe or a cigarette in my mouth, my lower jaw shakes. I hold my arms flexed, with the lower arm parallel to the floor, unless I make a conscious effort to change position. My head rarely moves unconsciously and I tend to follow objects with my eyes, although this does seem to be improving lately.

My larynx also appears to have suffered: I speak more quietly than before and am unable to laugh heartily or cough deeply. Also, during bowel movements, I seem to growl. If I swallow badly, which I do more frequently, my throat takes time to react—I continue to drink before replacing the glass and cough. As a result, I snort over the table. Also, I sigh deeply from time to time without reason.

My eyes have become more sensitive, often weeping due to cigarette smoke for several minutes and yet I rarely weep due to sad situations. I suffer from a constant excess of viscous saliva and sometimes drool. I am sure that I produce more saliva than previously and that it isn't simply a case of insufficient swallowing. Also, my face has a constant sheen of grease on it, despite frequent washing.

In the clinic I had great difficulty turning over in bed and although this has improved, when I go to bed, my head still remains raised above the pillow for more than half an hour. I never feel tired despite avoiding strenuous exercise and falling asleep takes at least 2 hours. This may be partly due to the fact that I feel more energy in the evening, wanting to talk (sometimes to myself) and making plans—I'm most alert between 10:30 and 11:00. The border between wake and sleep is uncertain and although I feel I have not slept, I know that

I have dreamt of things that must have been dreams even though they don't feel like it. For example, in my dreams, my right foot (that has few movement problems in reality) no longer works or I read long passages from a book and on waking discover that I haven't read the said pages (and I would not be able to read so much).

Another problem with getting to sleep is what I call "registration"—that is, the taking into my consciousness of every physical and emotional process. As a result, I notice that I am falling asleep and hence become more awake. This also affects my ability to imagine things, because I tell myself that I need to imagine something and then cannot do so. I tell myself to "register" things to remember them but then know I cannot—it is a very annoying habit. Also, I suffer from an unreasonable sense of guilt—whether about eating too much chocolate or not reading a sufficiently difficult passage.

I still find it very hard to make a decision, but it is better than when I was first ill. However, important things like changing position in bed, still take a long time to decide. But this is because I am afraid that a change in position will start my leg movement disturbances.

Along with my unnatural fears, all of these sensations are so strong that they are almost physical—and come from the middle of the back of my head.

I feel strongly that I am no longer who I once was. While I was previously known to tell the corniest jokes, nowadays I am surprised if I actually understand one. In the company of others, I never know what to say; for example, I could not have given this report orally as I would have done before. And the "waiting" for the movement disturbances always upsets me—I know that however well I feel, my problems will return. And that brings me back to the unreasonable fears I suffer along with an over-reaction to unexpected noise, when my heart races at the slightest sound.

Nowadays, when I listen to beautiful music, I always weep—something that would have been unheard of before. And I am constantly "singing internally" to myself—I will repeat the same melody and lyrics in parallel to doing something different. It carries on without me thinking about it and when I do, it still continues. It makes no difference and gives no relief if I actually externalize the song and sing aloud. It is not the normal problem of having a song stuck in your mind, but much more permanent with each note and lyric constantly there. As a general rule, it doesn't annoy me—I just let it continue. Another impulsive behavior I have is counting—if I hear any rhythmical noise, I need to count and often do it wrongly so that I can stop the counting.

I feel I laboriously balance my condition so that I don't get worse—or better. To wish for it to be better gives me the fear that it may worsen. And the negative success of my "registration" tells me to get angry when I know that my fears are unreasonable. But all in all, I remain very depressed about my condition and am sure that it is harmful to be so introspective.

One area of progress that would have been impossible 6 months ago however, is the ability I have had to fall in love again—albeit with the typical doubt and apprehensions that I feel.

COMMENT: This patient shows many interesting psychological symptoms, such as the loss of motivation, loss of ability to concentrate and make decisions, hallucinations, the presence of hyperconsciousness and excessive emotionality (weeping during music), as well as racing thoughts, as in the previous patients. He does not note a lethargic period, although he did have insomnia and diplopia. He was initially nauseous and had hallucinations, as in some of the earlier cases. He developed clear movement disorders, such as impaired balance, stooped posture, bradykinesia, and manipulative problems. Finally, this patient has respiratory issues, a "greasy face," and sialorrhea. Note that he is sure, like Dr. Delater, that he is producing excess saliva and not just having difficulty swallowing (see Chapter 7). These signs and the movement disorders are associated with parkinsonism, so it appears that this patient had some features of the amyostatic-akinetic type of EL. Similarly, the patient noted that his left arm "did not do what it was told." James Parkinson describes this phenomenon in his famous "Essay on the Shaking Palsy" as the limb "failing to obey the dictates of the will."

Case 6. Self-report by an anonymous British physician

This self-report, by an anonymous British physician, was published in the British medical journal *The Lancet*, in 1948. The author had been employed as a naval doctor, then went into general practice.

Sleepy sickness is perhaps one of the cruelest afflictions to be endured by man. Though myself a doctor, I know little about the pathology of the disease; and indeed I have no knowledge of its clinical course or ultimate end, beyond the sequence of events that have already befallen me. I make no inquiries, nor do I dip into periodicals and books dealing with the complaint; for it is foolish, in my estimation, to anticipate what may never happen.

"Creeping paralysis"—the title already given to another disease—would be an excellent name for this disability, which drags unrelentingly along its laborious course. It is quite impossible to say "I'm worse than I was a week or a month ago." It is necessary to look back much further to recall little things that could once be managed but are now impossible or very difficult.

I am supposed to have contracted the disease in 1924, when I was 29. I ran a temperature for a few days and saw double for a week. This diplopia rather alarmed me at the time, but a brother houseman reassured me by saying that this phenomenon indicated only fatigue of the eye muscles, which was to be expected in any febrile condition. Previously, the Navy had claimed me for 8 years, but now I went into general practice at a seaside town, where I joined the local sailing club.

It was while sailing that I got the first inkling that all was not well with my makeup. Several boats had reached a mark-buoy round which it was necessary to gybe—a tricky movement, which would have disturbed the most hardened seaman, for a general smash-up seemed inevitable. Suddenly my hand started to vibrate on the tiller; it was a most curious sensation though only momentary. I mastered myself, regained my grip, both mental and physical, and steered round the buoy without incident.

Another warning came a few days later at a public luncheon. I was on my feet, proposing a vote of thanks to the speaker, when my right hand started to vibrate again. I wavered a bit, rammed my hand into my trouser pocket, and continued. I don't think anyone else noticed the contretemps. Some time after this I noticed that it was becoming difficult to write, quite a short letter taking a considerable time; and my handwriting, which always had been a bit of a puzzle, become completely illegible. Soon I lost my nerve for the excitement of sailing. There is always a spice of danger in navigating, even in local waters; and competing in the single-handed race—which I myself had instituted—became for me a most alarming affair.

At this stage, I consulted my brother, a general practitioner, who arranged for me to see a London neurologist. The three of us rendezvoused at the great man's country house; and, without my knowing, he diagnosed my ailment over the teacups. Afterwards he took me for a stroll in the garden. I remember he asked me if my mouth seemed wetter than usual. I answered, no. Little did I realize that as the years went by excessive salivation was to become the greatest tribulation of my life. In the kindest and most gentle way he told me what I was suffering from. In a way, it was a relief to know something definite.

Things went from bad to worse, and I had difficulty in memorizing my patients' faces and what I had prescribed for them. Deciding to give up my practice and go back to the Navy—my first love—I went to the Admiralty for medical examination, and felt guilty enough at putting my signature to a written statement that I was free from physical disability. In this early stage I could easily have fooled the whole Royal College of Physicians. But life on a submarine depot-ship, spending hour after hour with nothing to do but just sit and think or perhaps listen to Service jargon, proved an impossibility for me. I lasted a couple of months, then collapsed and was invalided out of the Service.

This just about finished me, and I found it beyond my powers even to think of a job of work. In the backwater of a village, with my wife and child, life became happy; and in the winter months I enjoyed rough-shooting, though slow on the trigger. My age was now 34. Then tremor and salivation began to trouble me. The embarrassment of excessive salivation is comprehensible only by those who have suffered it; it is very trying to have one's mouth perpetually full of fluid, waiting to spill over at the slightest relaxation of facial muscles. My brother put me on a proprietary preparation of scopolamine, which for years acted like a charm, drying up the mouth, reducing tremor, and making me feel fairly well. But as time wore on, it lost its almost magical effect, which has never returned. I was now treated with a preparation of stramonium, which still has a remarkably consistent action. Unfortunately it takes an hour to act, and in that time there is an almost overpowering temptation to hurry things up by taking a little more. The result of an overdose is devastating: a bone-dry mouth, a feeble heart-beat, a feeling of distress, and hysteria producing an exaggerated sense of humor, though in the background all the time is a sober awareness. If, on the other hand, I take too little, salivation deluges me. It is remarkably hard to strike a happy mean, for the path between the two extremes is very narrow. Owing to the atropine in stramonium, the pupils dilate, and strong glasses are needed. Before a fire, the heat is sufficient to dry up the conjunctivae and the upper lid tends to stick to the eyeball. This is sometimes quite painful. The trouble is alleviated by a kettle steaming on the hob, or a dish of water placed before the fire.

Gradually difficulty in swallowing has manifested itself; it is impossible to get down any food without copious draughts of water, and even this does not always work. I never take a meal with any but my own family, for eating demands my whole attention. Though right-handed, I use a fork in the left hand (the less affected) for almost all varieties of food; a fork is much easier to manipulate than a spoon. Crisp dry food is the most readily masticated; anything that cloys is anathema. "Ryvita" [a rye cracker], recrisped in the oven, is ideal. Of a different texture, sponge-cake is also excellent, seeming to dissolve in the mouth. A satisfying meal entails an hour's hard work. One of the greatest irritations is the inability, through being unable to swallow quickly, to join in the conversation, however trite my unspoken comment. By the time I have swallowed, the talk has swung on to some fresh subject.

My speech has become indistinct. Until I got used to it, this caused me great annoyance. How maddening it is to receive a grotesquely irrelevant answer to some simple remark, from someone trying his best to understand. How much better it would be if he said that he did not comprehend. My latest affliction is inability to walk well—the "festinating gait." This is much worse indoors when my way is beset with many corners. Once on an open road I can get along with a certain ease; but there are ominous signs that this will not last. Curiously enough, it is easier to walk backwards than forwards.

For the last 20 years I have been writing, punching the typewriter with my left forefinger—the only digit of the ten that will perform this duty. Free-lancing is surely the most disappointing of all occupations. I must have had some 200 articles rejected; but slowly my name is getting known, for I seem just now to be selling two articles a month, and two plays have been accepted by the BBC.

This tremendous interest keeps me going but a snag—inevitably, I suppose—has recently developed. I can no longer type with any ease or dexterity, my one good finger refusing to function. This is really distressing but, as nearly always happens, there is a way out. In America they are manufacturing an electric typewriter, which at the softest touch does everything, even rolling on the paper and shifting the keyboard; but naturally it is expensive.

I have to fight my own peculiar demon—the devil of frustration. Everything is difficult to accomplish; little details which come like second nature to the normal person are a series of puzzles to me; and sometimes there is no solution. Putting on clothes, doing up shoe-laces, fastening shirt buttons, holding a cup of tea *without its slopping over—all these are obstacles in the routine of life. Some of these things have to be done for me.*

So here I am, at the age of 55, with difficulty in walking, talking, eating, writing, and typing, with a whole host of minor ailments; yet a happy man with dozens of compensations. How has this disease affected my character and temperament? All for the better, I think. I can bear the keenest disappointment with almost complete equanimity; this happens two or three times a week when those big buff envelopes, addressed by myself, pass through the letter-box, and also when some new disability asserts itself. I am now much more sympathetic and can better understand other people's foibles, peculiarities, bothers, and ailments.

My belief that man possesses a separate entity apart from his husk of a body has been greatly strengthened by my experiences. I sit, as it were, inside my carapace watching my person behaving in its vile fashion, while my being is a thing apart, held prisoner for a time. This rather queer sensation of being outside oneself has been exaggerated by my complaint; it is most comforting, and strengthens my faith that there is not complete extinction ahead, but a better deal in a new life.

COMMENT: This patient's account of his EL is very limited. He had an episode of fever and diplopia for 1 week in 1924 at age 29. It is interesting that, despite being a physician at this time, he had no knowledge of EL. At some later time, tremor of the right hand developed; rigidity, sialorrhea, and difficulty swallowing subsequently developed over a 25-year period. At age 55, he showed walking abnormalities. His reference to walking backwards probably represents retropulsion. Although he and his physicians assumed that he had PEP, he does not describe oculogyric crises, tics, dystonias, compulsions, or other features more compatible with PEP, and his mind does not seem to have been affected. His affliction had a rather early age of onset and pursued an unusually slow course for idiopathic Parkinson disease (PD), but such slowly progressive cases do occasionally occur. His putative EL was very nonspecific and may have simply been influenza. Thus, although diagnosed with EL/PEP, his true disease remains unknown (PD or PEP), and one wonders how many other cases similar to this were perhaps incorrectly diagnosed as EL (see Chapter 7).

Case 7. Self-report by Eleanore Carey

Eleanore Carey was a native of Elgin, Illinois. She entered, but did not complete, medical school at Cornell University. She wrote the following for *The American Mercury*, which was a magazine developed and initially edited by the renowned early 20th-century American journalist, H.L. Mencken. The magazine's first issue appeared in 1924, and its last in 1981. The article was entitled, *I Recover from Sleeping Sickness*.

"Wake up! Wake up! Open your eyes!" The old, familiar command gradually sank into my unconscious brain, and its meaning began to make itself clear. It seemed to me that life was nothing but a command to "wake up" when all I wanted in the world was to be left entirely alone and to be allowed to continue sleeping. What if I was almost dying of starvation because I could not be roused frequently enough to eat? Starvation was heaven compared to the ordeal of coming to consciousness, and I could see no reason why I should not be let alone to starve if I chose to do so.

I was at life's lowest ebb—ravaged by the dread and very often fatal malady known as encephalitis lethargica, or sleeping sickness. After 2 months of illness I was in little pain, in fact, I was very comfortable, provided they did not prod me nor stand me on my head, turn me over in bed nor dash cold water on my face to waken me. It was so heavenly just to be allowed to sleep, but these people around me seemed determined to prevent my being comfortable! When the idea finally crept through my sleeping brain that I must waken, it seemed to be a physical impossibility. I wanted to be obliging, but I just could not. It seemed to me to be just as difficult to come to consciousness as it would have been had I been buried in a pit as deep as the center of the earth, where the circular walls about me were of shiny, polished marble. There were no crevices for my fingers on its sides nor any places to put my feet, but I must climb out of that pit with my bare hands! This comparison constantly came to my mind during the length of my illness (Fig. 11.1). Perhaps it will give the reader a vague inkling of the dreadful lethargy which completely overpowers the victim of this disease and renders him impotent to make the effort to help himself.

Encephalitis lethargica is one of those strange diseases afflicting mankind, appearing in epidemic form of varying degrees of intensity, and the cause of which completely baffles the medical profession. The victim goes into a coma from which many never awake. There are some, however, who live through its initial stages only to emerge broken physically and mentally. And still there are a comparatively few others who come through the disease with a sharpened brain, keener mentally. But these few usually have one or more pronounced and unpleasant physical after-effects.

In 1923, an incipient epidemic made its appearance in New York, and I fell ill on the first of February of that year. In my case, the contention of some physicians that it was the after-effect of the Spanish influenza was logical, inasmuch as I had had the flu during the epidemic in 1918. That was 5 years before, but I remember well how in less than 24 hours I had nipped the attack in the bud, sending the disease into my system through the bloodstream.

Sleeping sickness is, in the beginning, very insidious. In my case there was first a severe pain in the back of my head, which refused to relent its torture in spite of the pain-eliminators I used. After a period of 3 weeks, during which time many other symptoms developed and I ran a high temperature, this pain traveled to the left shoulder, where it remained in agonizing intensity for approximately 6 weeks more.

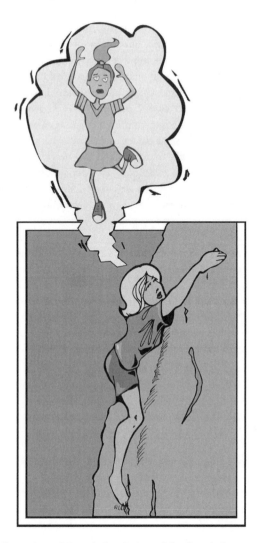

Figure 11.1 Illustration of Carey's description of the deep lethargy associated with encephalitis lethargica and her need to "climb out" because she needed to care for her daughter (drawn by Mrs. R. Shadle).

A detailed account of the many and varied symptoms which appear during these coming-down stages would be of no importance and is too lengthy to relate. One's life, however, is definitely divided—it comes to be regarded much as the soldiers must regard their lives—before and after the war. The sleeping-sickness patient thinks of life as before and after his sickness.

One of the foremost psychiatrists and neurologists of the present day has informed me that each case has different symptoms, ranging from practically nothing to violent convulsions, but that double vision, or the seeing of two or more objects in place of one, is a general symptom and practically all patients experience it, regardless of the severity of the case. It is one of the first definite and sure symptoms of the sickness, and often, as in my case, becomes a permanent after-effect. Today, after 11 years, I am told by different eye specialists, as well as the doctor himself, that the probabilities are that the defect will never be cured. It left certain eye muscles completely paralyzed, so that unless the object is far away, two objects are still visible. There seems to be no help in glasses nor in any treatment—all doctors conforming in their opinion as to the futility of material aid.

This same physician has said that a return to complete health is possible only in very mild cases. Those whose illness was severe will be afflicted with one or more of the after-effects probably throughout the rest of their lives to a greater or less degree, according to the patient's treatment of himself.

About the time the pain left my head and went into my shoulder I began to experience the first signs of sleepiness. It was more than mere sleepiness—it was like a drugged lethargy, a semiconsciousness filled with the hodge-podge thoughts of a nightmare.

I hear music—music in everything. The sound of people's voices, the rolling of a milk-wagon in early morning, and worst of all, the rumble and roar of the elevated trains as they passed near by—all these became bands, orchestras, and people singing—their voices registering all the way from baritone to high soprano. The music's persistency drove me to distraction, and the hideous hodge-podge and confusion which it caused seemed so real to me that the monotony made it a horror beyond description.

I had many visual illusions. I thought I was in a summer cottage, for instance, beside a lake where the music of chimes constantly sounded from a church steeple far away. I could even see the shadow of leaves on the floor from the moon-lighted window—and yet it was really winter and I was on the fifth floor of a New York hotel. In my delirium I took long journeys to far lands, where there were always terrible accidents, much death and destruction, and frightful scenes. The room in which I slept took on grotesque proportions—it was as large as a city block, and the objects in it were far, far away, when in reality they were no more than 6 feet from my bed.

The doctors who were called to diagnose my case finally called it sleeping sickness, and decided that the only "cure" was to leave the matter entirely to nature. They arranged for my care and for what little treatment was known to medical science. The fact that no longer would I have to force myself to consciousness at last reached my dormant mind and I relaxed, thanking the Lord for the chance just to sleep. Then came the coma so characteristic of the disease.

During the coma I experienced many dreams, or deliriums, many of which I can remember clearly still.

The raging fever consuming me night and day took what little flesh I had on my body and left me a literal skeleton. I weighed less than 80 pounds when I began the long and tedious climb out of the pit, but after the sickness itself had left and the fever subsided, it was only a few weeks before I noticeably commenced to gain weight rapidly.

I had slept for 3 months and a half—2,500 hours constantly, and many, many more in the ensuing months when the effort to get well became my chief aim in life.

My incentive to drag myself out of my coma was not thought out, or wondered about. It was an existing fact, brought to my consciousness with startling clarity by the presence of my small daughter, who was wholly dependent upon me for her welfare. I realized that I had to "snap out of" my illness and from the desire for sleep, and live again. There was no one to take care of her; if anything happened to me she would be lost, and the fear of this gave me the determination to live, and it became a question of whether or not I had the will power to go on living or would succumb to the ravages of the disease. This will power is of utmost importance for any recovery at all. The thought of death, the reader must remember, is not brought about by any melancholia or depression of spirit—it is the line of least resistance—the easiest and pleasantest way.

In my anxiety to force myself out of a deplorable condition I put aside by sheer will power the desire to lie down and sleep. I made myself take up the tasks of housekeeping when it seemed a physical impossibility to keep awake, and I clearly remember that many hundreds of times I fell asleep doing any one of the little menial tasks I took upon myself to perform.

My entire day was clouded by one obsession—the wish to sleep. It was torture—this continual forcing oneself to keep conscious, and a great part of that time I was not entirely conscious—going about in a daze. I termed the condition, somewhat aptly, I think, "groggy"—as it reminded me of the stories I had heard of prize-fighters continuing fighting long after they were really conscious of what they were doing. I had no control over the sleep that came, which was not unlike the stupor produced by some deadly drug. It seemed to strike first in the pit of the stomach and then gradually creep to the brain, take possession there and deaden my senses. And simultaneously it seemed as if a wave engulfed me—sweeping my entire body in a dreadful lethargy, almost literally paralyzing in its effects, so that both mind and body were lifeless.

These attacks during the first year of my recovery were practically continuous, causing me to be in this condition of lassitude the greater part of the time. And to make matters worse, domestic circumstances exactly the reverse of those which would tend to heal the exhausted nerves and devitalized body were all about me. My physician explained that these conditions were like the scratching of a raw sore—and sores cannot be healed by picking and irritation.

So I had to carry on getting well without rest, without relaxation—except for a brief heavenly visit to my blessed mother's home, who as at the beginning of life, soothed the way back toward health for me now.

I had laid my plans for a physical come-back. But I had not reckoned with another after-effect, which proved to be among the most difficult and distressing of all the results of that hideous illness. It was something entirely outside the pale *of my control, something about which at first I grieved considerably, but which later began to enrage and infuriate me.*

Acquaintances and even some closer friends of long standing began to look at me peculiarly. I was conscious of a sympathetic condescension—and at times almost an aversion—in their attitude. At first I was completely at a loss to know the reason, but an irate landlady, to whom, unfortunately, I owed some money, gave me the explanation. She accused me openly of being a drug addict and a sort of chronic inebriate, both of which conclusions were arrived at because of my sleepy appearance and the drowsiness which often overpowered me. She became vicious and embittered and would follow me from place to place, telling the people where I worked or lived these grotesque and brutal stories, and ill consequences would invariably follow. If she could find no other way to annoy me, even long after I left her, she would go to the school my daughter attended and follow her home to learn where we lived. I lost several positions, my employers apparently feeling that my "addiction to drugs" would be an evil influence in their organizations, and more than one landlady requested me to leave because she was suspicious.

Any number of people have asked me point-blank if I used any drug, or what I "have been drinking." And today, as in the days of 8 and 9 years ago, I am still the unfortunate victim of this vicious accusation. It seems as if I must, upon an introduction to anyone, immediately explain why I look like an addict of either drugs or liquor. But in many cases the explanations would be futile, since they would be regarded as elaborate alibis. It is maddening—particularly when it actually interferes with one's business and home life.

After a period of 3 years had gone by I returned to the physician who had taken care of me during my illness and protested this hideous condition, asking him if there was not some medicine or treatment he could prescribe that would alleviate the "grogginess." I made it clear to him that I was considerably unnerved at the constant direct or indirect implication that I was a drug addict or an inebriate. The only consolation I received from him was a sympathetic smile—and then he became angry. "It is a miracle that you are alive at all! Why do you care what people say? What must be the feelings of those others if you feel hurt that you are talked about? If you had decently died they would have only good things to say. Aren't you a bit ashamed to complain? There are hundreds of victims who would give anything to be as well as you are."

He was only telling the truth. I am indeed fortunate to be as well rid of the dreadful malady as I am, but I can only wonder what must be the feelings of those others who were not so fortunate. For even now there are times when I cannot keep awake, and these seizures and their results are a little short of agony.

I still go to sleep in the bathtub, often having slept there all night, to find on awaking in the cold gray dawn, that the hot water in which I fell asleep has grown bitter cold. Frequently I spend whole nights asleep at my desk, unable to rouse myself to get properly to bed. Dressing in front of my mirror I often lose consciousness for a few minutes, and I have dropped and broken so many hand-mirrors that I could never live long enough to live out the proverbial

7 years' bad luck. And when I have been unusually tired I have even fallen into a light sleep while waiting for traffic lights to change, or for a trolley-car, or even for a subway express—right at the edge of a crowded platform.

But these sleeping spells are not at all the same as those that come from being overtired. The patient is really in that semiconscious condition, known to many nervous people, that comes before they pass into a deep sleep. You are really conscious; there is a hodge-podge of dreams, unrelated, and not pertaining to anything in one's environment. The mind is confused and bewildered, and everything seems unreal. I find it difficult, particularly when I first rouse myself out of the lethargy, to remember directions. It seems impossible, for instance, to find the way into my bedroom, or to know which way to turn to get toward home if I am out.

On several occasions people have come up to me on the street and asked if I felt ill. It is about as humiliating a circumstance as I can imagine. The victim knows at once that he is suspected of having imbibed too freely or of having taken a drug. Embarrassment makes him seem the more guilty, and his bewilderment and mental confusion only help to confirm the mind of the observer.

That is probably the most detrimental after-effect of the disease and one which the physicians say can never be entirely cured. It can, however, be alleviated, so that it is never present unless the patient becomes overtired through either mental or physical exertion.

There are other after-effects of a physical nature which are more or less troublemaking, according to their intensity. One of the most astonishing is a glandular disturbance. This accounts for the increase in weight which seems to be a usual consequence of the disease. It also accounts for a complete right-about-face of many vital processes.

But the after-effect which in my own case has caused the greatest difficulty is the change in my appearance, which has made so many suspect that I take drugs or alcohol. As I have said, there seems to be no help for me. Surely I cannot go about the streets wearing a placard on my back and chest announcing to the inquisitive, the suspicious and the world in general, "I have had sleeping sickness. That is why I look this way!"

COMMENT: Ms. Carey's EL had some classic signs, such as extreme somnolence (progressing to coma) and diplopia. However, the somnolence is quite pervasive and is present throughout her illness. And her vivid description of the "lethargica" is far more detailed than any others that exist. Carey never had insomnia, as did most of the other cases described in this chapter, but she did have mental confusion (hallucinations). Carey's EL began with headache and, as in some of the previous cases, this was initially ascribed to influenza. The late changes in her physical appearance, suggestive of addiction, greatly disturbed her and perhaps were common, but have not generally been described. There is nothing in her initial condition that clearly resembles parkinsonism, although she appears to have had a chronic condition resembling PEP. Unfortunately, we do not know if her sequelae remained static, improved, or worsened.

Case 8. Self-report by American author Duff Gilfond

Duff Gilfond was born in the United States in 1902, the only child of parents who both managed small businesses. After a college education, she trained as a journalist and worked at regional newspapers, eventually becoming a renowned political correspondent. A regular contributor to the *New York Times* and the *New York Herald Tribune*, Gilfond was also the author of an acclaimed book about President Coolidge, *The Rise of Saint Calvin*. In 1930, she developed an incapacitating headache, which was only alleviated when she lay flat, and she also found that she had difficulty sleeping at night. She was eventually diagnosed with EL by an eminent neurologist, whom she refers to as "Dr. Bevely" in her book, *I Go Horizontal* (all the names she uses within her book, except her own, are fictitious). During her illness, she underwent many diagnostic tests, some more than once, in various hospitals, and was seen by at least 18 doctors. She was treated with hyoscine, which proved ineffective and unpleasant, resulting in acute hallucinations and unmanageable behavior, which fortunately ceased when the drug was discontinued. She also had an abortion because of her EL. After 7 years, she describes some easing of her headache on a day-to-day basis. Her book, *I Go Horizontal*, was published in 1940 as a record of the course of her illness and her experiences with the medical profession. The following brief account gives a flavor of her frustration with her situation and with the state of medical knowledge at the time.

My initial response to the headache was to talk to my physician-friend, Henry. Initially, he tried to persuade me that having a bad headache wasn't so unusual and that I had simply been lucky to have remained so healthy to date. Nevertheless, despite being a nonspecialist, when he saw me in such evident pain a few days later, he wondered if it could be encephalitis and called for the specialist, Dr. Pou. However, Dr. Pou was unable to make a satisfactory diagnosis and made a referral, first to a Dr. Brent, who was followed by Drs. Kelly and Palmer. This was the beginning of my frustrating relationship with the varied medical professions of the United States in the 1930s.

Despite extensive examinations, none of the physicians could explain my appalling pain and it was suggested that although my suffering was real, given that there was no apparent cause, I should ignore it and get on with my life. Desperate to be cured, I did my very best before once again collapsing under a dark "cloud" of misery that hid what had once been a "clear sky."

I searched for a doctor who would recognize that I was ill and finally heard about a well-regarded neurologist, a Dr. Bevely, whom I refer to as the Great Man. A very successful physician and professor, he was inundated with work and it took time and patience before I could finally meet him. Given that he then wanted to repeat medical tests that had already been undertaken without result, I was skeptical of starting with another expert. But I felt there was little choice and Bevely's assistant conducted the tests with the expectation that my symptoms would be explained by an eye problem or a brain tumor. However, 4 months after the onset of the illness, Dr. Bevely diagnosed encephalitis lethargica (EL).

In a footnote, Duff notes that she was still unwell when the book was finally ready for publication in 1940 but had, without doubt, continued to improve.

COMMENT: This case, of a young woman, offers primarily a limited description of a single symptom—headache—that persisted for at least 7 years, was constant and relieved only by lying supine in bed. At one point in her narrative she describes it as "pounding" or "hammering," and says that her head "throbbed." She briefly mentions insomnia, but then says she had no other symptoms or physical signs. There are no typical signs of EL or parkinsonism, and the rationale for the diagnosis of EL is not stated. Furthermore, she noted that some of the physicians she consulted questioned the diagnosis of EL, which is consistent with the idea that EL was markedly overdiagnosed (see Chapter 2). At the time, abortion was recommended for patients with EL who became pregnant (Neal, 1942). Gilfond also seems to suggest that it was relatively easy to find others who were suffering from chronic EL.

Although this woman's distress arouses our sympathy, her account, as in case 6, leaves us in doubt as to whether EL was an accurate diagnosis. We also need to recognize that part of the purpose of her book was to document her own frustrations with the medical community of her time.

OVERALL COMMENTS

In this chapter, we have collected the subjective accounts of eight individuals who were diagnosed with EL during the period 1919–1940. They describe their personal experiences in varying detail, each interpreting their symptoms in their own words. Five of the patients were physicians, and the descriptions provided are either by them directly, or based on their notes.

These self-reports, despite their differences, provide insights into the disease that may help with future diagnosis. Among the symptoms these patients report, several common elements stand out. Almost all had some degree of headache at the outset; fever and nausea were common. Severe drowsiness or sleepiness lasted from several weeks to a year or more, and was associated with vivid dreams, visual hallucinations, nightmares, and deliria. Typically, these patients described a sense of nervousness and inner agitation that often persisted into the chronic phase. Sialorrhea and visual symptoms such as double vision were also repeatedly mentioned. Parkinsonian signs were present in four of the cases (cases 1, 3, 5, and 6), but absent in the others. As for PEP, case 1 clearly developed it, whereas case 6 was diagnosed with PEP, but the symptoms rather resemble those of idiopathic PD.

In case 6 and in the Gilfond case, we question the diagnosis of EL/PEP. And, this of course leads to the question of accuracy in the diagnosis of EL in general. The variability in symptomatology that is discussed in Chapter 2 is quite evident among these cases, and leads again to the question of whether there really is a common underlying etiologic factor to all of these cases (see Chapter 12).

Finally, as highlighted in the recent book by Dr. Oliver Sacks on the relationship between music and the brain, *Musicophilia*, two self-reports (5 and 7) describe aspects of their syndrome related to music. Much of it was compulsive (e.g., constant humming, or hearing music everywhere), but music also brought pleasure and relief from some of the symptoms of EL.

REFERENCES CITED

Anonymous. (1922). *Epidemic (lethargic) encephalitis. Journal of the American Medical Association*, *78*, 407–409.

Anonymous. (1948). Effects of encephalitis lethargica. *Lancet*, 2, 904–905.

Carey, E. (1934). I recover from sleeping sickness. *The American Mercury*, 32, 165–169.

Delater, G. (1920). Auto observation d'encephalite lethargique. *Paris Medical*, *37*, 316–319.

Delater, G. (1948). Suite sur trent ans et fin d'une auto-observation d'encephalite lethargica. *Paris Medical*, *136*, 229–230.

Gilfond, D. (1940). *I Go Horizontal*. New York: Vanguard Press.

Mayer-Gross, W., & Steiner, G. (1921). Encephalitis lethargica in der selbstbeobachtung. *Zeitschrift fur die gesamte Neurologie und Psychiatrie*, *73*, 283–309.

Parsons, A. C., MacNalty, A. S., & Perdrau, J. R. (1922). *Report on Encephalitis Lethargica: Being an Account of Further Enquiries into the Epidemiology and Clinical Features of the Disease; Including the Analysis of over 1,250 reports on Cases Notified in England and Wales during 1919 and 1920, Together with Comprehensive Bibliography of the Subject*. London: His Majesty's Stationery Office.

12

FINAL THOUGHTS

Joel A. Vilensky and Sid Gilman

There are no real characteristics or physical signs by which the disease [EL] can be recognized, and as any function of the brain may be disturbed there may be a whole series of clinical manifestations.

Dr. F. Buzzard, cited in Hamer (1924, p. 26)

The idea of establishing a diagnostic scheme based upon symptoms was in his mind, untenable.

Referring to Dr. D.E Core, cited in Hamer (1924, p. 26)

DIAGNOSIS

The above quotations illustrate well the conundrum pertaining to a correct diagnosis of encephalitis lethargica (EL); that is, there appears to be no distinctive or pathognomonic symptom or sign (or set of them). Ziporyn (1992) said of another poorly defined syndrome, chronic fatigue syndrome, "Without an agreed-on definition, more sophisticated correlations and predictions become meaningless. If you don't know what chronic fatigue syndrome is, for example, how can you say what happens to people with chronic fatigue syndrome?" The same can clearly be said about EL, and this is why we have questioned whether EL represents a unitary condition and whether the presumed direct relationship between EL and PEP is real (as discussed in Chapter 7 and below).

As emphasized in the pre-1917 EL history chapter (Chapter 4), if von Economo's and Cruchet's initial cases had not been followed by the worldwide regional epidemics of EL, they would have remained curious historical/medical anomalies. The epidemics both supported the idea of EL as a clinical entity, and allowed clinicians to investigate its clinical aspects, etiology, and treatments. In contrast, at present, EL appears again to be a sporadic, nonepidemic disease for which an etiologic agent (or pathognomonic sign or symptom) still has not been identified. What does this mean for the diagnosis of EL today? Simply, *we suggest that it is impossible to be absolutely certain that any patient seen today with symptomatology resembling EL actually has the same syndrome that existed during the epidemic period.*

In the post-epidemic period chapter (Chapter 5), we suggested that the most parsimonious view of diagnosing EL today is to confine the diagnosis to those patients who show a constellation of symptoms and signs that are consistent with the somnolent-ophthalmoplegic type of EL defined by von Economo. We say this because these features led von Economo to consider EL to be a new disease entity, and it was only later, when EL epidemics occurred, that wide-ranging symptomatology was added to the differential diagnosis; eventually, nearly 30 different subtypes of EL were proposed to exist. Thus, we believe the term "encephalitis lethargica" should be used in a strict sense that remains consistent with the disease entity as originally recognized.

In other words, we suggest that patients who are diagnosed with EL today should show, shortly after an apparent "cold" (i.e., a few days to 1–2 weeks), prolonged lethargy and pseudosomnolence, diplopia, and ptosis, for which complete neurologic, radiologic, and serologic examinations have eliminated all known causes, such as tumor, stroke, other viral and bacterial agents, and the like. We believe that the presence of the initial cold-like signs and symptoms is as important as the later somnolent-ophthalmoplegic ones. Von Economo (1917) specifically stated, "We want to emphasize, however, that most of our cases started with the feeling of a cold, headache, and general malaise and possibly joint pain." For these (and only these) modern patients, a diagnosis of EL is reasonable, but certainly not definitive. Pertaining to extrapyramidal signs, such signs were not emphasized in any of the early reports on EL and only became significant with the later epidemics. Thus, we would accept such signs as supportive of an EL diagnosis, but not conclusive. Similarly, unexplained parkinsonian signs in a patient who did not previously or concurrently show somnolent-ophthalmoplegic signs and symptoms are not, in our view, an acceptable basis for a diagnosis for EL. Finally, the presence of oculogyric crises, which were not considered part of the constellation of signs and symptoms of acute EL during the epidemic period (see Chapter 5), is again supportive, but not sufficient, for a diagnosis of EL.

UNITY OF DISEASE

There seems little doubt that EL was overdiagnosed, probably significantly so, during the epidemic period. We presented quotes to this effect in Chapter 2 by Ford, and by Riley. Similarly, Hirsch, in 1920 asked, "What at the moment is not encephalitis lethargica?" Gottstein (1920, 1921; and see Foley 2009c) addressed this issue analytically in a 1921 doctoral thesis. He wondered whether "the etiology, clinical presentation, and pathological anatomy could distinguish EL from other disorders" and answered, no. Gottstein concluded that von Economo's criteria were not as specific as claimed, and he identified overlap between EL and influenza, as well as other encephalitides including polioencephalitis.

The Spanish influenza pandemic overlapped EL in time (although we do recognize that this overlap often did not extend to specific geographic regions because there were many regions in which EL and influenza epidemics did not occur simultaneously. In a previous publication (McCall et al., 2008), we pointed out some of the clinical problems with considering EL to be caused by influenza and these same issues are relevant to whether some influenza cases could have been misdiagnosed as EL. We noted that postinfluenzal encephalopathy is typically quite rare, appears 2–3 weeks after influenza, and complete recovery is the most common outcome. However, Foley concluded that "the 1918 influenza pandemic was exceptional in both its epidemiology and its clinical characteristics" (Foley 2009a, p. 144). He did not consider a neurovirulent effect to be one of its peculiarities, but there are clinical descriptions from the time that do suggest neurovirulent variants.

As detailed in Chapter 4, which was authored by Dr. Foley, there is a long historical record of EL-like complications associated with influenza—but there are also many problems in interpreting these data, often related to changes in semantics over time. Undoubtedly, the most comprehensive collection of data about the 1918 Spanish influenza epidemic, with substantial data from earlier influenza epidemics as well, is the massive almost 1,600-page, two-volume, 1934 report by Drs. D. and R. Thomson that was part of the *Annals of The Pickett-Thomson Research Laboratory*, London. Although published in both England and the United States, the volumes are not readily available and are rarely cited in articles and books on the 1918 influenza epidemic. These volumes are comparable in size and scope to the Matheson reports on EL. The Thompson volumes have an entire section devoted to nervous complications of influenza (see Table 12.1).

Although without modern serological testing to confirm influenza as a cause, it is impossible to know whether the EL-like influenza complications listed in Table 12.1 were truly due to influenza or to EL (or to both; cf. Foley 2009a,b,c), clearly these findings demonstrate that EL could easily have been misdiagnosed as influenza and vice versa. Our hypothesis, as suggested in various chapters of this book, is that EL was not a unitary condition and now we theorize that influenza (the Spanish influenza) was indeed often misdiagnosed as EL.

Table 12.1 EL-like Complications of the Spanish Inflenza

Reference	*Nervous complications of Influenza that Resemble EL Symptomatology*
Harris (1919)	"There is no acute malady after which disturbance of the nervous system is so frequent as after influenza, and none that has such varied nervous sequelae. There may be ptosis, paralysis of the external ocular muscles, or even complete third-nerve palsy" (p. 92–93); reported that paraesthesia of all sorts have been described as sequelae, including pins-and-needles sensation, vague pains, numbness, hyperesthesia, etc. And, "there is scarcely a nerve twig, or nerve trunk, that has not been known to suffer from influenza, with resulting local tenderness and trophic symptoms of skin or muscle persisting for variable periods" (p. 98); epilepsy can also occur.
Savage (1919)	Influenza, of all infectious diseases, is the most likely to be followed by mental disorder.
Chodak (1919)	Paralysis of soft palate
Meyerhof (1919)	Abducent nerve paralysis
Clark (1919); Maillard & Brune (1919)	Epilepsy
Nonne (1919)	Bulbar paralysis
Tanfari (1919)	Hemiplegia
Guillain & Libert (1920)	Paralysis of the serratus anterior
Porot & Senges (1920)	Facial paralysis
Ordway (1920)	Chorea
Whale (1922)	Pertaining to problems of phonation, "… general paresis of intrinsic laryngeal muscles is not the only form seen. Often the cricothyroid is spared, as if the poison had selective action on the recurrent laryngeal nerve. Or a lack of tension, with ample movements, suggesting that only the cricothyroid is affected, may occur" (p. 412).
Abrahams (1922)	Recorded several cases of transient Bell palsy and saw two cases of unilateral posterior thoracic neuritis with paralysis of the serratus anterior; one directly followed an acute attack of influenza, the other appearing a few weeks after convalescence. He reported that a high percentage of the more serious cases, whether fatal or not, showed marked involuntary jerkings and twitchings of one limb or of the head and neck or of one side of the abdomen or of the back (von Economo considered myoclonus of the abdomen to be a typical sign of EL; see Chapter 2).

(Continued)

Table 12.1 continued

Reference	Nervous complications of Influenza that Resemble EL Symptomatology
Boenninghaus (1924)	Described three cases of unilateral pharyngeal paralysis following influenza; in the first, the involvement of the pharynx was an isolated phenomenon; in the second, it was associated with facial paralysis on the same side; and in the third with paralysis of the tongue, palate, and vocal cord of the same side. Dysphagia was moderate in degree, but it was impossible to swallow solids without taking some fluid afterward; the diagnosis in each case was made by examination of the pharynx on phonation, when the posterior pharyngeal wall was seen to be drawn to the normal side.

Not surprisingly, this hypothesis was suggested during the EL epidemic period, but has been forgotten. Tucker (1918), in a study of 11 cases, found the relationship so striking that he concluded, "epidemic encephalitis lethargica is either a recrudescence or recurrence of influenza, or in some cases the expression of influenza per se" (p. 1449). Jelliffe (1922) considered EL to frequently be of "influenza origin." And Jordan (1927) said, "It seems, however, to be definitely established that while some cases of epidemic encephalitis follow closely on the heels of an attack of influenza, others originate independently and have no traceable connection with ordinary clinical influenza" (p. 1604). Thus, Jordan most closely predated our hypothesis, suggesting that some cases of EL are associated with influenza, whereas others are not.

Another author (Lucksch, 1928; and see Foley 2010c) even attributed postencephalitic parkinsonism (PEP) to the influenza epidemic:

> The most striking phenomenon of the most recent epidemic—besides the great mortality—is the frequent and grave participation of the central nervous system in the disease. Among these nervous changes, the chronic or so-called residual phenomena apparently have no predecessors of equal significance and frequency in former epidemics, at least not in the striking and repeated picture of parkinsonism and of the vegetative disturbances associated with it.

Thus, it seems possible that some of the cases diagnosed as EL were actually cases of a neurovirulent form of influenza. This view offers at least a partial explanation for the huge variation in symptomatology in EL, the contagiousness in some cases (Chapter 6), and certainly for some of the problems that we have highlighted in Chapter 7 pertaining to the putative relationship between EL and PEP.

Further support for the hypothesis that at least some of the epidemic-period EL cases were due to influenza is found in a 1927 book on infectious diseases of the nervous system by the eminent British epidemiologist, A.S. MacNalty (Chapter 6). He stated that "it seems reasonable to conclude that the virus of encephalitis lethargica first infects the upper respiratory passages, where it either may lurk and give rise to the carrier phase in the person infected or may pass on to attack the brain" (p. 156). He then quoted Dr. Willougby Gardner pertaining to the first manifestations of EL: "There is a slight swelling but very marked congestion of the fauces and pharynx: the color is a deep crimson, but sometimes is almost vermilion. There is comparatively little swelling of the tonsils, but whitish patches of exudates are to be seen on tonsils, fauces, pharynx... . These throats tend to become dry and are often associated with a red, bare, swollen and dryish tongue" (p. 156). This description of the initial signs and symptoms of EL can be directly related to a 1998 article by Yuen et al. that described the presenting symptoms and signs in 12 patients with serologically confirmed H5N1 infection. Of the 12, three initially had a sore throat and another two more had a "congested oropharynx." Other initial signs and symptoms were fever, vomiting, headache, cough, rhinorrhea, dizziness, and diarrhea. All of these are consistent with the initial signs and symptoms of EL (see Chapter 2).

In our discussion of chronic EL in Chapter 7 and in other chapters in this book, we have suggested that EL and PEP may not have been unitary phenomena. Earlier, we suggested that some of the EL cases diagnosed during the epidemic period were probably a neurovirulent form of influenza. We also call attention here to the very recent article (2009) by Dale et al. suggesting that hyperkinetic EL cases may be due to the development of autoantibodies to the extracellular domain of NR1/NR2 subunits of the N-methyl-D-aspartate receptor (NMDAR$_{Ab}$). In presenting this hypothesis, Dale et al. are implicitly accepting that the etiology of EL was not uniform.

CONCLUSION

Based on this and other information presented in this book, we believe we are justified in postulating the following pertaining to EL:

1. A unique syndrome was prevalent during the early part of the 20th century. Although we believe EL was significantly overdiagnosed, its independent diagnosis by experienced clinicians in many different countries makes it difficult to argue against it being a unique nosological entity. And, presumably, this uniqueness is related to a unique pathological agent or combination of agents, perhaps in conjunction with some genetic susceptibility. This agent or agents have yet to be defined.

2. The ever-increasing constellation of signs and symptoms that became associated with EL is compelling evidence in itself that EL was overdiagnosed. We have provided documentation to demonstrate

similar symptomatology between EL and some cases of influenza, suggesting that the latter condition may have been quite commonly misdiagnosed as EL in the epidemic period.

3. Acute EL was followed by the development of chronic sequelae in some cases, although probably many fewer than currently perceived. As noted by Neal (1925), those persons who developed mild cases of acute EL and recovered probably did not seek medical attention and were not considered in the data sets showing the percentage of EL cases that developed chronic sequelae. Postencephalitic parkinsonism could be a sequel of EL, but was not the only one (i.e., not all chronic EL was PEP).

4. Postencephalitic parkinsonism is generally considered to be a single disease entity that directly follows EL. We suggest that PEP is one presumptive chronic sequel to EL, but its relationship to EL is probably less direct than commonly believed, and development of PEP may depend on a constellation of etiologic factors of which EL is typically one. This view would be consistent with the fact that there is no other nonfamilial parkinsonian disorder that can be attributed to a single etiologic factor. We suggest that PEP, like idiopathic parkinsonism, is likely due to some complex interaction of genes and environment, in which EL was a factor.

We hope that our compilation and integration of the EL material provided here will enable a comprehensive data-based view of both the EL that occurred during the epidemic period and cases of EL that may be occurring sporadically now, and also allow a more effective response if an EL epidemic reappears in the future.

REFERENCES CITED

Dale, R. C., Irani S. R., Brilot, F., Pillai S., Webster, R., Gill, D., et al. (2009). N-Methyl-D-Aspartate receptor antibodies in pediatric dyskinetic encephalitis lethargic. *Annals of Neurology, 66,* 704–709.

Foley, P. B. (2009a). Encephalitis lethargica and influenza. I. The role of the influenza virus in the influenza pandemic of 1918/1919. *Journal of Neural Transmission, 116,* 143–150.

Foley, P. B. (2009b). Encephalitis lethargica and influenza. II. The influenza pandemic of 1918/1919 and encephalitis lethargic: epidemiology and symptoms. *Journal of Neural Transmission, 116,* 1275–1308.

Foley, P. B. (2009c). Encephalitis lethargica and influenza. III. The influenza pandemic of 1918/1919 and encephalitis lethargic: neuropathology and discussion. *Journal of Neural Transmission, 116,* 1309–1321.

Hamer, W. H. (1924). Poliomyelitis, encephalitis and influenza. *Annual Report of the Medical Officer of Health of the Administrative Council of London,* 20–32.

Hirsch, C. (1920). Zur vergleichenden Pathologie der Enzephalitis nebst kritschen Bermekungen zur Encaphliatis lethargic (epidemica)-Diagnose. *Berliner Klinische Wochesnschrift, 57,* 605–607.

Jelliffe, S. E. (1922). *The Nervous Syndromes of Influenza*. In F. G. Crookshank (Ed.), *Influenza: Essays by Several Authors* (pp. 351–377). London: William Heinemann (Medical Books) Ltd.

Jordan, E. O. (1927). The influenza epidemic of 1918: Encephalitis and influenza. *Journal of the American Medical Association, 89*, 1603–1606.

Lucksch, F. (1928). Pathologic anatomy of influenza: A review based chiefly on German sources. *Archives of Pathology, 5*, 448–491.

MacNalty, A. S. (1927). "*Epidemic Diseases of the Central Nervous System*. London, Faber&Gwyer.

McCall, S., Vilensky, J. A., Gilman, S., & Taubenberger J. K. (2008). The relationship between encephalitis lethargica and influenza: A critical analysis. *Journal of Neurovirology 14*, 177–185.

Neal, J. B., Jackson, H. W., & Appelbaum, E. (1925). A study of four hundred and fifty cases of epidemic encephalitis. *American Journal of Medical Sciences, 170*, 708–722.

Thomson, D., & Thomson, R. (1934). Influenza (Part II): With special reference to the complications and sequelae, bacteriology of influenza pneumonia, pathology, epidemiological data, prevention and treatment. *Annals of the Pickett-Thomson Research Laboratory, X*. London: Baillière, Tindall, and Cox.

Tucker, B. R. (1918). Epidemic encephalitis lethargic, or epidemic somnolence, or epidemic cerebritis, with report of cases and two necropsies. *Journal of the American Medical Association, 72*, 1448–1450.

von Economo, C. (1917). Encephalitis lethargica. *Wiener Klinische Wochenschrift, 30*, 581–585.

Yuen, K. Y., Chan, P. K. S., Peiris, M., Tsang, D. N. C., Que, T. L. Shortridge, K. F., et al. (1998). Clinical features and rapid viral diagnosis of human disease associated with avian influenza A H5N1 virus. *Lancet, 351*, 467–471.

Ziporyn, T. (1992). *Nameless Diseases*. New Brunswick, NJ: Rutgers University Press.

INDEX